DRUG DOSAGE IN LABORATORY ANIMALS
A HANDBOOK

DRUG DOSAGE IN LABORATORY ANIMALS
A HANDBOOK

Third Edition, Revised and Enlarged

R. E. Borchard
C. D. Barnes
L. G. Eltherington

Second Printing, 1991

THE TELFORD PRESS, INC.
Post Office Box 287. Caldwell, New Jersey 07006

Library of Congress Cataloging-in-Publication Data

Borchard, Ronald E.
    Drug dosage in laboratory animals : a handbook / by R.E. Borchard.
C.D. Barnes, and L.G. Eltherington. -- 3rd rev. and enlarged ed.
        p.   cm.
    Rev. ed. of: Drug dosage in laboratory animals / by C.D. Barnes
and L.G. Eltherington. 2nd rev. and enl. ed. [c1973].
    Includes bibliographical references.
    ISBN 0-936923-19-9
    1. Drugs--Dosage--Tables. 2. Laboratory animals--Tables.
3. Pharmacology, Experimental--Tables. I. Barnes. Charles D..
1935-   . II. Eltherington. L. G. (Lorne George) III. Barnes.
Charles D., 1935-   Drug dosage in laboratory animals. IV. Title.
    [DNLM: 1. Animals. Laboratory--tables. 2. Drugs--administration &
dosage--tables.   QV 50 B261d]
RM145.B65 1990
615.5'8--dc20
DNLM/DLC
for Library of Congress   89-20415
                                                                CIP

CONTENTS

The first and second editions of this handbook were favorably accepted and appeared to fill a "need" for many investigators. There were, however, two major criticisms concerning "a lot of blank pages" and omission of "favorite drugs". There is no question that, somewhere in the published literature, drug dosage information exists which could fill some of the blank spaces; we simply have not found the information. In our judgement, the value of the book, which contains over 7300 doses and 2278 references for over 440 drugs, far outweighs this justifiable criticism. We deliberately designed the format so that an investigator could add special interest drug and dosage information to create his own "personalized" handbook. The selection of drugs included or omitted from this handbook was governed by two considerations; first, our judgement as to general interest in the drug and second, our finding enough information about the drug to justify its inclusion.

We have expanded this third edition to include 230 new drugs, 1000 additional references and 2700 new doses. The sections on factors modifying drug response and anesthesia have also been expanded and brought up to date with 100 new anesthetic doses.

INTRODUCTION

This handbook provides pharmacodynamic and toxicologic dosage for drugs commonly used in biomedical research. Including typical representatives of the major drug groups was the primary consideration governing drug selection. Antimicrobial agents were omitted because: (1) animal dose information is available from the label information which accompanies veterinary preparations (dog, cat); (2) doses for other laboratory animal species are generally lacking; (3) doses vary with extent of infection and species of microorganism. A secondary selection criterion was the reported use of a drug in several animal species and via more than one route of administration. Some research compounds, and drugs with a specific or limited spectrum of use (for example, radiation-protective drugs), were deliberately omitted because they do not satisfy this requirement. A number of new drugs that show promise of future widespread use clinically, or as experimental tools, are included even though they do not yet meet the specified criterion.

Drug responses are classified according to (1) toxicity, (2) primary use or action, and (3) secondary uses or actions. To present efficiently as many doses as possible, it was sometimes necessary to classify a number of specific drug actions and uses under one general heading. For example, a "cardiovascular" category may include drug effects on cardiac output, regional blood flow, vascular resistance, mean arterial blood pressure, etc. A "behavior" classification may represent drug-induced alterations of conditioning, learning, sociological behavior and spontaneous motor activity. Where available space and sufficient information permits, single drug effects or uses are listed separately. Since the dosage entries are referenced, the technique of grouping drug effects and uses allows tabulation of more doses in a limited space, thus reducing the handbook size without sacrificing completeness. Toxicological data are included to provide information relating to the upper part of a drug dose-response curve, thereby assisting the investigator in choosing a maximally effective dose that produces minimal toxicity. In some instances lethal doses were obtained for an animal species or route of administration for which no pharmacodynamic information was found. Lethal doses are presented in the following order of importance: (1) LD_{50}-lethal dose 50%, the dose, calculated statistically, sufficient to kill 50 percent of the population; (2) MLD-minimum lethal dose, the dose reported sufficient to kill a single member of an experimental group; and (3) LD-lethal dose, the dose which has been reported to kill an unspecified number of an experimental group.

Drugs are listed in alphabetical order according to the nomenclature suggested by the USAN (United States Adopted Names) and the *USP Dictionary of Drug Names*, 1988. Secondarily, the tenth edition of the *Merck Index* was consulted. Wherever possible, three common and/or trade names are included and cross-indexed with the official name. All *in vivo* doses are expressed as milligrams per kilogram of body weight (mg/kg) of the "commonly used" salt, except where otherwise indicated.

The introductory material, discussing factors modifying drug response and anesthesia, is a simplified presentation of basic pharmacological and rational anesthetic principles necessary for maximum data validity in acute animal experiments. Biomedical research literature contains much contradictory information which may be partially explained by differences in anesthetic agents or techniques and indifference to basic pharmacological principles in the design and interpretation of experiments.

Table I contains a list of injectable anesthetic doses and combinations commonly used in seven species of laboratory animals. For reasons discussed in the previous and later sections, these injectable anesthetics are recommended *only* for chronic or recovery experiments. Inhalation agents are suggested as the only rational means of providing general anesthesia for acute, non-recovery experiments.

Appendix A presents hormone maintenance and replacement doses which have been reported to be effective following surgical removal of endocrine glands. The material is referenced, and tabulated under the surgical name of the animal following gland removal, e.g., hypophysectomized.

In vitro concentrations, expressed as milligrams per 100 ml of bathing solution (mg%), except where indicated otherwise, are included for use of investigators studying drug effects on isolated organs or tissue. The information is presented in a tabular form and space has been allowed for addition of new concentrations and responses of particular interest to the investigator. Similar to the *in vivo* material, all concentrations refer to the "commonly used" salt. Non-referenced concentrations are from laboratory teaching experiments, familiar to the authors, in which the bathing or perfusing solution was aerated with 95% oxygen and 5% carbon dioxide and maintained at 37°C.

A publication (1157) cited in the second edition of *Drug Dosage in Laboratory Animals* has provided valuable information on classical techniques for studying isolated preparations.

FACTORS MODIFYING DRUG RESPONSES

Rational drug administration to laboratory animals involves two major considerations: (1) pharmacological action, i.e., influence of the drug on the animal and (2) drug disposition, i.e., influence of the animal's *milieu interieur* upon uptake, distribution and elimination of the drug. The tabular portion of this handbook provides dosage information related to pharmacological action and this introduction will briefly consider physiological and pharmacological factors which influence drug disposition.

PHYSIOLOGICAL FACTORS

Age. A young animal, especially newborn, exhibits differences from the adult in drug absorption, distribution, metabolism, excretion and sensitivity. For example, hepatic enzyme systems responsible for the biotransformation of barbiturates are deficient in the newborn (1245) resulting in increased drug effect. Nonmetabolized drugs may reproduce a greater effect because of decreased renal function or increased access to receptor sites, for example, greater blood-brain barrier permeability. The neonate has a relatively larger volume of total body water due to extracellular fluid, but a smaller intracellular fluid volume than mature animals, which will affect drug concentrations in those compartments.

Endocrine. Any major hormonal imbalance may be expected to influence drug action. Adrenal insufficiency attenuates the vascular effect of catecholamines and hypothyroidism enhances the respiratory depression of narcotic analgesics. Animals that exhibit circadian rhythms, such as the mouse, may demonstrate marked difference in drug response related to the day-night time of administration (1246). Metabolizing enzymes are stimulated by androgens, but depressed by progestins and adrenal medullary secretions. Thyroid secretions may stimulate or depress certain drug metabolizing systems.

Health. Animals used for drug studies, especially those who are to receive general anesthesia, should be in the laboratory environment at least two weeks prior to the experiment. Observation of dietary habits, character of stool and general physical status should exclude "sick" animals. A procedure for the preoperative evaluation of dogs (1247) could be modified and applied to the pre-experimental preparation of any laboratory animal.

Nutrition. A starved animal with depleted glycogen stores will experience greater response from cardiovascular and central nervous system drugs. Likewise dehydration, with subsequent hypovolemia and altered volume of drug distribution, may result in enhanced drug toxicity.

Sex. Drug disposition differences between males and females of some species (especially rats) are probably related to hormonal differences. For example, in male rats barbiturate sleeping times may be increased by administration of female sex hormones to equal those of the female (1248).

Species. Quantitative and even qualitative differences in drug disposition have been shown to exist between species and even within different strains of the same species. They are apparently related to different rates and/or pathways of drug biotransformation. For example, the dog is unable to metabolize codeine to morphine and rapidly demethylates ephedrine, whereas the rat excretes part of the administered codeine as morphine and hydroxylates ephedrine as the primary inactivating pathway (1249, 1250). Drugs, such as the opioids and aspirin-like antiinflammatory agents, which are biotransformed by glucoronidation in most species, are excreted slowly in cats, since they have a natural deficiency in glucoronyl transferase enzyme (2274). These species differences are reflected in the dosage regiments suggested.

Temperature. The influence of body temperature on drug effects may be subtle and unknown or quite striking (1251). Mild hypothermia in the dog (32-33°C) results in a 30 percent decrease of metabolism while moderate temperature decline (28-30°C) elicits a 50 percent decrease in metabolism, heart rate and blood flow (1252). Hyperthermia produces an elevation of metabolic rate and cardiac output. Changes in body temperature, easily monitored by rectal or esophageal thermometer, may result from: (1) heat loss secondary to anesthesia-induced vasodilation, (2) heat gain from a warm environment, drug effects and excessive draping, (3) tracheal cannulation and subsequent loss, especially in the dog, of a considerable part of its heat-regulating system.

Temperament. Drug disposition in the conscious animal will be markedly influenced by the animal's reaction to handling and manipulation. Variations in the duration and intensity of auditory, visual and musculo-cutaneous stimulation will result in central-nervous-system-induced cardiovascular changes that may alter drug disposition. The use of trained animals will reduce but not eliminate these variations. Likewise, a struggling, frightened animal requires a larger dose of anesthetic agent for induction which, particularly with the use of injectable agents, may result in a drug overdose.

PHARMACOLOGICAL FACTORS

An excellent comprehensive discussion of the many pharmacological factors which influence drug disposition may be found in a recent textbook (1253, 2106, 2280). A factor of great importance apparent from any consideration of drug disposition is drug interaction. The following discussion of the pharmacological factors important in the uptake, distribution and elimination of drugs will attempt to provide examples of drug interactions that influence drug disposition.

Route of Administration. Drugs may be administered enterally, or parenterally. The former involves the gastrointestinal (GI) tract and hence the oral, sublingual and rectal route, while the latter bypasses the GI tract and refers to all other routes. Route of administration is important in consideration of speed of onset, intensity, and duration of drug action.

ORAL ADMINISTRATION (PO)

The oral route of administration in animals is often used for the study of chronic drug effects or to determine factors relating to efficiency of gastrointestinal absorption. For acute experiments, this route frequently results in slow or unpredictable absorption of the drug and is seldom used except in industrial screening. In some animal species (mouse, guinea pig, rat, and rabbit), the passage of a stomach tube is relatively easy. Other species (cat, dog, and monkey) react violently to attempts at intubation.

PARENTERAL ADMINISTRATION

Aseptic technique is important for all injections. Sterile needles and syringes should be used and needles must be sharp. The injection site should be disinfected; 70% isopropyl alcohol is recommended.

Intravenous (IV). This route is often preferred for administering compounds in solution. Its primary advantage is that the investigator is able to slowly titrate the amount of drug needed (determined roughly by considering the animal's weight, age, sex, etc.) to elicit a particular response. Also, some drugs which are tissue irritants can be safely administered intravenously. The skin over the vein should be shaved and, if possible, pulled taut to prevent the vein from moving. Application of small amounts of a rubefacient such as xylene will elicit vasodilation and facilitate injection. The skin and vein should be pierced in separate thrusts of the needle to avoid running the needle through the vein and producing a subsequent hematoma. A practical disadvantage of IV injection in cats, dogs, and monkeys is that usually two persons are required for the procedure.

Intraperitoneal (IP). This method of injection is one of the most popular means of administering non-irritating chemicals. The peritoneum of the abdominal cavity presents a large absorptive area, and as long as the needle is placed in the midline below the umbilicus and directed approximately 45° cephalad, there is little danger of piercing the abdominal viscera. This technique may usually be performed by one person, even with cats and dogs, but provides a relatively slow onset of drug effect compared to IV injection. Two major problems are associated with the method. One is the dose is administered as a bolus; since it is not possible to titrate the drug, an overdose may be administered to a sensitive animal. Secondly, most of the absorbed material enters the portal circulation and there may be significant hepatic inactivation of the compound before reaching its site(s) of action. Another consideration with the intraperitoneal route is the volume of fluid injected. Volume is especially important in small animals such as mice, rats, and guinea pigs, and can produce volume effects which may be manifested as physiologic changes unrelated to the pharmacologic properties of the drug being studied. There is evidence that even the concentration of the solution used may considerably alter experimental results, e.g., LD_{50}.

Intramuscular (IM). A drug may be given intramuscularly in an aqueous solution, and aqueous suspension, or in a solution or suspension in oil. The drugs are administered directly into the muscle where they spread out along the muscle fibers and fasciae. This distribution affords a large absorbing surface and results in gradual absorption. The IM route of administration of a repository dosage form, such as an oil suspension, is particularly useful when a prolonged effect is desired. Some irritating substances are administered IM in aqueous form, since absorption can be fairly rapid and complete.

Subcutaneous (SC). The subcutaneous route is used only for administering non-irritating drugs. This technique may result in a slow absorption of some drugs, especially vasoconstrictor agents. Compounds which cause local vasodilation, such as some local anesthetics, often incorporate a vasoconstrictor to slow down absorption. The site of SC injection may be quite important. For example, drugs which are administered to elicit an action on the central nervous system and are metabolized by liver enzymes should be injected into subcutaneous areas which do not drain into the portal circulation. A common site of SC injection is the back of the neck. In this area there is usually ample loose skin which can be raised, eliminating the possibility of an intradermal injection. Aspiration of the syringe before injection will assure that the needle is not lying in a blood vessel. A modification of SC administration is pellet implantation under the skin of the back (for example, desoxycorticosterone acetate).

Intrathoracic. Injection of drugs high in the seventh intercostal space in a route of administration second in rapidity of onset only to the IV method. There are objections to this route of administration due to the possibility of irritating lungs and pleura, but such irritation is probably insignificant in acute experiments. The amount injected should be less than that used by routes other than IV.

With substances which do not pass the blood brain barrier two routes of administration for delivering the drug to the nervous tissue are common. Intracerebroventricular (ICV).

Intracerebroventricular (ICV). This route of administration is one of the most commonly used to introduce drugs to the nervous system which cross the blood brain barrier poorly. For this technique a guide tube is usually placed into one of the lateral ventricals under steriotaxic control and fixed to the skull with screws and dental cement. The drug is then introduced in small volumes with a needle or cathetor directed into the ventrical by the guide tube. Though most species will tolerate the implanting of a chronic guind tube, considerable diligence is needed to prevent the introduction of infection. The distribution of the drug throughout the ventricals is fairly rapid but to reach sites distant from the ventrical relies soley on diffusion and so a gradient is established which can make determining effective dose arduous.

Intrathecal (IT). When drug application to a portion of the spinal cord is desired, this is often the route of choice. It usually involves introducing a small catheter into the atlo-occipital opening just under the dura and then thredding it down along the surface of the cord to the level desired. The drug is then introduced in a small volume into the cerebrospinal fluid of the subdural skill and practiced but is much less likely to produce damage than the introduction of a needle through the intervertebral space.

Drug Absorption. The two major factors affecting the amount and rate of drug absorption are:

A. Drug Factors
    1. Charge and lipid solubility
    2. Concentration gradient
    3. Geometry and functional grouping
    4. Molecular size
    5. Particle size and physical state
    6. Solubility and rate of dissolution
B. Barrier Factors
    1. Absorbing surface area
    2. Bowel activity
    3. Enzymatic activity
    4. Stomach emptying time
    5. pH of the compartment
    6. Vascularity and blood flow of the compartment

Membrane (barrier) permeabilities (for example, gut to blood, blood to urine and urine to blood) depend upon the transport process, whether it is passive, as in the case of diffusion and filtration, or active. Most drugs are salts of weak acids or bases and are passively transported across membranes based upon the pH-partition hypothesis--i.e., only lipid-soluble, unionized molecules can move down a concentration gradient. The stomach has a low pH and consequently weak acids, such as the barbiturates, exist primarily in the unionized state and are absorbed at a rate dependent upon their lipid solubility. However the narcotic analgesics, such as morphine, are weak bases and absorbed poorly from the stomach. Drug interactions can markedly influence absorption; for example, epinephrine produces vasoconstriction thus delaying the absorption of local anesthetics; narcotic and sedative-hypnotic drugs produce respiratory depression and delay the uptake of inhalation anesthetics; alkalosis will decrease the amount of phenobarbital entering the brain and increase the amount excreted in the urine.

Protein Binding. Many drugs are bound to plasma proteins, especially albumin. Only the free drug in the plasma can pass to receptor sites and elicit a pharmacological effect. Any attempt to describe intensity of drug action in terms of blood concentrations will be frustrated, unless the degree of protein binding is known. The binding percentage of some drugs varies with the drug plasma concentration. Competitive protein binding has been demonstrated between muscle relaxants and local anesthetics (1254) and a large number of other drugs (1253). A knowledge of protein binding is mandatory for the investigator who is studying drug-receptor interactions by the use of agonist-antagonist drug combinations.

Distribution. Once a drug enters the circulation a constant distribution and redistribution occurs until it is finally eliminated from the body. Blood flow, protein binding and the blood-tissue partition ratio initially determine drug distribution to receptor, storage (fat, bone, etc.) and biotransformation-excretion sites. This is followed by redistribution of the drug from primary receptor and storage sites to secondary and/or biotransformation-excretion sites. The short duration of thiopental anesthesia is due to a combination of metabolism and redistribution of the drug from brain to muscle and fat (1255). Changes in the distribution of cardiac output, such as in shock, would shunt blood from liver, muscle and fat and produce higher plasma and hence brain levels, resulting in a more intense and longer-lasting anesthetic state. Renal and/or liver disease would likewise alter drug disposition and result in intensified drug action.

Biotransformation. The term detoxification was formerly used to describe drug metabolism but was discarded when it became apparent that some drugs are metabolically *activated* in the body. For example, the antidepressant activity of imipramine is mediated by its metabolite desmethylimipramine (1256). Most drug biotransformation occurs in liver microsomes and involves microsomal enzyme, cytochrome p-450, reduced nicotinamide adenine dinucleotide (NADPH) and molecular oxygen. This system is reviewed in several excellent papers (1253, 1257, 1258). Only brief generalizations will be presented here. Acceleration of drug metabolism by "enzyme induction" has been demonstrated in animals following the repeated administration of barbiturates, analgesics, tranquilizers, antihistamines, sex hormones, oral antidiabetic drugs, anti-inflammatory agents and many others (1259). While prior drug exposure may be controlled by the investigator to some extent, the fact that insecticides, herbicides and various other hydrocarbon compounds are capable of inducing enzyme synthesis, or possibly blocking enzyme activity, creates a potential source of variation in drug disposition between and within animal species. For example, narcotic analgesics, diethyl ether, chloramphenicol and antidepressant drugs have been shown to inhibit hepatic enzymes (1259). Use of chloramphenicol as a laboratory antibiotic prolongs barbiturate sleep in dogs and cats (1260).

A more immediate effect on drug metabolism is the inhibition of microsomal enzyme systems by a variety of drugs such as sulfonamides (and other antimicrobials), phenylbutazone, and cimetidine. Toxic effects depend on the plasma drug plateau concentrations established after enzyme inhibition.

Excretion. Most drug elimination occurs via the kidney except in the case of inhalation agents and a few compounds that are excreted into the bile. Even the metabolic products of some of the halogenated inhalation anesthetics are excreted in the urine (1261) and their metabolism can be "induced" by other drugs. They in turn have the ability to "induce" enzymes responsible for metabolizing other drugs such as phenobarbital (1262).

Factors which govern drug absorption and distribution also play a role in determining urinary excretion. Since reabsorption of weak acids and bases from the urine also depends upon the pH-Partition Hypothesis, urine acidification will facilitate clearance of amphetamine and ephedrine while favoring reabsorption of barbiturates and salicylates. Respiratory acidosis, secondary to hypoventilation in spontaneously breathing anesthetized animals, or respiratory alkalosis produced by mechanical hyperventilation, may have profound effects on the absorption, distribution and excretion of some drugs.

An increasing number of investigators are using drugs in experimental animals, some in only a "minor" way (for anesthesia) and other for purposes of pharmacological investigation. This introductory material is designed to provide a general background for understanding the many variables that interact to govern the magnitude, onset and duration of drug action. The following section, on anesthetic principles and techniques, will emphasize factors governing the uptake, distribution and elimination of anesthetic agents.

ANESTHESIA

Anesthetic principles and techniques used in biomedical research have been reviewed (1263, 2279). Unfortunately, the review fails to distinguish the marked differences between the anesthetic technique for acute (non-recovery) experiments and that for chronic (recovery) experiments. The two experimental conditions require vastly different techniques and anesthetic considerations. General anesthesia may be produced by injection of drugs such as barbiturates, chloralose, urethane, etc. or by inhalation of agents such as the anesthetic gases, nitrous oxide and cyclopropane or the volatile hydrocarbons diethyl ether, isoflurane, halothane and methoxyflurane. Principles of drug disposition, discussed in the introduction, especially apply to the injectable agents since there is a continuous distribution, redistribution, metabolism and excretion of, for example, pentobarbital, and this results in a continual change in brain concentration and hence anesthetic state. For chronic experiments, a changing state of anesthesia presents no problem providing that overdose is avoided and analgesia and immobility are maintained. Similarly, injectable agents for preanesthetic medication or use as adjuncts to general anesthesia may be rationally used in recovery experiments but these same drugs, as well as injectable general anesthetic agents, provide a varying intensity of drug effect as a background for collection of experimental data. Interpretation of data derived from acute experiments using barbiturate type anesthesia is difficult because of the animal's constantly changing homeostatic background. The description of barbiturate anesthesia as "an hormonal physiologic situation" (1264) should perhaps be applied to the use of any injectable anesthetic. The popularity of α-chloralose for cardiovascular and neurophysiological studies is based upon the drug's apparent lack of reflex and cardiovascular depression compared to the barbiturates. In one study of left ventricular dynamics following a small single dose of chloralose (60 mg/kg, IV), it was demonstrated that the heart rate, blood pressure and cardiac output of dogs did not change from awake values over a three-hour period (1265). However, when attempts were made to keep a constant "level" of anesthesia by infusion of chloralose (330 mg/kg, IV) over a three-hour period, there were marked fluctuations in cardiovascular parameters (1266). Unfortunately, any attempt to maintain a constant brain concentration of injectable anesthetic by means of I.V. infusion and using some "sign of anesthesia level" such as depression of corneal pain or other reflexes is doomed to result in wide fluctuations of the anesthetic state. In a study of five injectable anesthetics, using I.V. infusion and a variety of "signs of anesthesia," it was found that only walking and freedom from ataxia appeared in the same order with all drugs tested and furthermore, a sign of "deep anesthesia" such as depression of the patella reflex often persisted until the animal was capable of spontaneous movement (1267). To further diminish the possibility of achieving a constant anesthetic state, the same author showed that acute tolerance occurs--during a single exposure to the five injectable anesthetics studied; the central nervous system appears to adapt to the presence of the drug (1268). This means that even assuming a constant brain concentration could be maintained (a very difficult task when one considers the many dynamic factors we have discussed which affect drug disposition), the anesthetic "level" will change with time.

Inhalation anesthesia and the avoidance of injectable preanesthetic drugs appear to offer the closest approximation to a constant anesthetic state for acute experiments. In chronic experiments where data is collected under anesthesia several times, anesthetic stability via inhalation agents is mandatory. The uptake and distribution of inhalation anesthetics has been recently reviewed (1269). The great advantage of inhalation compared to injection anesthesia is that once equilibrium has been established, alveolar, arterial and brain concentrations are equal. Therefore, monitoring alveolar (end-tidal) concentration, and maintaining it constant by altering inspired concentration, assures a constant brain concentration and hence anesthetic "level" except for one problem. A study (1270) showed that cardiovascular adaptation in man occurs over a five-hour period of anesthesia with cyclopropane, diethyl ether, fluroxene and halothane. Perhaps this reflects an acute tolerance similar to that seen with the injection anesthetics (1268). However, the same study reported unpublished observations that no time-related cardiovascular adaptation occurs with halothane in the dog. These observations would have to be extended to other animal species before one could be certain that laboratory animals do not show acute tolerance to inhalation anesthetics. A publication from the same laboratory (1270) reported that no circulatory adaptation occurs in man anesthetized with isoflurane, a volatile hydrocarbon anesthetic that is not metabolized in the body.

The concept of minimum alveolar concentration (MAC), i.e., the alveolar concentration of inhalation agent required to prevent gross muscular movement in response to a painful stimulus, was introduced in 1963 (1271). MAC has been determined in a number of laboratory animals, including the rat (1272), and provides a technique for maintaining a constant "level" of inhalation anesthesia within and between experiments, thus markedly reducing the variability of experimental data which has been traditionally obtained on a constantly changing anesthetic background.

Utilization of the MAC technique for acute experiments in laboratory animals involves expensive apparatus for dispensing and monitoring inhalation agents, but in our opinion this expense, when compared to that of other "routine" laboratory supplies such as polygraphs, stimulators, oscilloscopes, etc., is justified on the basis of more precise control over anesthesia and the subsequent greater validity of collected data. A reflection of this view is demonstrated in a neurophysiological study (1273) where the authors state that inhalation anesthesia more closely approximates a "normal" brain state, produced by an *encephale isole* preparation, than do animals under barbiturate anesthesia.

It is important to note that morbidity and mortality, in animals that must recover from anesthesia, is much greater following use of injectable agents, especially pentobarbital, than following use of inhalation agents. This is probably due to the long recovery time, accompanied by heat loss, pneumonia, etc., aggravated by lack of post-operative care.

No matter whether an inhalation or injectable general anesthetic is chosen, there is a good possibility that the agent will add unknown variables to the experiment. Perhaps the most outstanding example of anesthesia interfering with experimental results concerned the initial investigations of the sensory pathways between peripheral receptors and the cerebral cortex. Under anesthesia, the pathways seemed to be quite simple, but later research showed that while primary pathways for afferent stimuli, such as those in the thalamus, were unaffected by deep anesthesia, the secondary reticular pathways were depressed. Another example of anesthetic interference is a report by Gutman and Chainovitz (815). Small doses of pentobarbital, light anesthesia with ether or nitrous oxide, or injection of morphine, converted blood pressure responses to painful stimuli in the rabbit from pressor to depressor. Chlorpromazine, an anesthetic adjunct, attenuated the reaction but did not convert it. The authors also mentioned that the same induced reversal of blood pressure response occurred when stimulating the mesencephalic reticular formation. Finally, Page and McCubbin (809) concluded from their experiments that the greatly augmented depressor activity of ganglionic blocking agents in dogs following pentobarbital anesthesia probably depends upon nearly complete inhibition of parasympathetic, cardioinhibitory activity and partial suppression of sympathetic compensatory reflexes by the action of pentobarbital. The above examples serve to demonstrate the problems which may arise from using anesthetic or anesthetic adjuncts which modify the physiological parameters under investigation.

The final part of this section provides suggestions regarding the use of general anesthesia in acute animal experiments. Seemingly insignificant or self-evident procedures are included, as these are often overlooked by an investigator:

Blood volume. Measurement of central venous pressure (CVP) and urine output will allow infusion of salt solutions to replace losses from bleeding, tissue trauma and other causes of dehydration.

Empty stomach. Animals should be fasted for at least twelve hours prior to administration of the anesthetic as a safeguard against the possibility of vomiting during the experiment and the subsequent aspiration of the material into the lungs.

Rapport. "Making friends" with the animal will contribute much to a smooth anesthetic induction. Attempting to anesthetize a frightened, struggling animal, often made that way by undue restraint, may have fatal consequences due to the use of more anesthetic than normally required.

Route of administration. Injectable anesthetics should be administered intravenously whenever possible. This allows titration of a maximally effective dose. Intrathoracic, subcutaneous and intraperitoneal injections may also be utilized for administration of injectable anesthetics but possess the disadvantage that a bolus injection may be lethal to a sensitive animal.

Temperature maintenance. Whenever possible, the esophageal or rectal temperature of anesthetized animals should be monitored. If the temperature is known, a heating pad can be used as required to maintain a constant body temperature.

The smaller laboratory species are more susceptible to heat loss because of their relatively larger surface area. This phenomenon also helps explain the relatively larger anesthetic (as well as other drugs) doses required by the smaller species.

Unobstructed airway. Placing a tracheal cannula or endotracheal tube in an anesthetized animal provides a patent airway and permits aspiration of accumulated secretions which might impair respiratory exchange.

Ventilation. All general anesthetics and many of the drugs used for preanesthetic medication and during anesthesia are respiratory depressants. Adequate ventilation cannot be assessed by "extent of chest wall expansion and the persistence of bright red arterial blood" as has been reported. Only measurement of end-tidal or arterial carbon dioxide tension ($PaCO_2$) and maintenance within a normal range assures adequate ventilation. Hypoxemia with resultant metabolic acidosis can be avoided with certainty only by measuring and correcting and deficits in arterial oxygen tension (PaO_2) and pH. Acid-base changes can profoundly change the disposition of both injected and inhaled drugs by altering ionization, receptor sensitivity, tissue perfusion, metabolic and excretory mechanisms, etc. A sophisticated review of anesthesia and ventilation is presented in an earlier publication (1277).

ANESTHETIC DOSES

The following pages present a list of injectable anesthetics and preanesthetic medications which have been successfully used in various animal species. In some instances two or more agents are listed to be used in combination. For example, atropine, morphine, and pentobarbital have been used in combination to produce anesthesia in a dog. In this case, the atropine and morphine are administered 30 and 29 minutes, respectively, prior to the pentobarbital. These two premedication agents serve to reduce the incidence of parasympathetic secretions and provide analgesia prior to administering the pentobarbital. Following the tables is a list of the major advantages and disadvantages associated with some of the more widely used anesthetic agents.

ABBREVIATIONS
Used in Drug Dosage Tables

μg	microgram
μMol	micromole
BID	twice daily
d	day
ED	effective dose
g	gram
h	hour
IG	intragastric
IA	intra-arterial
IC	intracardiac
ICV	intracerebroventricular
IM	intramuscular
IP	intraperitoneal
IT	intrathecal
IV	intravenous
kg	kilogram
L	liter
LD	lethal dose
LD_{50}	lethal dose - 50%
M	meter
MED	minimum effective dose
mg	milligram
MLD	minimum lethal dose
mMol	millimole
ng	nanogram
nMol	nanomole
PC	per cutaneous
PO	per os (orally)
Q	every
QID	4 times daily
SC	subcutaneous

TABLE 1
Anesthetic Doses

Species	Anesthetic [a]	Time [b] (min.)	Route [a]	Dose (mg/kg)	Reference
Mouse	Amobarbital		IV	54	65
	Barbital		IV	234	65
	Chloral Hydrate		IP	400	LM[c]
	α-Chloralose		IP	114	204
	Chlorobutanol (in 50% alcohol)		IP	175	LM
	Droperidol(2%)-Fentanyl(0.04%)		IP	[d]0.02-0.05	LM
	Etomidate		IP	22-25	2274
	Hexobarbital		IV	47	392
	Ketamine		IV	50	2279
	Ketamine		IP	100-200	2279
	Ketamine		IM	400	2279
	Pentobarbital		IV	35	111
	Phenobarbital		IV	134	65
	Probarbital		IP	75	66
	Secobarbital		IV	30	63
	Thiamylal		IV	25-50	2275
	Thiopental		IV	25	111
	Tribromoethanol		IV	120	66
	Urethane		IP	1500	1912
Rat	⌈Acepromazine		IP	12⌉	1540
	⌊Ketamine		IP	120⌋	
	Amobarbital		IV	55	63
	Barbital		IP	190	125
	Chloral Hydrate		IP	300	197
	α-Chloralose		IP	55	205
	α-Chloralose		IV	100	1425
	Diallybarbituric Acid		SC	60	66
	Droperidol(2%)-Fentanyl(0.04%)		IM	[d]0.3	2279
	Droperidol(2%)-Fentanyl(0.04%)		IP	[d]0.13	LM
	Hexobarbital		IP	75	393
	Inactin		IP	100	1842
	Ketamine		IP	100	1430
	Ketamine		IM	100	2267

[a]Other routes of administration may be found with additional dosage information in the main body of the handbook.
[b]The numbers refer to time elapsed (in minutes) before the injection of the following drug.
[c]LM means that the dose was obtained from a pharmacology teaching manual.
[d]Dose is given as ml/kg.
[e]mg/kg/min infusion

TABLE 1 (continued)

Species	Anesthetic [a]	Time [b] (min.)	Route [a]	Dose (mg/kg)	Reference
Rat (cont'd)	Ketamine		IP	40-160	2279
	Methohexital		IP	37.5	2265
	Pentobarbital		IV	25	111
	[Pentobarbital		IP	35]	1164
	Chloral Hydrate		IP	160]	
	[Pentobarbital		IP	10]	2266
	Ketamine		IP	75]	
	Phenobarbital		IP	40	2265
	Phenobarbital		IV	100	589
	Probarbital		SC	225	66
	Secobarbital		IV	17.5	63
	Thiopental		IV	25	111
	Tiletamine-Zolazepam (1:1)		IM	20-30	2274
	Tribromoethanol		IP	550	547
	Urethane		IP	780	127
	Urethane		SC	1200	1167
	[Xylazine		IM	6]	1958
	Ketamine		IM	80]	
Guinea Pig	Amobarbital		IV	50	63
	Chloral Hydrate		IP	400	1164
	Chlorobutanol (in 50% alcohol)		IP	175	LM
	Droperidol(2%)-Fentanyl(0.04%)		IM	[d]0.66-0.88	2279
	Droperidol(2%)-Fentanyl(0.04%)		IP	0.8	LM
	Ketamine		IM	44-256	2279
	Pentobarbital		IP	30	2279
	Pentobarbital		IM	15-30	2279
	Pentobarbital		IV	30	111
	[Pentobarbital		IP	35]	1164
	Chloral Hydrate		IP	160]	
	Phenobarbital		IP	100	LM
	Secobarbital		IV	20	63
	Thiopental		IV	20	111
	Tribromoethanol		IV	100	66
	Urethane		IP	1500	LM
Rabbit	Amobarbital		IV	40	72
	Barbital		IV	175	LM
	α-Chloralose		IV	120	LM
	Chloral hydrate		IV	200	2279
	Diallylbarbituric Acid		IV	50	LM
	Droperidol(2%)-Fentanyl(0.04%)		IM	[d]0.22	2274

TABLE 1 (continued)

Species	Anesthetic [a]	Time [b] (min.)	Route [a]	Dose (mg/kg)	Reference
Rabbit (cont'd)	Hexobarbital		IV	25	LM
	Ketamine		IV	15-20	2279
	Ketamine		IM	44	2279
	⌈ Morphine	30	SC	10 ⌉	LM
	⌊ Chlorobutanol (in 50% alcohol)		PO	175 ⌋	
	Paraldehyde		IV	300	7
	Pentobarbital		IV	30	111
	Pentobarbital		IP	40	2279
	Pentobarbital		IV	25-40	2279
	Phenobarbital		IV	200	590
	Probarbital		IP	66	66
	Secobarbital		IV	22.5	72
	Thiamylal		IV,IP	45-50	2275
	Thiopental		IV	20	111
	Thiopental		IV	20-50	2279
	Tribromoethanol		IV	80	66
	Urethane		IV	1000	LM
	⌈ Urethane		IP	700 ⌉	305
	⌊ Pentobarbital		IP	40 ⌋	
	Xylazine		IM	5	2279
	⌈ Xylazine		IM	5 ⌉	1733
	⌊ Ketamine		IM	50 ⌋	
Cat	Amobarbital		IV	11	24
	Barbital		IV	200	LM
	Chloral Hydrate		PO	250	LM
	α-Chloralose		IV	75	208
	⌈ α-Chloralose		IV	50 ⌉	747
	⌊ Urethane		IV	50 ⌋	
	⌈ α-Chloralose		IV	80 ⌉	748
	⌊ Pentobarbital		IV	12 ⌋	
	⌈ α-Chloralose		IV	80 ⌉	154
	⌊ Pentobarbital		IV	6 ⌋	
	Diallylbarbituric Acid		IV	36	291
	Hexobarbital		IV	25	66
	Ketamine		IM	11-33	2272
	Ketamine		IV	11-22	LM
	⌈ Ketamine		IM	6.6-22 ⌉	LM
	⌊ Acepromazine		IV,IM	0.22-0.55 ⌋	
	⌈ Ketamine		IM	6.6-22 ⌉	LM
	⌊ Diazepam		IV,IM	0.33-1.1 ⌋	
	⌈ Ketamine	10-15	IM	10-15 ⌉	1686
	⌊ Pentobarbital		IV	30 ⌋	
	⌈ Ketamine		IM	6.6-22 ⌉	LM
	⌊ Xylazine		IM	0.44 ⌋	

TABLE 1 (continued)

Species	Anesthetic [a]	Time [b] (min.)	Route [a]	Dose (mg/kg)	Reference
Cat (cont'd)	Pentobarbital		IP	20 ⎤	2228
	Barbital		IP	200 ⎦	
	Methohexital		IV	11	2273
	Paraldehyde		IV	300	7
	Pentobarbital		IV	25	111
	Phenobarbital		IP	180	LM
	Secobarbital		IV	25	63
	Thiamylal		IV	17.6	2275
	Thiamylal		i.thoracic	25	2275
	Thiopental		IV	28	24
	Tiletamine-Zolazepam (1:1)		IM	6-13	2274
	Tribromoethanol		IV	100	557
	Urethane		IV	1250	LM
	Urethane		IP	400 ⎤	749
	α-Chloralose		IP	50 ⎦	
	Urethane		IP	280 ⎤	750
	Diallylbarbituric Acid		IP	70 ⎦	
	Urethane		IP	360 ⎤	408
	Diallylbarbituric Acid		IP	90 ⎦	
	Urethane		IP	250 ⎤	LM
	Pentobarbital		IP	30 ⎦	
Dog	Acepromazine	10-15	IM	0.55 ⎤	
	Ketamine	5	IM	11-22	2274
	Thiamylal		IV	To effect ⎦	
	Amobarbital		IV	50	LM
	Barbital		IV	220	LM
	Barbital		IV	250 ⎤	LM
	Thiopental		IV	15 ⎦	
	Barbital		IV	220 ⎤	422
	Pentobarbital		IV	15 ⎦	
	Chloral Hydrate		IV	125	LM
	α-Chloralose		IV	100	209
	Dial-urethane		IV	[d]10	2269
	Droperidol(2%)-Fentanyl(0.04%)		IM	[d]0.05-0.15	LM
	Droperidol(2%)-Fentanyl(0.04%)		IV	[d]0.03-0.09	LM
	Etomidate		IV	1.5-3	2274
	α-Chloralose		IV	100 ⎤	2268
	α-Chloralose		IV	[e]0.17 ⎦	
	Morphine		IM	2 ⎤	1368
	α-Chloralose		IV	100 ⎦	
	Morphine	30	SC	1 ⎤	490
	α-Chloralose		IV	100 ⎦	
	Morphine	60	SC	1 ⎤	753
	α-Chloralose		IV	80 ⎦	

TABLE 1 (continued)

Species	Anesthetic [a]	Time [b] (min.)	Route [a]	Dose (mg/kg)	Reference
Dog (cont'd)	⎡ α-Chloralose		IV	50 ⎤	LM
	⎣ Thiopental		IV	15 ⎦	
	⎡ Morphine	30	SC	10 ⎤	LM
	⎣ Chlorobutonal				
	(in 50% alcohol)		PO	225 ⎦	
	Morphine		SC	1	966
	Thiopental		IV	20	LM
	Hexobarbital		IV	30	66
	Methohexital		IV	11	2273
	Paraldehyde		IV	300	7
	⎡ Pentobarbital		IP	30 ⎤	497
	⎣ Pentobarbital		IV	e6 ⎦	
	⎡ Pentobarbital		IV	10 ⎤	2027
	⎣ α-Chloralose		IV	80 ⎦	
	⎡ Morphine	30	SC	10 ⎤	751
	⎣ Pentobarbital		IV	20 ⎦	
	⎡ Morphine	30	IM	2 ⎤	747
	⎣ Pentobarbital		IV	15 ⎦	
	⎡ Morphine	60	IM	3 ⎤	458
	⎣ Pentobarbital		IV	12 ⎦	
	⎡ Atropine	30	SC	1 ⎤	
	⎢ Morphine	30	SC	10	LM
	⎣ Pentobarbital		IV	30 ⎦	
	Phenobarbital		IV	80	591
	⎡ Phenobarbital		IV	200 ⎤	LM
	⎣ Thiopental		IV	15 ⎦	
	⎡ Promazine	5	IV,IM	4.4 ⎤	LM
	⎣ Ketamine		IM	17.6 ⎦	
	⎡ Promazine	5	IV,IM	4.4 ⎤	LM
	⎣ Ketamine		IV	to effect ⎦	
	Secobarbital		PO	40	63
	Thiamylal		IV	17.6	2275
	Tiletamine-		IM	6-13	2274
	Zolazepam (1:1)				
	Thiopental		IV	25	716
	Tribromoethanol		IV	125	557
	Urethane		IV	1000	413
	⎡ Urethane		IP	500 ⎤	2270
	⎣ α-Chloralose		IP	50 ⎦	
	⎡ Urethane		IV	480 ⎤	
	⎢ α-Chloralose		IV	48	752
	⎣ Morphine		IV	2 ⎦	
	⎡ Morphine	60	SC	2 ⎤	
	⎢ Urethane		IV	250	742
	⎣ α-Chloralose		IV	60 ⎦	

TABLE 1 (continued)

Species	Anesthetic [a]	Time [b] (min.)	Route [a]	Dose (mg/kg)	Reference
Dog (cont'd)	Morphine	60	SC	3	LM
	Urethane		IV	50	
	α–Chloralose		IV	13	
	Diallylbarbituric Acid		IV	8	
	Morphine	30	SC	5	LM
	Urethane		PO	1500	
	Xylazine	5	IV	1	2274
	Ketamine		IV	10	
Monkey	Amobarbital		IV	40	63
	Dial-Urethane		IV	[d]0.7	2271
	Droperidol(2%)- Fentanyl(0.04%)		IM	[d]0.11	2279
	Ketamine		IV	28-45	2279
	Ketamine		IM	7-40	2279
	Ketamine	10-15	IM	18	2274
	Thiamylal		IV	15	
	Pentobarbital		IV	20-33	2279
	Pentobarbital		IP	30	2279
	Pentobarbital		IV	25	111
	Phenobarbital		IP	100	161
	Secobarbital		IV	17.5	63
	Tiletamine- Zolazepam (1:1)		IM	3	2274
	Thiamylal		IV	25	2275
	Xylazine	10-15	IM	6	2279
	Ketamine		IV	To effect	
	Xylazine		IM	6	2279
	Ketamine		IM	7-40	

[a]Other routes of administration may be found with additional dosage information in the main body of the handbook.

[b]The numbers refer to time elapsed (in minutes) before the injection of the following drug.

[c] LM means that the dose was obtained from a pharmacology teaching manual.

[d]Dose is given as ml/kg.

[e]mg/kg/min infusion

TABLE 2
Advantages and Disadvantages for Anesthetic Agents and Adjuncts

Agent	Advantages	Disadvantages
1. Injection Anesthetics	Inexpensive, easy to use, rapid onset.	Constantly changing anesthetic state. Poor reproducibility.
α-Chloralose	Less reflex depression than barbiturates. Catecholamine release may support circulation (1266).	Low water solubility. Inject warm or in a 10% solution with propylene glycol 200.
Dial (Ciba)*	More rapid onset and less toxic than urethane alone. Less reflex depression than with barbiturate alone.	Urethane toxicity limits use to acute experiment.
Droperidol-Fentanyl	IV use not generally required. Analgesic; can antagonize opioid component (fentanyl).	Cardiac and respiratory depression. Transient behavioral changes. Thermo-regulatory upset; vomition, defecation.
Etomidate	Potent hypnotic, wide margin of safety, rapid induction.	Not analgesic in subanesthetic doses.
Ketamine	IV use not generally required. Large margin of safety; no cardiovascular nor respiratory depression. Analgesic.	Poor relaxation and poor recovery; convulsive, hallucinogenic. Retention of reflexes. Used in combination with phenothiazines, benzodiazepines and xylazine to overcome disadvantages.
Methohexital	Very short duration (<15 min, may be a disadvantage). Recovery from metabolism (use in low fat animal).	IV use required; short duration; violent recovery possible. Metabolism required; low margin of safety.
Pentobarbital	Rapid onset. High water solubility.	IV use required generally. Marked cardiovascular and reflex depression. Extravascular → severe inflammation, sloughing.
Thiamylal	Short duration (15-30 min). Recovery from redistribution (metabolism later). Good anesthesia and relaxation.	Longer duration in animals with low body fat. IV use generally required. Cardiovascular and respiratory depression; low margin of safety.
Thiopental	Short duration (15-30 min). Useful to induce anesthesia prior to inhalation agents.	Solution rapidly decomposes. Fat solubility → remains in the body a long time (1255).

*Contains: Urethane, 400 mg/ml.
Diallylbarbituric Acid, 100 mg/ml.

TABLE 2 (continued)

Agent	Advantages	Disadvantages
Tiletamine-Zolazepam	Similar to ketamine-diazepam combinations.	
Urethane	Little reflex depression. High water solubility. Long duration.	Liver and bone marrow toxicity. Used only in acute experiments.

2. __Inhalation Anesthetics__

Agent	Advantages	Disadvantages
Inhalation Anesthetics	Constant and reproducible anesthesia, therefore less data variability.	More skill required. Some need expensive equipment. Alveolar tension difficult to monitor in animal smaller than rat (1272).
Cyclopropane	Rapid induction. Easy to measure--as difference from oxygen (1274).	Explosive, circulatory adaptation. Tendency to laryngospasm.
Diethyl Ether	Respiratory stimulation. Good muscle relaxation.	Slow induction and slow recovery. Explosive and stimulates secretions. Long duration in body fat. Circulatory adaptation occurs.
Floroxene	Cardiovascular stimulation. Little respiratory depression.	Irritating and explosive over 4%. Circulatory adaptation. Metabolized in the body.
Halothane	Rapid induction, rapid recovery, Non-explosive and potent.	Expensive. Cardiovascular depression and adaptation. Sensitization of myocardium to catecholamines. Poor analgesia; metabolized. Need precision vaporizers. Malignant hyperthermia implications.
Isoflurane	Low metabolism. Non-explosive. No circulatory → adaptation "constant" anesthetic state. Rapid induction, rapid recovery.	Expensive. Cardiorespiratory depression. Need precision vaporizers.
Methoxy-flurane	Potent and non-explosive. Non-irritating to respiratory tract. Good analgesia (post-anesthetic) and muscle relaxation. Precision vaporizers not needed.	Slow induction and slow recovery. Alveolar-arterial gradient. High fat solubility → long duration in body. High oxygen flows to vaporize. Highly metabolized. Ages rubber equipment.
Nitrous Oxide	Not metabolized. Easily measured (1275) and used (1278). Analgesic, additive to other anesthetics.	Only analgesia in safe concentrations. Need muscle relaxants to prevent movement. Hypoxia and diffusion hypoxia.

TABLE 2 (continued)

Agent	Advantages	Disadvantages
3. Adjuncts to Anesthesia	Facilitate induction and maintenance of anesthesia, improve safety.	Injectable drugs and not advised for acute experiments.
Atropine	Decreases respiratory secretion and vagal bradycardia.	Ganglionic blockade and CNS effects.
Benzo-diazepine Tranquilizers (Diazepam)	Used with several anesthetics, especially dissociative types (e.g., ketamine). Improves induction and recovery; better relaxation (allows intubation).	
Phenothazine Tranquilzers (Chlor-promazine)	Preanesthetic sedation. Reduces dose of anesthetic required.	Many pharmacological actions, especially cardiovascular depression. Prolonged recovery.
Curare	Immobility with minimal anesthesia or with nitrous oxide. "Ordinary doses" do not enter brain (1276).	Release histamine. Need artificial ventilation. Must use analgesics.
Succinyl-choline	Rapid onset and short duration. Can titrate I.V. Immobility with minimal anesthesia.	Increased serum K^+. Implicated in malignant hyperthermia. Other cholinergic actions. Must use analgesics.
Narcotics (Morphine)	Analgesia and sedation facilitate anesthesia. Use as only anesthetic if support ventilation.	Release histamine. Respiratory depression causing delay in induction of inhalation anesthesia.
Xylazine	Preanesthetic sedation; reduces dose of anesthetic; analgesic. Emetic action (especially in cats; may be a disadvantage). Antagonized by α_2 blockers (e.g., yohimbine)	Cardiorespiratory depression; emesis; severe CNS depression.

DRUG DOSAGE TABLES

ACETALDEHYDE

(Ethanal, Acetic Aldehyde, Ethylaldehyde)

mg/kg		Mouse	Rat	Guinea Pig	Rabbit	Cat	Dog	Monkey	
Lethal Dose	IV				Y300 [3]	300 [4]			
Y-LD$_{50}$	IP		500 [2]						
Z-MLD	IM								
	SC	Y560 [1]	Y640 [1]		Y1200 [3]				
	PO		Y1900						
Hypnotic	IV						8.5 [4]		
	IP				700 [4]				
	IM				700 [4]				
	SC				700 [4]				
	PO								
Sympathomimetic	IV					10 [5]	10		
	IP								
	IM								
	SC								
	PO								
	IV								
	IP								
	IM								
	SC								
	PO								

IN VITRO

mg %	Cardiac	Vascular	Gut	Uterine	Visceral	Skeletal	Trachea	

ACETAMINOPHEN
(Datril, Phenaphen, Tylenol)

mg/kg		Mouse	Rat	Guinea Pig	Rabbit	Cat	Dog	Monkey
Lethal Dose	IV							
Y-LD$_{50}$	IP							
Z-MLD	IM							
	SC							
	PO							
Nephrotoxic	IV							
	IP	400 1279	710 1280					
	IM							
	SC							
	PO							
Hepatotoxic	IV							
	IP	600 1281	500 1282					
	IM							
	SC							
	PO							
Anti-inflammatory	IV							
	IP							
	IM							
	SC							
	PO		1195 1283					
Analgesic [a]Q8h [b]Freund's adjuvant	IV							
	IP							
	IM							
	SC							
	PO		b 200 1284				a 10 2272	
Inhibit acetic acid writhing	IV							
	IP							
	IM							
	SC							
	PO		305 1291					
	IV							
	IP							
	IM							
	SC							
	PO							
	IV							
	IP							
	IM							
	SC							
	PO							

ACETANILIDE

(N–Phenylacetamide, Antifebrin, Acetylaniline)

mg/kg		Mouse	Rat	Guinea Pig	Rabbit	Cat	Dog	Monkey	
Lethal Dose	IV					13.5_{11}	300_{11}	300_7	
Y–LD_{50}	IP	$Y820_{946}$	Y800						
Z–MLD	IM								
	SC	1300_6							
	PO	1840_7	$Y800_8$	1500_7	1500_{11}	250_{11}	700_{12}		
Toxic	IV						62_7	275_7	
	IP								
	IM								
	SC	1200_7							
	PO	1840_7	500_{10}		1200_7		700_7	600_7	
Analgesic	IV								
antipyretic	IP	110_{946}	400_9						
	IM								
	SC								
[a]total mg	PO					$^a125$	$^a500$		
	IV								
	IP								
	IM								
	SC								
	PO								

IN VITRO

mg %	Cardiac	Vascular	Gut	Uterine	Visceral	Skeletal	Trachea	

ACETAZOLAMIDE

(Diamox, Acetamox, Vetamox)

mg/kg		Mouse	Rat	Guinea Pig	Rabbit	Cat	Dog	Monkey
Lethal Dose	IV							
Y-LD$_{50}$	IP							
Z-MLD	IM							
	SC							
	PO							
Renal	IV						30 [1286]	
	IP							
	IM							
	SC		0.15 [1285]					
^{a}Q8h	PO					7[a] [2272]	7[a] [2272]	
Choroid	IV		50 [1287]			30 [1289]		
plexus effects	IP		20 [1288]					
	IM							
	SC							
	PO							
Hypocalcemic	IV							
	IP							
	IM							
	SC							
	PO		10 [1290]					
Anticonvulsant	IV							
	IP	100 [1292]						
	IM							
	SC							
	PO							
	IV							
	IP							
	IM							
	SC							
	PO							
	IV							
	IP							
	IM							
	SC							
	PO							
	IV							
	IP							
	IM							
	SC							
	PO							
	IV							
	IP							
	IM							
	SC							
	PO							

mg/kg		Mouse	Rat	Guinea Pig	Rabbit	Cat	Dog	Monkey
Lethal Dose Y-LD$_{50}$ Z-MLD	IV							
	IP							
	IM							
	SC							
	PO							
Hyperkinetic	IV	2.5 [1293]	1 [1293]					
	IP							
	IM							
	SC							
	PO							
Inhibit enkephalinase	IV		10 [1294]					
	IP	1 [1294]						
	IM							
	SC							
	PO							
Analgesic	IV		5 [1294]					
	IP							
	IM							
	SC							
	PO							
Antidiarrheal	IV		5 [1294]					
	IP							
	IM							
	SC							
	PO							
Behavioral	IV	10 [1294]						
	IP	50 [1294]						
	IM							
	SC							
	PO							
	IV							
	IP							
	IM							
	SC							
	PO							
	IV							
	IP							
	IM							
	SC							
	PO							
	IV							
	IP							
	IM							
	SC							
	PO							

ACETYLCHOLINE
(Miochol, Acecoline, Arterocoline)

mg/kg		Mouse	Rat	Guinea Pig	Rabbit	Cat	Dog	Monkey
Lethal Dose Y-LD$_{50}$ Z-MLD	IV	Y20 [13]	Y22 [13]		Y0.3			
	IP	Y>125 [904]						
	IM							
	SC	Y170 [13]	Y250			Y10 [15]		
	PO	Y3000 [13]	Y2500 [13]					
Parasympatho-mimetic	IV	0.004 [1197]	0.002 [855]	0.006 [1295]	0.01	0.01	0.01	
	IP							
	IM							
	SC				1 [14]			
	PO							
Nicotinic (atropinized animal)	IV				0.1	0.1	0.1	
	IP							
	IM							
	SC							
	PO							
Writhing	IV							
	IP	3 [1296]						
	IM							
	SC							
	PO							

IN VITRO

mg %	Cardiac	Vascular	Gut	Uterine	Visceral	Skeletal	Trachea
Guinea Pig	0.025		0.01	0.02	0.02 [16]		0.04 [1157]
Rabbit	0.003 [16]	0.0025 [1298]	0.02 [16]	0.05 [16]	0.07 [16]		
Dog		0.003 [16]	0.1 [16]	0.03 [16]		0.0009 [1800]	
Rat	3.815 [1297]		0.0002 [1157]	0.01 [1157]		1 [1157]	

ACETYLCYSTEINE
(Mucomyst, NAC, Respaire)

mg/kg		Mouse	Rat	Guinea Pig	Rabbit	Cat	Dog	Monkey
Lethal Dose	IV							
Y-LD$_{50}$	IP							
Z-MLD	IM							
	SC							
	PO							
Protect against	IV							
acetaminophen	IP	653 1300	400 1282					
hepatotoxicosis	IM							
	SC							
	PO	1200 1301						
	IV							
	IP							
	IM							
	SC							
	PO							
	IV							
	IP							
	IM							
	SC							
	PO							
	IV							
	IP							
	IM							
	SC							
	PO							
	IV							
	IP							
	IM							
	SC							
	PO							
	IV							
	IP							
	IM							
	SC							
	PO							
	IV							
	IP							
	IM							
	SC							
	PO							
	IV							
	IP							
	IM							
	SC							
	PO							

ADENOSINE

(My-B-Den, 9-ß-D-Ribofuranosidoadenine, Adenine, Riboside)

mg/kg		Mouse	Rat	Guinea Pig	Rabbit	Cat	Dog	Monkey
Lethal Dose	IV	[a]1000 [1318]						
$Y-LD_{50}$	IP							
$Z-MLD$	IM							
[a]LD_{100}	SC							
	PO							
Cardiovascular	IV		[a]0.15 [1319]					
	IP							
[a]mg/kg/min	IM							
	SC							
	PO							
Decrease	IV							
endotoxin	IP	500 [1322]						
mortality	IM							
	SC							
	PO							
	IV							
	IP							
	IM							
	SC							
	PO							

IN VITRO

mg %	Cardiac	Vascular	Gut	Uterine	Visceral	Skeletal		
Guinea Pig	0.0267 [1320]							
Dog	0.0027 [1321]							

ALBUTEROL

(Proventil, Ventolin, Salbutamol)

mg/kg		Mouse	Rat	Guinea Pig	Rabbit	Cat	Dog	Monkey	
Lethal Dose	IV								
Y-LD$_{50}$	IP								
Z-MLD	IM								
	SC								
	PO								
Cardiovascular	IV				0.001 $_{1427}$				
	IP								
	IM								
	SC								
	PO								
Erythropoietic	IV				[b]0.05 $_{2190}$				
	IP								
	IM								
[a]daily	SC	[a]2.5 $_{1855}$			5 $_{2190}$				
[b]mg/kg/min	PO								
	IV								
	IP								
	IM								
	SC								
	PO								
	IV								
	IP								
	IM								
	SC								
	PO								
	IV								
	IP								
	IM								
	SC								
	PO								
	IV								
	IP								
	IM								
	SC								
	PO								
	IV								
	IP								
	IM								
	SC								
	PO								
	IV								
	IP								
	IM								
	SC								
	PO								

ALCOHOL, ANHYDROUS

(Ethanol, Ethyl Alcohol)

mg/kg		Mouse	Rat	Guinea Pig	Rabbit	Cat	Dog	Monkey
Lethal Dose $Y\text{-}LD_{50}$ $Z\text{-}MLD$	IV	Y1953 [27]				3945 [33]	5365 [35]	
	IP	Y7260 [1323]	Y5000 [29]	Y5560 [4]				
	IM							
	SC	Y8285 [27]					7000	
	PO	Y9488 [27]	Y13,600 [4]		Y9500 [29]		6000	
Alter brain chemistry	IV							
	IP		4475 [31]					
	IM							
	SC							
	PO		6000 [1342]					
Behavioral	IV						3000 [981]	
	IP	1000 [1324]	3000 [1329]					
	IM							
	SC							
	PO	3160 [935]					2000 [895]	500 [1325]
CNS $^{a}ED_{50}$	IV		1000 [1208]		690 [34]			
	IP	a3000 [1323]	2250 [1334]					
	IM							
	SC							
	PO							
Paralytic (anesthetic)	IV							
	IP	4000 [28]		4000 [4]		4000 [4]		
	IM							
	SC							
	PO	8835 [1123]	6000 [1180]	4000 [4]	5000 [4]	4000 [4]		
Hypocalcemic	IV							
	IP							
	IM							
	SC							
	PO		4000 [1207]			2000 [1207]		
Metabolic effects $^{a}mg/kg/hr$	IV						a100 [1339]	
	IP	4000 [1326]						
	IM							
	SC							
	PO	6000 [1327]	5000 [1328]					
Dependence	IV							
	IP	1250 [1330]	1000 [1335]					
	IM							
	SC							
	PO							
Endocrine effects $^{a}intragastric$	IV							
	IP	2800 [1331]	2000 [1340]					
	IM							
	SC							
	PO	23,400 [1332]						a2500 [1333]

mg/kg		Mouse	Rat	Guinea Pig	Rabbit	Cat	Dog	Monkey
Thermoregulatory	IV							
	IP	2000 1336	2000 1337					
	IM							
	SC							
	PO							
Affect circadian rhythm	IV							
	IP	2000 1338						
	IM							
	SC							
	PO							
Teratogenic	IV							
	IP							
	IM							
	SC							
	PO		6000 1341					
	IV							
	IP							
	IM							
	SC							
	PO							
	IV							
	IP							
	IM							
	SC							
	PO							
	IV							
	IP							
	IM							
	SC							
	PO							
	IV							
	IP							
	IM							
	SC							
	PO							
	IV							
	IP							
	IM							
	SC							
	PO							
	IV							
	IP							
	IM							
	SC							
	PO							

ALINIDINE
(ST 567-BR)

mg/kg		Mouse	Rat	Guinea Pig	Rabbit	Cat	Dog	Monkey	
Lethal Dose	IV								
Y-LD$_{50}$	IP								
Z-MLD	IM								
	SC								
	PO								
Cardiac	IV						[1] 1343		
	IP								
	IM								
	SC								
	PO								
	IV								
	IP								
	IM								
	SC								
	PO								
	IV								
	IP								
	IM								
	SC								
	PO								

IN VITRO

mg %	Cardiac	Vascular	Gut	Uterine	Visceral	Skeletal		
Guinea Pig	[a]2.8×10^{-5}*							
Dog	8.5×10^{-8}**							
[a]molar								
solution								

*2163   **1343

ALLOBARBITAL

(Diallylbarbituric acid, Dial, Malilum)

mg/kg		Mouse	Rat	Guinea Pig	Rabbit	Cat	Dog	Monkey
Lethal Dose	IV				70 109			
Y-LD$_{50}$	IP				Z100 128	100 290		
Z-MLD	IM							
	SC		Y110 68		100 109			
	PO			30 76	Z125 128			
Anesthetic	IV				50	36 291		
	IP					70 292		
	IM							
	SC	60 66						
	PO							
	IV							
	IP							
	IM							
	SC							
	PO							
	IV							
	IP							
	IM							
	SC							
	PO							

IN VITRO

mg %	Cardiac	Vascular	Gut	Uterine	Visceral	Skeletal		

ALLOXAN

(Mesoxalylurea, Mesoxalylcarbamide)

mg/kg		Mouse	Rat	Guinea Pig	Rabbit	Cat	Dog	Monkey	
Lethal Dose	IV	Y200 36	300 37		200 7		100 41		
Y-LD$_{50}$	IP	Y350 36							
Z-MLD	IM								
	SC								
	PO								
Diabetogenic	IV	75 1344	40 38						
	IP		200 39						
	IM								
	SC		200 40						
	PO					750 7			
	IV								
	IP								
	IM								
	SC								
	PO								
	IV								
	IP								
	IM								
	SC								
	PO								
	IV								
	IP								
	IM								
	SC								
	PO								
	IV								
	IP								
	IM								
	SC								
	PO								
	IV								
	IP								
	IM								
	SC								
	PO								
	IV								
	IP								
	IM								
	SC								
	PO								
	IV								
	IP								
	IM								
	SC								
	PO								

ALLYLGLYCINE
(DL-2-Amino-4-pentanoic acid)

mg/kg		Mouse	Rat	Guinea Pig	Rabbit	Cat	Dog	Monkey	
Lethal Dose	IV								
Y-LD$_{50}$	IP	218.75 [1354]							
Z-MLD	IM								
	SC								
	PO								
Seizures	IV								
	IP	[a]115.13 [1354]					495 [1354]		
	IM								
[a]ED$_{50}$	SC								
	PO								
	IV								
	IP								
	IM								
	SC								
	PO								
	IV								
	IP								
	IM								
	SC								
	PO								
	IV								
	IP								
	IM								
	SC								
	PO								
	IV								
	IP								
	IM								
	SC								
	PO								
	IV								
	IP								
	IM								
	SC								
	PO								
	IV								
	IP								
	IM								
	SC								
	PO								
	IV								
	IP								
	IM								
	SC								
	PO								

ALPHAPRODINE

(Nisentil, Nu 1196, Prisilidene)

mg/kg		Mouse	Rat	Guinea Pig	Rabbit	Cat	Dog	Monkey	
Lethal Dose	IV	Y54 [42]		Y18 [42]	Y18.5				
Y-LD$_{50}$	IP	Y73 [42]	Y22 [42]						
Z-MLD	IM								
	SC	Y98 [42]	Y23 [42]						
	PO		Y90 [43]						
Analgesic	IV								
	IP								
	IM								
	SC		3 [43]				20		
	PO		10 [43]						
Cardiovascular	IV				1.5 [43]		1 [42]		
and	IP								
respiratory	IM								
	SC								
	PO								
Increase	IV						1 [43]		
intestinal	IP								
tone	IM								
	SC								
	PO								
	IV								
	IP								
	IM								
	SC								
	PO								
	IV								
	IP								
	IM								
	SC								
	PO								
	IV								
	IP								
	IM								
	SC								
	PO								
	IV								
	IP								
	IM								
	SC								
	PO								
	IV								
	IP								
	IM								
	SC								
	PO								

ALPROSTADIL

(Prostin VR, Prostaglandin E$_1$, PGE$_1$)

mg/kg		Mouse	Rat	Guinea Pig	Rabbit	Cat	Dog	Monkey	
Lethal Dose	IV								
Y-LD$_{50}$	IP								
Z-MLD	IM								
	SC								
	PO								
Cardiovascular	IV						[a]0.002 2155		
[a]total mg/min	IP	0.05 2158					[b]0.25 2155		
[b]total μg IA	IM						[c]0.0001		
[c]mg/kg/min	SC								
i. cardiac	PO								
Thermoregulatory	IV					[a]0.3 2161			
	IP		0.5 2160			[b]0.5 2161			
[a]total mg	IM								
[b]total μg ICV	SC								
	PO								
Anticonvulsant	IV	[a]57.6 2122							
[a]total μg ICV	IP	[b]3.75 2122							
(vs strychine)	IM								
[b]total μg ICV	SC								
(vs picrotoxin)	PO								

IN VITRO

mg %	Cardiac	Vascular	Gut	Uterine	Visceral	Skeletal		
Monkey		3.54x10^{-5}*						

*2162

AMANTADINE
(Symmetrel, Amazolon, Mantadix)

mg/kg		Mouse	Rat	Guinea Pig	Rabbit	Cat	Dog	Monkey
Lethal Dose	IV							
Y-LD$_{50}$	IP	[a]50 1348						
Z-MLD	IM							
[a]LD$_{10}$	SC							
	PO							
Induce	IV							
tremors	IP	[a]146 1346						
	IM							
[a]ED$_{50}$	SC							
	PO							
Depress	IV							
microsomes	IP		50 1345					
	IM							
	SC							
	PO							
Block	IV							
amphetamine	IP	150 1347						
hyperactivity	IM							
	SC							
	PO							
	IV							
	IP							
	IM							
	SC							
	PO							
	IV							
	IP							
	IM							
	SC							
	PO							
	IV							
	IP							
	IM							
	SC							
	PO							
	IV							
	IP							
	IM							
	SC							
	PO							
	IV							
	IP							
	IM							
	SC							
	PO							

AMIDEPHRINE

(Fentrinol, Nalde, Dricol)

mg/kg		Mouse	Rat	Guinea Pig	Rabbit	Cat	Dog	Monkey
Lethal Dose Y-LD$_{50}$ Z-MLD	IV	190 $_{840}$						
	IP						4.8 $_{840}$	
	IM							
	SC	Y1990 $_{840}$						
	PO	Y>6000 $_{840}$						
Cardiovascular	IV		0.01 $_{1351}$		4 $_{840}$	0.01 $_{840}$		
	IP	0.3 $_{840}$						
	IM							
	SC							
	PO	5 $_{840}$						
Cardiac	IV		1 $_{1350}$					
	IP							
	IM							
	SC							
	PO							
	IV							
	IP							
	IM							
	SC							
	PO							
	IV							
	IP							
	IM							
	SC							
	PO							
	IV							
	IP							
	IM							
	SC							
	PO							
	IV							
	IP							
	IM							
	SC							
	PO							
	IV							
	IP							
	IM							
	SC							
	PO							

AMILORIDE

(Midamor, Arumil, Colectril)

mg/kg		Mouse	Rat	Guinea Pig	Rabbit	Cat	Dog	Monkey
Lethal Dose	IV							
Y-LD$_{50}$	IP							
Z-MLD	IM							
	SC							
	PO							
Cardiovascular	IV		30 1352					
	IP							
	IM							
	SC							
	PO							
Diuretic	IV							
	IP							
	IM							
	SC		0.1 1285					
	PO							
	IV							
	IP							
	IM							
	SC							
	PO							

IN VITRO

mg %	Cardiac	Vascular	Gut	Uterine	Visceral	Skeletal	
Dog	0.230 1353						

Γ-AMINOBUTYRIC ACID

(4-Aminobutanoic acid, GABA)

mg/kg		Mouse	Rat	Guinea Pig	Rabbit	Cat	Dog	Monkey
Lethal Dose	IV							
Y-LD$_{50}$	IP							
Z-MLD	IM							
	SC							
	PO							
Cardiovascular	IV				3 $_{208}$	10 $_{208}$	3 $_{208}$	
	IP							
	IM							
	SC							
	PO							
CNS	IV					0.1 $_{357}$	100 $_{358}$	
(inhibition)	IP							
	IM							
	SC	2500 $_{999}$						
	PO							
Behavioral	IV	1000 $_{359}$						
	IP							
	IM							
	SC							
	PO	400 $_{359}$						
Decrease	IV							
picrotoxin	IP	4120 $_{1354}$						
convulsions	IM							
	SC							
	PO							
	IV							
	IP							
	IM							
	SC							
	PO							
	IV							
	IP							
	IM							
	SC							
	PO							
	IV							
	IP							
	IM							
	SC							
	PO							
	IV							
	IP							
	IM							
	SC							
	PO							

AMINOPHYLLINE
(Theophylline Ethylenediamine, Aminophyllin, Phyllocontin)

mg/kg		Mouse	Rat	Guinea Pig	Rabbit	Cat	Dog	Monkey
Lethal Dose Y-LD$_{50}$ Z-MLD	IV		Z190 [77]		Y150 [45]			
	IP							
	IM							
	SC	Z140 [7]						
	PO	Y540						
Cardiovascular [a]Q8h [b]Q12h	IV		150 [44]		35 [46]	35 [46]	[a]10 [2273]	
	IP							
	IM						[a]10 [2273]	
	SC							
	PO		100 [44]			[b]5 [2272]	[b]10 [2272]	
Diuretic [a]Q8h [b]Q12h	IV						20	
	IP							
	IM						[a]10 [2273]	
	SC							
	PO		20 [44]			[b]6.6 [2273]	[a]10 [2273]	
Respiratory [a]Q8h [b]Q12h	IV						[a]10 [2273]	
	IP		3 [1355]					
	IM						[a]10 [2273]	
	SC							
	PO					[b]6.6 [2273]	[a]10 [2273]	
Antithrombotic [a]mg/kg/min	IV						[a]0.02 [1356]	
	IP							
	IM							
	SC							
	PO							
Renal vascular [a]mg/min IA	IV						[a]2.5 [1357]	
	IP							
	IM							
	SC							
	PO							

IN VITRO

mg %	Cardiac	Vascular	Gut	Uterine	Visceral	Skeletal	Respiratory	
Langendorff (Perfusion)	[a]5							
Guinea Pig [a] total mg							5.478 [1358]	

AMINOPTERIN

(4-Aminofolic acid, 4-Amino-PGA)

mg/kg		Mouse	Rat	Guinea Pig	Rabbit	Cat	Dog	Monkey	
Lethal Dose	IV								
Y-LD$_{50}$	IP	[a]10 $_{1359}$							
Z-MLD	IM								
[a]LD$_{10}$	SC								
	PO								
Antileukemia	IV								
(optimal dose)	IP	[a]0.3 $_{1359}$							
	IM								
[a]alternate days	SC								
	PO								
	IV								
	IP								
	IM								
	SC								
	PO								
	IV								
	IP								
	IM								
	SC								
	PO								
	IV								
	IP								
	IM								
	SC								
	PO								
	IV								
	IP								
	IM								
	SC								
	PO								
	IV								
	IP								
	IM								
	SC								
	PO								
	IV								
	IP								
	IM								
	SC								
	PO								
	IV								
	IP								
	IM								
	SC								
	PO								

4-AMINOPYRIDINE

mg/kg		Mouse	Rat	Guinea Pig	Rabbit	Cat	Dog	Monkey	
Lethal Dose	IV								
Y-LD$_{50}$	IP								
Z-MLD	IM								
	SC								
	PO								
Antagonize	IV					[a]0.6 2277			
ketamine	IP								
	IM								
[a]used with	SC								
yohimbine	PO								
Antagonize	IV						[a]0.3 2274		
xylazine	IP								
	IM								
[a]used with	SC								
yohimbine	PO								
Antagonize	IV					[a]0.15 2274			
barbiturates	IP								
	IM								
[a]used with	SC								
yohimbine	PO								

IN VITRO

mg %	Cardiac	Vascular	Gut	Uterine	Visceral	Skeletal	Nervous Tissue	
Rabbit		0.0376 1360						
Cat							0.0094*	

*1361

AMINOPYRINE

(Dipirin, Amidopyrine, Pyramidon)

mg/kg		Mouse	Rat	Guinea Pig	Rabbit	Cat	Dog	Monkey	
Lethal Dose	IV	Y184 49	Z135 51						
Y-LD$_{50}$	IP		Y248 52						
Z-MLD	IM								
	SC	Y350 49			417 56		300 57		
	PO	Y1850 49	Y1700	Z925 4	Z750 4				
Analgesic,	IV				50 50		[a]30-100 2275		
antipyretic,	IP	150 50							
anti-	IM								
inflammatory	SC		200 50						
[a]total mg	PO	300 7	650 50	130 35			[a]265 24		
Hypothermic	IV								
	IP				100 4				
	IM				100 4				
	SC		150 54		100 4				
	PO		30 905						
Decreased	IV					10 847			
dorsal root	IP								
potential	IM								
	SC								
	PO								

IN VITRO

mg %	Cardiac	Vascular	Gut	Uterine	Visceral	Skeletal		

AMIODARONE

(Cordarone, Ancoron, Miodaron)

mg/kg		Mouse	Rat	Guinea Pig	Rabbit	Cat	Dog	Monkey
Lethal Dose	IV							
Y-LD$_{50}$	IP							
Z-MLD	IM							
	SC							
	PO							
Cardiac	IV		50 [1362]					
	IP		50 [1363]					
	IM							
[a]daily	SC				[a]20 [1364]			
	PO							
	IV							
	IP							
	IM							
	SC							
	PO							
	IV							
	IP							
	IM							
	SC							
	PO							
	IV							
	IP							
	IM							
	SC							
	PO							
	IV							
	IP							
	IM							
	SC							
	PO							
	IV							
	IP							
	IM							
	SC							
	PO							
	IV							
	IP							
	IM							
	SC							
	PO							
	IV							
	IP							
	IM							
	SC							
	PO							

AMITRIPTYLINE
(Amitid, Amitril, Elavil, Endep)

mg/kg		Mouse	Rat	Guinea Pig	Rabbit	Cat	Dog	Monkey
Lethal Dose	IV	Y27 [58]			Y9.9 [58]			
Y-LD$_{50}$	IP	Y76 [58]	Y72 [58]					
Z-MLD	IM							
	SC	Y328 [58]	Y1290 [58]				50 [1210]	
	PO	Y289 [58]	Y530 [58]					
Anti-depressant	IV							
	IP	1 [58]	20 [59]					
	IM							
[a] total mg	SC		10 [1365]					
	PO	1 [58]	30 [1365]			[a]5-10 [2272]	1-2 [2272]	
Adrenolytic,	IV						1.2 [58]	
hypothermic	IP	30 [59]	30 [59]					
	IM							
	SC							
	PO	10 [1071]	10 [1071]					
Behavioral	IV					5 [850]		3 [949]
	IP	8 [1155]	5.1 [848]					
	IM						0.1 [1370]	
	SC							
	PO							10 [949]
EEG	IV				2 [835]	0.2 [949]		3 [949]
	IP							
	IM							
	SC							
	PO							
CNS	IV	6.6 [838]			10 [950]	10 [850]		
	IP	13 [1371]				50 [1367]		
	IM							
	SC	4.4 [1296]				20 [837]	50 [1210]	
	PO							
GABA	IV							
binding	IP							
	IM							
[a] daily	SC		[a]10 [1366]					
	PO							
Cardiovascular	IV					[a]0.75 [1367]	[a]0.5 [1368]	
	IP		34.67 [1373]					
	IM							
[a] mg/kg/min	SC							
	PO							
Decreased	IV							
shock-induced	IP							
fighting	IM							
[a] ED$_{50}$	SC							
	PO	[a]40.5 [1372]						

mg/kg		Mouse	Rat	Guinea Pig	Rabbit	Cat	Dog	Monkey	
Corneal lesions	IV								
	IP								
	IM								
	SC								
	PO		1.8 1374						
	IV								
	IP								
	IM								
	SC								
	PO								
	IV								
	IP								
	IM								
	SC								
	PO								
	IV								
	IP								
	IM								
	SC								
	PO								

IN VITRO

mg %	Cardiac	Vascular	Gut	Uterine	Visceral	Skeletal		
Dog	0.05 1369							

AMMONIUM CHLORIDE

(Ammonium Muriate, Sal Ammoniac, Salmiac)

mg/kg		Mouse	Rat	Guinea Pig	Rabbit	Cat	Dog	Monkey	
Lethal Dose	IV			240_{62}					
Y-LD_{50}	IP								
Z-MLD	IM								
	SC	500							
	PO								
Diuretic	IV								
	IP		250_{61}						
	IM								
	SC								
	PO		250			$50\text{-}200_{2275}$	$50\text{-}200_{2275}$		
Medullary stimulant	IV	150_4	150_4	150_4	150_4	150_4	150_4	150_4	
	IP								
	IM								
	SC								
	PO								
Expectorant	IV								
	IP								
	IM								
	SC								
	PO					25*	25*		

*2275

IN VITRO

mg %	Cardiac	Vascular	Gut	Uterine	Visceral	Skeletal		

AMOBARBITAL

(Amytal, Dexamyl, Talamo, Tuinal)

mg/kg		Mouse	Rat	Guinea Pig	Rabbit	Cat	Dog	Monkey	
Lethal Dose	IV	Z135 63	Z90 63	Z80 63	Y75 70	54	61 64		
Y-LD50	IP	200 64	Y115	Z120 63	90 66	Z120 63			
Z-MLD	IM		Z230 4						
	SC	Z280 63	190 68	Z170 63	Z150 63				
	PO		400 63		Y575 71	Y110	125 63		
Anesthetic	IV	54 65	55 63	50 63	40 72	11 24	50	40 63	
	IP	65 66	100 4	60 63	54 66	75	65		
	IM				50	100 4			
	SC	130 63	150	85 63	70 66	100 4	105		
	PO	160 1125	225 69		90 66	100	175 66		
Spinal cord	IV					30			
depressant	IP								
	IM								
	SC								
	PO								
Behavioral	IV						1 947		
	IP		5 932						
	IM								
	SC		15 952						
	PO						8 951		
Sedative	IV	1-3 2274	1-3 2274	1-3 2274	1-3 2274			1-3 2274	
	IP								
	IM								
	SC								
	PO	4.4-11 2274	4.4-11 2274	4.4-11 2274	4.4-11 2274	4.4-11 2274	4.4-11 2274	4.4-11*	
	IV								
	IP								
	IM								
	SC								
	PO								
	IV								
	IP								
	IM								
	SC								
	PO								
	IV								
	IP								
	IM								
	SC								
	PO								
	IV								
	IP								
	IM								
	SC								
	PO								

*2274

AMPHETAMINE
(Benzedrine, Alentol, Ortedrine)

mg/kg		Mouse	Rat	Guinea Pig	Rabbit	Cat	Dog	Monkey
Lethal Dose Y-LD$_{50}$ Z-MLD	IV	Y25 [73]			25 [52]		10 [1375]	
	IP	Y120 [74]	Y125 [80]					
	IM							
	SC	270 [75]	Y160 [81]					
	PO	22 [73]	Y60.5 [82]		Y85		Z20 [83]	
Sympathomimetic	IV			0.5	0.5	0.5	0.5	
	IP	90 [936]	10 [7]					
	IM							
	SC		80 [83]					
	PO							
CNS stimulant	IV		0.1 [1379]		0.75 [87]	1.5	2.5	
	IP							
	IM					1-4 [2275]	1-4 [2275]	
	SC	5 [76]	3 [84]			1.5 [24]	1.69 [942]	
	PO		2					
Antagonize reserpine	IV							
	IP	2.5 [78]						
	IM							
	SC							
	PO	4 [79]						
Increase spontaneous motor activity	IV							
	IP	4 [954]	4 [937]					
	IM							
	SC	1.6 [1101]	0.68 [85]					5 [89]
	PO	4.6 [1391]	1.25 [936]				0.2-4 [2275]	
Behavioral [a]BID, 10 d	IV					5 [853]	4.3 [1116]	
	IP	2 [874]	2 [834]			7 [1100]	[a]5 [1378]	
	IM							0.3 [1377]
	SC		3 [1376]				1 [895]	
	PO		3 [934]			2 [953]		
Dopamine neuron action	IV		1 [1380]					
	IP	5 [1393]						
	IM							
	SC							
	PO							
Alter brain chemistry [a]BID, 10 d	IV							
	IP	15 [1347]	1 [1381]			[a]5 [1378]		
	IM							
	SC		1.75 [1382]					
	PO						0.8 [1311]	
Anorexic [a]total mg/d i. cranial	IV		[a]0.05 [1383]					
	IP	4.6 [1392]						
	IM							
	SC							
	PO	4.6 [1391]	10 [2275]				2.5-10 [2275]	

mg/kg		Mouse	Rat	Guinea Pig	Rabbit	Cat	Dog	Monkey	
Ocular	IV					0.05 [1385]			
	IP					[a]0.5 [1385]			
	IM								
[a]total mg ICV	SC		1 [1384]						
	PO								
Hyperphagia and obesity	IV		[a]0.5 [1386]						
	IP								
	IM								
[a]total mg ICV	SC								
	PO								
Self administration	IV		0.145 [1387]					0.43 [1388]	
	IP								
	IM								
	SC								
	PO							0.3 [1389]	
Decrease tissue uptake of norepinephrine	IV					10 [91]			
	IP	10 [910]							
	IM								
	SC								
	PO								
Increase digestion time	IV								
	IP		10 [7]						
	IM								
	SC								
	PO								
Hyperthermic reaction	IV				4 [1182]				
	IP		5 [1136]		15 [820]	15 [820]			
	IM								
	SC		10 [942]						
	PO								
Cardiovascular	IV					0.2 [888]	0.25 [883]		
	IP								
	IM								
	SC								
	PO								

IN VITRO

mg %	Cardiac	Vascular	Gut	Uterine	Visceral	Skeletal	CNS	
Anti-5HT			10 [92]					
Rabbit			2 [1157]				0.135[1390]	

AMRINONE
(Inocor, WIN 40680)

mg/kg		Mouse	Rat	Guinea Pig	Rabbit	Cat	Dog	Monkey	
Lethal Dose	IV								
Y-LD$_{50}$	IP								
Z-MLD	IM								
	SC								
	PO								
Cardiac	IV						1-10 $_{2274}$		
	IP								
	IM								
	SC								
	PO						2-10 $_{2274}$		
	IV								
	IP								
	IM								
	SC								
	PO								
	IV								
	IP								
	IM								
	SC								
	PO								

IN VITRO

mg %	Cardiac	Vascular	Gut	Uterine	Visceral	Skeletal		
Guinea Pig	0.9135 $_{1394}$							
Cat	3.654 $_{1396}$							
Dog	10 $_{1395}$							

ANGIOTENSIN

(Angiotonin, Hypertensin)

mg/kg		Mouse	Rat	Guinea Pig	Rabbit	Cat	Dog	Monkey	
Lethal Dose	IV		8 [93]						
Y-LD$_{50}$	IP								
Z-MLD	IM								
	SC								
	PO								
Cardiovascular	IV		0.0001 [1397]		0.0001 [93]	0.0001 [93]			
	IP						[a]0.0001 [1398]		
[a]total mg IA	IM								
	SC					0.0005 [93]			
	PO								
Renal	IV						[a]0.06 [1399]		
vascular	IP								
[a]total µg IA	IM								
	SC								
	PO								
Increase	IV								
serum	IP		[a]1 [1400]						
aldosterone	IM								
[a]ng/min	SC								
	PO								

IN VITRO

mg %	Cardiac	Vascular	Gut	Uterine	Visceral	Skeletal	Nictitating Membrane	
Contractile	0.0001 [1224]	0.001 [93]	0.001 [93]				0.003 [1236]	

ANILERIDINE

(Leritine, Alidine, Apodol)

mg/kg		Mouse	Rat	Guinea Pig	Rabbit	Cat	Dog	Monkey	
Lethal Dose	IV	[a]Y25 [58]							
Y-LD$_{50}$	IP	[a]Y53 [58]	[a]Y45 [58]						
Z-MLD	IM								
[a] as base	SC	[a]Y100 [58]	[a]Y163 [58]						
	PO	[a]Y128 [128]	[a]Y175 [58]						
Analgesic	IV								
	IP								
	IM							[a]1.25 [58]	
[a] as base	SC		[a]5 [58]				[a]5 [58]		
	PO		[a]12 [58]				[a]5 [58]		
Cardiovascular	IV					2 [94]	2 [94]		
	IP								
	IM								
	SC								
	PO								
Respiratory depression	IV					4 [94]	4 [94]		
	IP								
	IM								
	SC								
	PO								
	IV								
	IP								
	IM								
	SC								
	PO								
	IV								
	IP								
	IM								
	SC								
	PO								
	IV								
	IP								
	IM								
	SC								
	PO								
	IV								
	IP								
	IM								
	SC								
	PO								
	IV								
	IP								
	IM								
	SC								
	PO								

ANTIPYRINE

(Phenazone, Analgesine, Phenylone)

mg/kg		Mouse	Rat	Guinea Pig	Rabbit	Cat	Dog	Monkey	
Lethal Dose	IV				700 [109]				
Y-LD$_{50}$	IP	Z1000 [4]							
Z-MLD	IM	Z1000 [4]							
	SC	Y1000 [109]		1000 [109]	1250 [109]	700 [109]			
	PO	Y1800 [109]	Y1800 [18]	1400 [109]			750 [109]		
Analgesic,	IV								
antipyretic	IP	197 [1045]			100 [4]	100 [4]			
	IM				100 [4]	100 [4]			
^{a}total mg	SC		600 [21]		100 [4]	100 [4]			
	PO		220 [18]		500 [4]	500 [4]	^{a}1000 [97]		
Anti-	IV								
inflammatory	IP								
	IM								
	SC								
	PO			100 [55]					
	IV								
	IP								
	IM								
	SC								
	PO								

IN VITRO

mg %		Cardiac	Vascular	Gut	Uterine	Visceral	Skeletal		

APOMORPHINE

mg/kg		Mouse	Rat	Guinea Pig	Rabbit	Cat	Dog	Monkey
Lethal Dose	IV		40 [95]				Y80	
Y-LD$_{50}$	IP							
Z-MLD	IM							
	SC							
	PO							
Emetic	IV					30 [96]	0.075	
	IP					[a]0.25 [1401]		
	IM							
[a]ICV	SC					30 [96]	0.31 [938]	
	PO						200 [4]	
Morphine	IV							
antagonist	IP							
	IM							
	SC	10 [1417]					1	
	PO							
CNS stimulant	IV		10 [95]			10-40 [1199]		
	IP							
	IM							
	SC							
	PO							
Bulbocapnine	IV	5 [1156]				10 [1156]		
antagonist	IP							
	IM							
	SC							
	PO							
Inhibit	IV		0.0096 [1380]					
dopamine	IP							
neurons	IM							
	SC		0.012 [1402]					
	PO							
Behavioral	IV	3.2 [1415]			4 [1405]			
	IP	10 [1416]	0.016 [1403]					
	IM							0.0321*
	SC	0.5346 [1407]	0.1 [1404]					
	PO							
Thermoregulatory	IV				4 [1405]			
	IP	1 [1413]	0.1 [1408]					
	IM							
	SC	1 [1414]						
	PO							
	IV							
	IP							
	IM							
	SC							
	PO							

*1406

37

APOMORPHINE (continued)

mg/kg		Mouse	Rat	Guinea Pig	Rabbit	Cat	Dog	Monkey	
Cardiovascular	IV					1 1409	b 0.6 1412		
	IP					a0.07 1409			
	IM								
aICV	SC								
btotal μg IA	PO								
	IV								
	IP								
	IM								
	SC								
	PO								
	IV								
	IP								
	IM								
	SC								
	PO								
	IV								
	IP								
	IM								
	SC								
	PO								

IN VITRO

mg %	Cardiac	Vascular	Gut	Uterine	Visceral	Skeletal	CNS	
Rat							0.0267*	
Rabbit							0.0003**	

*1410   **1411

ASPIRIN

(Acetylsalicylic acid, Acetonyl, Bufferin, Easprin, Empirin)

mg/kg		Mouse	Rat	Guinea Pig	Rabbit	Cat	Dog	Monkey
Lethal Dose Y-LD$_{50}$ Z-MLD	IV				Z700 [4]			
	IP	Y495 [17]	Y500 [19]					
	IM							
	SC					Z700 [23]		
	PO	Y1100 [18]	Y1500 [20]		Y1800 [18]		Y3000	
Analgesic, antipyretic [a] total mg [b] Q12h [c] Q48h	IV							
	IP	25 [908]		269 [22]				
	IM							
	SC	22 [908]	20 [948]					
	PO	100 [908]	450 [21]	300 [923]	[a]500 [4]	[c]10 [2272]	[b]10 [2272]	100 [25]
Toxic dose (convulsant)	IV							
	IP	100 [1316]						
	IM							
	SC							
	PO	250 [1317]					750 [4]	
Block bradykinin broncho- constriction	IV			2 [26]				
	IP		125 [908]					
	IM							
	SC							
	PO							
CNS [a] total mg	IV						[a]5 [947]	
	IP	100 [1115]						
	IM							
	SC							
	PO	250 [930]						
Gastro- intestinal toxicosis	IV						100 [1304]	
	IP							
	IM							
	SC		78 [1146]					
	PO		200 [1302]				100 [1303]	
Anticoagulant	IV						1 [1307]	
	IP	20 [1305]						
	IM							
	SC							
	PO	100 [1318]	10 [1306]					
Cardiovascular	IV		3.75 [1309]					
	IP							
	IM							
	SC							
	PO		75 [1308]					
Anti- inflammatory [a] Q72h	IV		308.4 [1310]					
	IP							
	IM							
	SC							
	PO		452 [1283]			[a]40 [2273]	50 [1311]	

mg/kg		Mouse	Rat	Guinea Pig	Rabbit	Cat	Dog	Monkey	
Urinary	IV		15.7 [1310]						
	IP								
	IM								
	SC								
	PO		30 [1312]						
	IV								
	IP								
	IM								
	SC								
	PO								
	IV								
	IP								
	IM								
	SC								
	PO								
	IV								
	IP								
	IM								
	SC								
	PO								

IN VITRO

mg %	Cardiac	Vascular	Gut	Uterine	Visceral	Skeletal		
Rat	5 [1313]							
Guinea Pig		5.4 [1314]						
Rabbit		18 [1315]						

ATENOLOL

(Tenormin, ICI 66082)

mg/kg		Mouse	Rat	Guinea Pig	Rabbit	Cat	Dog	Monkey
Lethal Dose Y-LD$_{50}$ Z-MLD	IV							
	IP							
	IM							
	SC							
	PO							
Cardiovascular	IV				0.7 [1427]		1 [1428]	
	IP							
	IM							
	SC							
	PO							
Renin secretion [a]mg/kg/min IA	IV						0.3 [1429]	
	IP						[a]0.002 [1429]	
	IM							
	SC							
	PO							
	IV							
	IP							
	IM							
	SC							
	PO							
	IV							
	IP							
	IM							
	SC							
	PO							
	IV							
	IP							
	IM							
	SC							
	PO							
	IV							
	IP							
	IM							
	SC							
	PO							
	IV							
	IP							
	IM							
	SC							
	PO							
	IV							
	IP							
	IM							
	SC							
	PO							

ATROPINE
(Atropisol)

mg/kg		Mouse	Rat	Guinea Pig	Rabbit	Cat	Dog	Monkey	
Lethal Dose Y-LD$_{50}$ Z-MLD	IV	Y90 [100]			71 [107]	Z30 [109]	100 [104]		
	IP	Y250 [101]	Y280 [101]	Y400 [101]			175 [104]		
	IM								
	SC	Y900 [101]	750 [101]	450 [104]	375 [107]	140 [104]	225 [104]		
	PO	Y400 [102]	Y750 [101]	Y1100 [101]	1450 [107]				
Anticholinergic	IV	1 [1197]	0.55 [1310]		2	2 [109]	1		
	IP	0.33 [915]	0.5 [103]						
	IM	10 [1440]		5	0.11 [101]				
	SC	0.05 [101]	3 [101]			0.6 [110]	0.5		
	PO	0.55 [101]	10 [101]						
Preanesthesic medication	IV								
	IP								
	IM					1 [557]	2.75 [557]		
	SC	0.05 [97]	0.05 [97]	0.05 [97]	0.05 [97]	0.05 [557]	0.1	0.05 [97]	
	PO			1 [105]					
CNS (EEG)	IV				3 [108]	4 [112]			
	IP		6 [1158]			4 [112]			
	IM							1.5 [945]	
	SC		5 [1159]				7.2 [1160]		
	PO								
Behavioral	IV				0.5 [1161]		1 [915]	0.3 [3363]	
	IP	10 [1116]	15 [106]			3.5 [1100]			
	IM					1.5 [945]		1.5 [945]	
	SC	10 [856]	5 [941]			10 [944]	0.5 [1162]		
	PO	20 [935]				50 [945]			
Gastrointestinal	IV		0.1 [1431]			0.01 [1444]	0.1 [1433]		
	IP		1 [1430]						
	IM								
	SC		6 [1432]						
	PO		5.4 [1435]						
Cardiovascular	IV		50 [1436]				0.1 [1438]		
	IP								
	IM								
	SC								
	PO								
Mydriatic	IV	5 [1443]							
	IP								
	IM								
	SC	1 [1439]							
	PO								
Block oxotremorine effects	IV								
	IP	0.1 [1441]	3 [1434]						
	IM								
	SC	0.1 [1442]							
	PO								

ATROPINE (continued)

mg/kg		Monkey	Rat	Guinea Pig	Rabbit	Cat	Dog	Monkey	
Decrease	IV								
dopamine	IP						50 1240		
uptake	IM								
(brain)	SC								
	PO								
Protect	IV								
against	IP								
organo-PO$_4$	IM								
toxicosis	SC	25 1950							
	PO								
Anticonvulsant	IV								
	IP								
	IM								
	SC	3 2165							
	PO								
Opioid	IV								
interactions	IP	4 1457							
	IM								
	SC	10 1417							
	PO								
Central	IV								
anticholinergic	IP	5 1458							
	IM								
(anti-Parkinson)	SC								
	PO								
	IV								
	IP								
	IM								
	SC								
	PO								

IN VITRO

mg %	Cardiac	Vascular	Gut	Uterine	Visceral	Pancreas	Renal	
Anticholinergic	0.1		0.01 101	0.1	0.01			
Anti-5HT G. Pig			1 92					
Anti-5HT Rat			0.5 92					
Langendorff	[a]0.05 1157							
Rat			0.0029 1430			1.7x10^{-5}*		
Rabbit		0.289 1315					0.0289**	
Guinea Pig	0.029 2164		5.79x10^{-5}*					
[a]total mg								

*1434   **1437

AZACYCLONOL
(Frenquel, Psychosan, Ataractan)

mg/kg		Mouse	Rat	Guinea Pig	Rabbit	Cat	Dog	Monkey
Lethal Dose Y-LD$_{50}$ Z-MLD	IV	Y177 [115]					45 [117]	
	IP	Y220 [115]						
	IM							
	SC	Y350 [115]						
	PO	Y650 [115]						
Decreased spontaneous motor activity	IV	93 [116]						
	IP							
	IM							
	SC	213 [116]						
	PO	520 [116]						
Hexobarbital sleep potentiation	IV							
	IP	78 [117]						
	IM							
	SC	71 [116]						
	PO	100 [118]						
Cardiovascular	IV						32 [117]	
	IP							
	IM							
	SC							
	PO	300 [119]						
Hypothermic	IV							
	IP							
	IM				10 [120]			
	SC							
	PO							
Antagonize ritalin motor effects	IV							
	IP							
	IM							
	SC							
	PO	300 [1447]						
	IV							
	IP							
	IM							
	SC							
	PO							
	IV							
	IP							
	IM							
	SC							
	PO							
	IV							
	IP							
	IM							
	SC							
	PO							

AZAPETINE
(Ilidar)

mg/kg		Mouse	Rat	Guinea Pig	Rabbit	Cat	Dog	Monkey
Lethal Dose	IV	Y27 [210]			Y28 [210]		Y50 [210]	
	IP	Y210 [210]						
	IM	Y600 [421]						
	SC	Y725 [210]						
	PO	Y460 [210]						
Adrenolytic (cardiac)	IV						32 [422]	
	IP							
	IM							
	SC							
	PO							
Analgesic Hypothermic	IV							
	IP							
	IM							
	SC		100 [421]					
	PO							
Cardiovascular	IV						1 [421]	
	IP							
	IM							
	SC							
	PO						10 [421]	
Antifibrillatory	IV						3 [421]	
	IP							
	IM							
	SC							
	PO							
	IV							
	IP							
	IM							
	SC							
	PO							
	IV							
	IP							
	IM							
	SC							
	PO							
	IV							
	IP							
	IM							
	SC							
	PO							
	IV							
	IP							
	IM							
	SC							
	PO							

AZATHIOPRINE

(Imuran, Azanin, Imurel)

mg/kg		Mouse	Rat	Guinea Pig	Rabbit	Cat	Dog	Monkey
Lethal Dose	IV							
Y-LD$_{50}$	IP							
Z-MLD	IM							
	SC							
	PO							
Potentiate	IV							
UV-induced	IP							
skin tumors	IM							
	SC							
[a]Daily	PO	[a]50 $_{1445}$						
Suppress	IV							
immune	IP							
response	IM							
[a]5 d, then	SC							
3-4 mg/kg	PO	80 $_{1446}$				2.2 $_{2272}$	[a]10 $_{2275}$	
	IV							
	IP							
	IM							
	SC							
	PO							
	IV							
	IP							
	IM							
	SC							
	PO							
	IV							
	IP							
	IM							
	SC							
	PO							
	IV							
	IP							
	IM							
	SC							
	PO							
	IV							
	IP							
	IM							
	SC							
	PO							
	IV							
	IP							
	IM							
	SC							
	PO							

BACLOFEN

(Lioresal, Baclon)

mg/kg		Mouse	Rat	Guinea Pig	Rabbit	Cat	Dog	Monkey
Lethal Dose	IV							
Y-LD$_{50}$	IP							
Z-MLD	IM							
	SC							
	PO							
Anticonvulsant	IV							
	IP		5 $_{1448}$					
	IM							
	SC							
	PO							
Analgesic	IV							
	IP							
	IM							
	SC	10 $_{1449}$	4 $_{1453}$					
	PO							
Motor	IV					0.5 $_{1451}$		
impairment	IP	20 $_{1450}$						
	IM							
	SC	10 $_{1455}$						
	PO	200 $_{1450}$						
Neurotoxic	IV							
(rotorod)	IP	[a]16.4 $_{1452}$						
	IM							
[a]TD$_{50}$	SC							
	PO							
Hypothermia	IV							
	IP	5 $_{1454}$						
	IM							
	SC							
	PO							
	IV							
	IP							
	IM							
	SC							
	PO							
	IV							
	IP							
	IM							
	SC							
	PO							
	IV							
	IP							
	IM							
	SC							
	PO							

BARBITAL
(Barbitone, Diethylmalonylurea, Veronal)

mg/kg		Mouse	Rat	Guinea Pig	Rabbit	Cat	Dog	Monkey
Lethal Dose	IV	440 [27]			350 [66]			
Y-LD_{50}	IP	Y760 [122]	300 [66]		375 [128]			
Z-MLD	IM							
	SC	340 [66]	330 [66]		350 [66]	300		
	PO	600	400		Z275 [129]	275 [66]	350 [66]	
Anesthetic	IV	234 [65]			175	200	220	
	IP	300 [124]	190 [125]				250	
	IM							
	SC		200 [126]		100 [66]			
	PO		190 [125]		110 [66]	150 [66]		
Hypnotic	IV	275 [956]			130			
	IP		145 [127]					
	IM							
[a]total mg	SC	25 [958]						
	PO					[a]200 [24]	[a]550 [24]	
Behavioral	IV						125	0.6-10*
	IP	70 [1131]	240 [1095]					
	IM							
	SC							
	PO	100 [935]					2000 [30]	
Anticonvulsant	IV							
	IP	15.2 [955]						
	IM							
	SC	100 [957]						
	PO		30 [959]					
	IV							
	IP							
	IM							
	SC							
	PO							
	IV							
	IP							
	IM							
	SC							
	PO							
	IV							
	IP							
	IM							
	SC							
	PO							

*1178

BARIUM CHLORIDE

mg/kg		Mouse	Rat	Guinea Pig	Rabbit	Cat	Dog	Monkey	
Lethal Dose	IV		Z20 [53]		17 [86]	50 [86]	26 [86]		
Y-LD$_{50}$	IP	Y500							
Z-MLD	IM								
	SC		Y178 [82]	55 [86]	55 [82]	38 [82]	15 [86]		
	PO		335 [82]		170 [82]		90		
Cardiovascular	IV			10			7.5		
	IP								
	IM								
	SC		35 [82]						
	PO								
	IV								
	IP								
	IM								
	SC								
	PO								
	IV								
	IP								
	IM								
	SC								
	PO								

IN VITRO

mg %	Cardiac	Vascular	Gut	Uterine	Visceral	Skeletal	
Spasmogenic	5	2	3 [88]		10		
Guinea Pig			4 [1157]				

BEMEGRIDE
(Megimide, Mikedimide, Eukraton)

mg/kg		Mouse	Rat	Guinea Pig	Rabbit	Cat	Dog	Monkey
Lethal Dose Y-LD$_{50}$ Z-MLD	IV	Y20 [111]	Y16.3 [121]	Y26.5 [131]	Y25 [121]			
	IP	Y45 [111]	Y23.5 [121]					
	IM							
	SC	Y43 [121]	Y30.5 [962]					
	PO	Y100 [111]						
Analeptic	IV	10 [111]		10 [131]	1 [132]	14 [97]	10 [133]	
	IP	10 [961]	30 [123]	15 [961]		14 [97]	20 [97]	
	IM							
	SC	25 [964]						
	PO							
Convulsant	IV	20.1 [121]	9.5 [121]	18.5 [131]	5.5 [121]	4.5 [134]		
	IP	20 [961]	20 [130]	17.5 [961]				
	IM							
	SC	43 [121]						
	PO							
CNS (EEG)	IV	10 [963]			3 [963]	2 [854]		
	IP							
	IM							
	SC							
	PO	25 [960]						
Decrease presynaptic inhibition	IV				10 [1103]			
	IP							
	IM							
	SC							
	PO							
	IV							
	IP							
	IM							
	SC							
	PO							
	IV							
	IP							
	IM							
	SC							
	PO							
	IV							
	IP							
	IM							
	SC							
	PO							
	IV							
	IP							
	IM							
	SC							
	PO							

BENACTYZINE
(Suavitil, Parasan, Cafron)

mg/kg		Mouse	Rat	Guinea Pig	Rabbit	Cat	Dog	Monkey
Lethal Dose Y-LD$_{50}$ Z-MLD	IV				15 [135]			
	IP	115 [135]	115 [135]	115 [135]	115 [135]			
	IM							
	SC	Y250 [136]						
	PO	Y350 [119]						
Behavioral	IV				1 [132]	4.7 [145]	1.8 [915]	
	IP	22 [137]	50 [106]					
	IM				0.1 [967]			
	SC	50 [138]	20 [143]		1.5 [941]	6 [135]		
	PO							
Barbiturate sleep potentiation	IV				5 [141]			
	IP	5 [141]						
	IM							
	SC	5 [142]		30 [142]	25 [142]			
	PO			50 [142]				
Anticonvulsant	IV				1 [132]			
	IP	10 [139]		15 [132]				
	IM	2 [140]						
	SC							
	PO							
Anticholinergic	IV				0.5 [135]	0.1 [135]		
	IP	6 [915]	24 [144]					
	IM							
	SC	2 [819]						
	PO							
EEG	IV				0.5 [969]	2 [968]		
	IP							
	IM							
	SC							
	PO							
	IV							
	IP							
	IM							
	SC							
	PO							
	IV							
	IP							
	IM							
	SC							
	PO							
	IV							
	IP							
	IM							
	SC							
	PO							

BENSERAZIDE

(Madopa, Madopar)

mg/kg		Mouse	Rat	Guinea Pig	Rabbit	Cat	Dog	Monkey	
Lethal Dose	IV								
Y-LD$_{50}$	IP								
Z-MLD	IM								
	SC								
	PO								
Anorexic	IV								
	IP								
	IM		75 1383						
	SC								
	PO								
Inhibit	IV								
L-dopa	IP								
piloerection	IM								
and exopthalmos	SC	50 1456							
	PO								
Reverse	IV								
dopamine	IP	0.5 1670							
antagonism	IM								
of reserpine	SC								
	PO								
Potentiate	IV								
5HTP hyper-	IP	5 1760							
motility and	IM								
anticonvulsive	SC								
action	PO								
Anti-5HTP, anti-	IV								
chlorimipramine	IP	50 2189							
	IM								
	SC								
	PO								
	IV								
	IP								
	IM								
	SC								
	PO								
	IV								
	IP								
	IM								
	SC								
	PO								
	IV								
	IP								
	IM								
	SC								
	PO								

BENZTROPINE

(Cogentin, Cogentinol, Cobrentin)

mg/kg		Mouse	Rat	Guinea Pig	Rabbit	Cat	Dog	Monkey
Lethal Dose Y-LD$_{50}$ Z-MLD	IV	Y25 $_{58}$						
	IP							
	IM							
	SC	Y103 $_{58}$	Y353 $_{58}$					
	PO	Y94 $_{58}$						
Anticholinergic	IV				0.2 $_{839}$	1 $_{58}$		
	IP	10 $_{1458}$						
	IM							
	SC	0.95 $_{839}$	1.9 $_{839}$					
	PO							
Antagonize tremorine	IV							
	IP	1.5 $_{58}$						
	IM							
	SC							
	PO							
Increased EEG arousal threshold	IV				0.2 $_{831}$			
	IP							
	IM							
	SC							
	PO							
Dopamine release	IV							
	IP		25 $_{1381}$					
	IM							
	SC							
	PO							
Potentiate naloxone- induced jumping	IV							
	IP	1 $_{1457}$						
	IM							
	SC							
	PO							
	IV							
	IP							
	IM							
	SC							
	PO							
	IV							
	IP							
	IM							
	SC							
	PO							
	IV							
	IP							
	IM							
	SC							
	PO							

BEPRIDIL

(Bepadin, Vascor, Angopril)

mg/kg		Mouse	Rat	Guinea Pig	Rabbit	Cat	Dog	Monkey	
Lethal Dose	IV								
Y-LD$_{50}$	IP								
Z-MLD	IM								
	SC								
	PO								
Cardiovascular	IV						[1] 1459		
	IP								
	IM								
	SC								
	PO								
	IV								
	IP								
	IM								
	SC								
	PO								
	IV								
	IP								
	IM								
	SC								
	PO								

IN VITRO

mg %	Cardiac	Vascular	Gut	Uterine	Visceral	Skeletal		
Rat	0.0037 1461							
Guinea Pig	0.0367 1320							
Rabbit		0.3665 1460						

BETHANECHOL
(Duvoid, Myotonachol, Urecholine)

mg/kg		Mouse	Rat	Guinea Pig	Rabbit	Cat	Dog	Monkey
Lethal Dose	IV							
Y-LD$_{50}$	IP							
Z-MLD	IM							
	SC							
	PO							
Stimulate	IV		[a]0.01 [1431]				[b]0.08 [1462]	
pepsin and	IP							
acid secretion	IM							
[a]mg/kg/min	SC							
[b]mg/kg/hr	PO							
Cardiac	IV							
	IP							
	IM							
	SC							
[a]total μg IA	PO						[a]2.5 [1398]	
Respiratory	IV		[a]12.5 [1463]					
	IP							
	IM							
[a]mg/ml ICV	SC							
	PO							
Cholinergic	IV							
[a]total mg,	IP							
Q8h	IM							
	SC							
	PO						[a]2.5-5 [2273]	5-25 [2273]
Bladder	IV							
contraction	IP							
	IM							
[a]total mg	SC						1 [2275]	0.05 [2272]
	PO						[a]2.5-5 [2272]	0.5-1 [2272]

IN VITRO

mg %	Cardiac	Vascular	Gut	Uterine	Visceral	Skeletal		
Rat	0.1967 [1297]							

BETHANIDINE

(Betanidine, Benoxine, Benzaidin)

mg/kg		Mouse	Rat	Guinea Pig	Rabbit	Cat	Dog	Monkey	
Lethal Dose	IV	Y12 [171]							
Y-LD$_{50}$	IP	Y150 [171]							
Z-MLD	IM								
	SC	Y260 [171]							
	PO	Y520 [171]							
Sympatholytic	IV				0.5 [171]	0.3 [171]	0.65 [171]	10 [171]	
	IP								
	IM								
	SC					2.5 [171]			
	PO					2.5 [171]	5 [171]		
Neuromuscular	IV					15 [171]	15 [171]	15 [171]	
block	IP								
	IM								
	SC					100 [171]			
	PO								
	IV								
	IP								
	IM								
	SC								
	PO								

IN VITRO

mg %	Cardiac	Vascular	Gut	Uterine	Visceral	Skeletal		
Adrenolytic		[a]0.065 [171]						
Sympathomimetic		[a]0.3 [171]			1 [171]			
[a]total mg								

BICUCULLINE

mg/kg		Mouse	Rat	Guinea Pig	Rabbit	Cat	Dog	Monkey
Lethal Dose Y-LD$_{50}$ Z-MLD	IV							
	IP							
	IM							
	SC							
	PO							
Potentiate peptide release	IV						1 [1465]	
	IP							
	IM							
	SC							
	PO							
Behavioral	IV							
	IP		2 [1466]					
	IM							
	SC							
	PO							
Urinary bladder effects	IV		0.3 [1467]					
	IP							
	IM							
	SC							
	PO							
Sympathetic	IV					0.25 [1469]		
	IP		1 [1468]					
	IM							
	SC							
	PO							
Convulsive	IV	0.4 [1470]						
	IP							
	IM							
	SC	25 [1470]						
	PO							
Cardio-respiratory [a]total μg i. cranial	IV					[a]10 [1471]		
	IP							
	IM							
	SC							
	PO							
Cardiovascular	IV					1 [1472]		
	IP							
	IM							
	SC							
	PO							
Motor neuron effects	IV					0.1 [1451]		
	IP							
	IM							
	SC							
	PO							

BICUCULLINE (continued)

mg/kg	IV	Mouse	Rat	Guinea Pig	Rabbit	Cat	Dog	Monkey
	IP							
	IM							
	SC							
	PO							
	IV							
	IP							
	IM							
	SC							
	PO							
	IV							
	IP							
	IM							
	SC							
	PO							
	IV							
	IP							
	IM							
	SC							
	PO							

IN VITRO

mg %	Cardiac	Vascular	Gut	Uterine	Visceral	Skeletal	CNS	
Rat							3.67 1464	

58

BLEOMYCIN

(Blenoxane)

mg/kg		Mouse	Rat	Guinea Pig	Rabbit	Cat	Dog	Monkey
Lethal Dose	IV							
Y-LD$_{50}$	IP							
Z-MLD	IM							
	SC							
	PO							
Pulmonary	IV	80 $_{1473}$						
fibrosis	IP							
model	IM							
[a]i. tracheal	SC	100 $_{1473}$						
	PO		[a]4 $_{1474}$					
	IV							
	IP							
	IM							
	SC							
	PO							
	IV							
	IP							
	IM							
	SC							
	PO							
	IV							
	IP							
	IM							
	SC							
	PO							
	IV							
	IP							
	IM							
	SC							
	PO							
	IV							
	IP							
	IM							
	SC							
	PO							
	IV							
	IP							
	IM							
	SC							
	PO							
	IV							
	IP							
	IM							
	SC							
	PO							

BOMBESIN

mg/kg		Mouse	Rat	Guinea Pig	Rabbit	Cat	Dog	Monkey	
Lethal Dose	IV								
Y-LD$_{50}$	IP								
Z-MLD	IM								
	SC								
	PO								
Gastrointestinal	IV								
	IP	[a]6.81 [1475]							
[a]total μg	IM	[b]0.027 [1475]							
[b]total μg IT	SC	[c]0.002 [1475]							
[c]Total μg ICV	PO								
	IV								
	IP								
	IM								
	SC								
	PO								
	IV								
	IP								
	IM								
	SC								
	PO								

IN VITRO

mg %	Cardiac	Vascular	Gut	Uterine	Visceral	Skeletal		
Rat			0.00073 [1476]					
Guinea Pig			0.00008 [1476]					

BRADYKININ
(Kallidin)

mg/kg		Mouse	Rat	Guinea Pig	Rabbit	Cat	Dog	Monkey
Lethal Dose	IV							
Y-LD$_{50}$	IP							
Z-MLD	IM							
	SC							
	PO							
	IV							
	IP							
	IM							
	SC							
	PO							
	IV							
	IP							
	IM							
	SC							
	PO							
	IV							
	IP							
	IM							
	SC							
	PO							

IN VITRO

mg %	Cardiac	Vascular	Gut	Uterine	Visceral	Skeletal		
Guinea Pig			0.002 1157					
Rat		0.9 1204						

BREMAZOCINE

mg/kg		Mouse	Rat	Guinea Pig	Rabbit	Cat	Dog	Monkey
Lethal Dose	IV							
$Y-LD_{50}$	IP							
$Z-MLD$	IM							
	SC							
	PO							
Behavioral	IV							
	IP							
	IM							0.003 [1477]
	SC	0.25 [1483]						
	PO							
Renal	IV							
	IP							
	IM							
	SC		0.2 [1478]					0.00006*
	PO							
Sedative	IV							
	IP							
	IM							
	SC	0.74 [1482]						0.0018*
	PO							
Analgesic	IV							
	IP							
	IM							
$^aED_{50}$	SC	0.3 [1484]	0.19 [1482]	^{a}0.018 [1482]				0.02 [1479]
	PO							
CNS	IV				0.05 [1481]			
	IP							
	IM							
	SC		0.25 [1480]					
	PO							
	IV							
	IP							
	IM							
	SC							
	PO							
	IV							
	IP							
	IM							
	SC							
	PO							
	IV							
	IP							
	IM							
	SC							
	PO							

*1479

BRETYLIUM
(Bretylol, Ornid, Darenthin)

mg/kg		Mouse	Rat	Guinea Pig	Rabbit	Cat	Dog	Monkey	
Lethal Dose Y-LD$_{50}$ Z-MLD	IV	Y20 [148]							
	IP	Y49 [149]							
	IM								
	SC	Y72 [148]							
	PO	Y400 [148]						>400 [149]	
Sympatholytic	IV	12.5 [148]	5 [150]		10 [1133]	15 [153]	5 [154]		
	IP								
	IM								
	SC								
	PO		400 [148]					200 [148]	
Neuromuscular block	IV								
	IP								
	IM								
	SC					100 [148]		50 [148]	
	PO								
Increased norepinephrine in liver, heart and kidney	IV								
	IP			50 [152]					
	IM								
	SC								
	PO								
Diuretic	IV								
	IP								
	IM								
	SC		100 [151]						
	PO								
Prevent guanethidine depletion of heart catecholamines	IV		5 [150]						
	IP								
	IM								
	SC								
	PO								
Bronchiolar dilatation	IV								
	IP								
	IM								
	SC			20 [1081]					
	PO								
Cardiovascular Reflex	IV						10 [1177]		
	IP		10 [1243]						
	IM								
	SC								
	PO								
	IV								
	IP								
	IM								
	SC								
	PO								

mg/kg		Mouse	Rat	Guinea Pig	Rabbit	Cat	Dog	Monkey	
	IV								
	IP								
	IM								
	SC								
	PO								
	IV								
	IP								
	IM								
	SC								
	PO								
	IV								
	IP								
	IM								
	SC								
	PO								
	IV								
	IP								
	IM								
	SC								
	PO								

IN VITRO

mg %	Cardiac	Vascular	Gut	Uterine	Visceral	Skeletal	CNS	
Finkleman 812			0.3 148					
Rabbit		0.1 148					0.0414*	
Guinea Pig	0.5		20 148	15 148				
Rat Diaphragm						40 148		

*1390

BROMADOLINE

(Bromamid, Promanylpromide, U-47931E)

mg/kg		Mouse	Rat	Guinea Pig	Rabbit	Cat	Dog	Monkey
Lethal Dose	IV							
Y-LD$_{50}$	IP							
Z-MLD	IM							
	SC							
	PO							
Analgesic	IV							
	IP							
	IM							
^{a}ED$_{50}$	SC	^{a}3.27 $_{1482}$	^{a}2.55 $_{1482}$					
	PO							
Sedative	IV							
(rotorod	IP							
test)	IM							
	SC	23.3 $_{1482}$						
	PO							
	IV							
	IP							
	IM							
	SC							
	PO							
	IV							
	IP							
	IM							
	SC							
	PO							
	IV							
	IP							
	IM							
	SC							
	PO							
	IV							
	IP							
	IM							
	SC							
	PO							
	IV							
	IP							
	IM							
	SC							
	PO							
	IV							
	IP							
	IM							
	SC							
	PO							

BROMOCRIPTINE

(Parlodel, Pravidel)

mg/kg		Mouse	Rat	Guinea Pig	Rabbit	Cat	Dog	Monkey
Lethal Dose Y-LD$_{50}$ Z-MLD	IV							
	IP							
	IM							
	SC							
	PO							
Cardiovascular	IV				0.04 [1485]			
	IP							
	IM							
	SC							
	PO							
CNS depression	IV		0.5 [1486]					
	IP	5 [1488]						
	IM							
	SC							
	PO							
CNS stimulation	IV							
	IP	20 [1488]						
	IM							
	SC							
	PO							
Renal	IV							
	IP		1 [1487]					
	IM							
	SC							
	PO							
	IV							
	IP							
	IM							
	SC							
	PO							
	IV							
	IP							
	IM							
	SC							
	PO							
	IV							
	IP							
	IM							
	SC							
	PO							
	IV							
	IP							
	IM							
	SC							
	PO							

BUFOTENINE

(Mappine, N-N-dimethylserotonin)

mg/kg		Mouse	Rat	Guinea Pig	Rabbit	Cat	Dog	Monkey
Lethal Dose $Y\text{-}LD_{50}$ $Z\text{-}MLD$	IV							
	IP		125 [155]					
	IM							
	SC							
	PO							
Behavioral	IV				1 [157]		1 [160]	10 [161]
	IP	5 [156]	5 [156]					
	IM							10 [161]
	SC		5 [156]					
	PO							
Cardiovascular	IV				0.1 [158]	0.1 [158]	0.05 [158]	
	IP		0.1 [155]					
	IM							
	SC							
	PO							
EEG (synchroniza-tion)	IV				0.08 [159]	5 [842]		
	IP							
	IM							
	SC				2.5 [156]			
	PO							
	IV							
	IP							
	IM							
	SC							
	PO							
	IV							
	IP							
	IM							
	SC							
	PO							
	IV							
	IP							
	IM							
	SC							
	PO							
	IV							
	IP							
	IM							
	SC							
	PO							
	IV							
	IP							
	IM							
	SC							
	PO							

mg/kg		Mouse	Rat	Guinea Pig	Rabbit	Cat	Dog	Monkey	
Lethal Dose Y-LD$_{50}$ Z-MLD	IV								
	IP								
	IM								
	SC	Y195 [162]							
	PO								
Catatonic	IV						40 [169]		
	IP	125 [163]	50 [165]			20 [1156]		10 [170]	
	IM								
	SC	70 [164]			100 [970]	40 [971]			
	PO								
Cardiovascular	IV					8 [167]			
	IP								
	IM								
	SC		75 [166]						
	PO								
Antagonize 5-HT and catecholamines	IV				90 [167]	30 [168]	60 [167]		
	IP								
	IM								
	SC								
	PO								
Convulsant	IV								
	IP								
	IM							40 [161]	
	SC								
	PO								
EEG	IV					25 [842]			
	IP								
	IM								
	SC								
	PO								
	IV								
	IP								
	IM								
	SC								
	PO								
	IV								
	IP								
	IM								
	SC								
	PO								
	IV								
	IP								
	IM								
	SC								
	PO								

BUPIVACAINE

(Marcaine, Sensorcaine, Carbostesin)

mg/kg		Mouse	Rat	Guinea Pig	Rabbit	Cat	Dog	Monkey
Lethal Dose	IV							
Y-LD$_{50}$	IP							
Z-MLD	IM							
	SC							
	PO							
Analgesic	IV							
	IP							
	IM							
	SC		25 1453					
	PO							
	IV							
	IP							
	IM							
	SC							
	PO							
	IV							
	IP							
	IM							
	SC							
	PO							

IN VITRO

mg %	Cardiac	Vascular	Gut	Uterine	Visceral	Skeletal		
Guinea Pig	0.288 1461							

BUPRENORPHINE
(Buprenex, Temgesic)

mg/kg		Mouse	Rat	Guinea Pig	Rabbit	Cat	Dog	Monkey	
Lethal Dose	IV								
Y-LD$_{50}$	IP								
Z-MLD	IM								
	SC								
	PO								
Analgesic	IV								
	IP								
	IM								
^{a}ED$_{50}$	SC	^{a}0.43 1489	0.5 1490	^{a}0.003 1482				1 1491	
	PO								
Renal	IV								
	IP								
	IM								
	SC		0.01 1492						
	PO								
Behavioral	IV							0.55 1497	
	IP								
	IM							0.0035*	
	SC		0.3 1493						
	PO								
Thermoregulatory	IV								
	IP								
	IM								
	SC	0.1 1495	0.001 1496						
	PO								
Blocks naloxone	IV								
	IP								
	IM								
	SC	10 1498							
	PO								
	IV								
	IP								
	IM								
	SC								
	PO								
	IV								
	IP								
	IM								
	SC								
	PO								
	IV								
	IP								
	IM								
	SC								
	PO								

*1494

BUTORPHANOL

(Stadol, Torbutrol, Torate)

mg/kg		Mouse	Rat	Guinea Pig	Rabbit	Cat	Dog	Monkey	
Lethal Dose	IV								
Y-LD$_{50}$	IP								
Z-MLD	IM								
	SC								
	PO								
Diuretic	IV								
	IP								
	IM								
	SC		20 1499						
	PO								
Analgesic	IV								
	IP								
[a]ED$_{50}$	IM								
[b]Q8h	SC	[a]0.17 1489	0.027 1500	[a]0.043 1482		[b]0.05 2272			
	PO								
Self	IV							0.01 1497	
administration	IP								
	IM								
	SC								
	PO								
Thermoregulatory	IV								
	IP								
	IM								
	SC	1.9 1495							
	PO								
Sedative	IV								
	IP								
	IM								
	SC	26 1482							
	PO								
	IV								
	IP								
	IM								
	SC								
	PO								
	IV								
	IP								
	IM								
	SC								
	PO								
	IV								
	IP								
	IM								
	SC								
	PO								

CAFFEINE
(Coffeine, Guaranine, Methyltheobromine)

mg/kg		Mouse	Rat	Guinea Pig	Rabbit	Cat	Dog	Monkey
Lethal Dose	IV	Y100 [172]	Y105 [172]		90 [109]	Z90 [109]	Y175 [183]	
Y-LD$_{50}$	IP	250	Y245 [109]	Z235 [109]		Z190 [109]		
Z-MLD	IM				200 [182]			
[a] housed	SC	185 [195]	Y250 [178]	Z220 [109]	275 [182]	150 [109]	110 [182]	
individually	PO	[a]Y1200 [960]	Y200		355 [182]	Z125 [109]	Z145 [109]	
CNS	IV				25	40 [854]		
(stimulant)	IP	7.5 [174]	50 [179]					
	IM	20 [175]				[a]125 [24]	125 [24]	
[a] total mg	SC	20 [176]	15 [180]			[a]125 [24]	50 [24]	
	PO	100 [960]	30 [1504]			[a]65-500*	10-25 [2275]	
Antiserotonergic	IV			30 [92]				
	IP	20 [177]	40 [181]					
	IM							
	SC		40 [181]					
	PO							
Behavioral	IV				58.25 [1503]			
	IP	16 [1131]	10 [1501]					200 [185]
	IM						5 [1502]	
	SC	20 [940]						
	PO	200 [935]	100 [973]			25 [953]		
Analeptic	IV				40		50	
	IP							
[a] total mg	IM							
	SC	200 [964]						
	PO					[a]65-500*	10-25 [2275]	
EEG	IV				[a]450 [974]	10 [184]		
	IP							
[a] total mg	IM							
	SC							
	PO							
Decurarization	IV					[a]210 [7]		
	IP							
[a] total mg	IM							
	SC							
	PO							
Cardiovascular	IV							
	IP		5 [1319]					
	IM							
[a] total mg	SC							
	PO					[a]65-500*	10-25 [2275]	
Teratogenic	IV							
	IP							
	IM							
	SC							
	PO		14 [1506]					

*2275

CAFFEINE (continued)

mg/kg		Mouse	Rat	Guinea Pig	Rabbit	Cat	Dog	Monkey	
Neuroendocrine	IV								
	IP		40 1507						
	IM								
	SC								
	PO								
	IV								
	IP								
	IM								
	SC								
	PO								
	IV								
	IP								
	IM								
	SC								
	PO								
	IV								
	IP								
	IM								
	SC								
	PO								

IN VITRO

mg %	Cardiac	Vascular	Gut	Uterine	Visceral	Skeletal		
Anti-5HT			10 92					
Langendorff	a1 1157							
Dog	19.4 1505							
a total mg								

CALCIUM CHLORIDE

mg/kg		Mouse	Rat	Guinea Pig	Rabbit	Cat	Dog	Monkey	
Lethal Dose	IV		Z169 186		274 109	249 109	274 109		
Y-LD$_{50}$	IP		Y500 187						
Z-MLD	IM								
	SC				472 109	249 109	274 109		
	PO		Y4000 187		1384 109				
Convulsant	IV								
	IP								
	IM								
	SC		1000 188						
	PO								
Magnesium	IV				150				
sulfate	IP								
antagonist	IM								
	SC								
	PO								
Cardiac	IV		[a]10 1508			[b]50-100	[b]200-500		
[a]total mg/hr	IP								
[b]i. cardiac	IM								
as 10% soln.	SC								
	PO								

IN VITRO

mg %		Cardiac	Vascular	Gut	Uterine	Visceral	Skeletal		

CAPSAICIN

mg/kg		Mouse	Rat	Guinea Pig	Rabbit	Cat	Dog	Monkey
Lethal Dose	IV							
Y-LD$_{50}$	IP							
Z-MLD	IM							
	SC							
	PO							
Cardiovascular	IV					[a]0.01 1510		
	IP							
	IM							
[a]total mg ICV	SC							
	PO							
Respiraratory	IV			0.001 1419				
effects	IP							
	IM							
	SC							
	PO							
Colonic	IV			0.0003 1419				
relaxation	IP							
	IM							
	SC							
	PO							
Endocrine	IV							
	IP							
	IM							
	SC		50 1511					
	PO							
Corneal	IV							
lesions	IP							
	IM							
	SC	50 1512						
	PO							
	IV							
	IP							
	IM							
	SC							
	PO							
	IV							
	IP							
	IM							
	SC							
	PO							
	IV							
	IP							
	IM							
	SC							
	PO							

CAPTOPRIL
(SQ 14225, Capoten, Lopirin)

mg/kg		Mouse	Rat	Guinea Pig	Rabbit	Cat	Dog	Monkey	
Lethal Dose	IV								
Y-LD$_{50}$	IP								
Z-MLD	IM								
	SC								
	PO								
Cardiovascular	IV		5 [1513]		2 [1514]		[a]0.5 [1515]		
	IP								
	IM								
[a]mg/kg/min	SC								
	PO		10 [1516]				31 [1517]		
Affect salt intake	IV								
	IP								
	IM								
	SC								
	PO		30 [1518]						
Affect renal blood flow	IV						0.2 [1519]		
	IP								
	IM								
	SC								
	PO								
	IV								
	IP								
	IM								
	SC								
	PO								
	IV								
	IP								
	IM								
	SC								
	PO								
	IV								
	IP								
	IM								
	SC								
	PO								
	IV								
	IP								
	IM								
	SC								
	PO								
	IV								
	IP								
	IM								
	SC								
	PO								

CARBACHOL
(Carbamylcholine, Lentin, Carcholin)

mg/kg		Mouse	Rat	Guinea Pig	Rabbit	Cat	Dog	Monkey
Lethal Dose	IV	Y0.3 [13]	Y0.1 [13]	0.045 [189]				
Y-LD$_{50}$	IP							
Z-MLD	IM							
	SC	Y3 [13]	Y4 [13]	0.08 [190]				
	PO	Y15 [13]	Y40 [13]					
Cholinergic	IV		0.0201 [1521]		0.002 [14]	0.03	0.03	
	IP							
	IM							
	SC		1 [1435]		0.1 [14]		0.01 [14]	
	PO				2 [14]		0.25 [14]	
Induce	IV							
writhing	IP	3 [1296]						
	IM							
	SC							
	PO							
Cardiovascular	IV		[a]0.5 [1520]					
	IP							
	IM							
[a]total μg ICV	SC							
	PO							

IN VITRO

mg %	Cardiac	Vascular	Gut	Uterine	Visceral	Skeletal	Renal	
Guinea Pig	0.008 [1157]		0.04 [1157]					
Rat	0.548 [1522]			0.02 [1157]				
Langendorff	[a]0.1 [1157]							
Rabbit							0.0182*	
[a] total mg								

*[1437]

CARBAMAZEPINE

(Epitol, Tegretol, Biston)

mg/kg		Mouse	Rat	Guinea Pig	Rabbit	Cat	Dog	Monkey
Lethal Dose	IV							
Y-LD$_{50}$	IP							
Z-MLD	IM							
	SC							
	PO							
CNS	IV							
	IP		100 $_{1523}$					
	IM							
	SC							
	PO							
Affect	IV							
muscle	IP					100 $_{1524}$		
tone	IM							
	SC							
	PO							
	IV							
	IP							
	IM							
	SC							
	PO							
	IV							
	IP							
	IM							
	SC							
	PO							
	IV							
	IP							
	IM							
	SC							
	PO							
	IV							
	IP							
	IM							
	SC							
	PO							
	IV							
	IP							
	IM							
	SC							
	PO							
	IV							
	IP							
	IM							
	SC							
	PO							

CARBIDOPA

(Lodosyn, Lodosin, MK 486)

mg/kg		Mouse	Rat	Guinea Pig	Rabbit	Cat	Dog	Monkey	
Lethal Dose	IV	165 1525							
Y-LD$_{50}$	IP								
Z-MLD	IM								
	SC								
	PO								
Inhibit	IV								
L-dopa	IP								
metabolism	IM								
	SC								
	PO	37 1292							
Inhibit	IV								
L-dopa	IP								
effects	IM								
	SC	80 1456							
	PO								
Analgesic	IV	10 1525							
	IP								
	IM								
	SC								
	PO								
Increase	IV								
gestation	IP								
	IM								
[a]BID + Dopa,	SC		[a]20 1703						
200 BID	PO								
	IV								
	IP								
	IM								
	SC								
	PO								
	IV								
	IP								
	IM								
	SC								
	PO								
	IV								
	IP								
	IM								
	SC								
	PO								
	IV								
	IP								
	IM								
	SC								
	PO								

CARISOPRODOL

(Rela, Soma, Somadril, Carisoma)

mg/kg		Mouse	Rat	Guinea Pig	Rabbit	Cat	Dog	Monkey
Lethal Dose Y-LD$_{50}$ Z-MLD	IV	165 $_{191}$	Y450 $_{115}$		Y124 $_{845}$			
	IP							
	IM							
	SC							
	PO		Y1320 $_{115}$					
Analgesic	IV	10 $_{191}$			10 $_{191}$			
	IP							
	IM							
	SC							
	PO		130 $_{117}$	100 $_{192}$				
Block EEG desynchroni- zation from afferent nerve stimulation	IV				10	10 $_{193}$		
	IP							
	IM							
	SC							
	PO							
Spinal cord depressant	IV					10 $_{841}$	30 $_{191}$	
	IP							
	IM							
	SC	100 $_{142}$						
	PO	225 $_{1146}$	305 $_{975}$					
Barbiturate sleep potentiation	IV							
	IP							
	IM							
	SC				100 $_{142}$			
	PO			100 $_{142}$				
Paralytic	IV				15.7 $_{845}$	5 $_{845}$		
	IP							
	IM							
	SC							
	PO							
	IV							
	IP							
	IM							
	SC							
	PO							
	IV							
	IP							
	IM							
	SC							
	PO							
	IV							
	IP							
	IM							
	SC							
	PO							

CENTCHROMAN

mg/kg		Mouse	Rat	Guinea Pig	Rabbit	Cat	Dog	Monkey
Lethal Dose Y-LD_{50} Z-MLD	IV							
	IP	Y400 1526						
	IM							
	SC							
	PO	Z1600 1526	Z1600 1526					
Anti-inflammatory $^aED_{50}$	IV							
	IP							
	IM							
	SC							
	PO	^{a}96 1526	^{a}36 1526					
Antibradykinin	IV			1 1526				
	IP							
	IM							
	SC							
	PO							
Respiratory stimulation	IV					5 1526		
	IP		80 1526					
	IM							
	SC							
	PO							
Cardiovascular (hypotension)	IV					5 1526		
	IP							
	IM							
	SC							
	PO							
	IV							
	IP							
	IM							
	SC							
	PO							
	IV							
	IP							
	IM							
	SC							
	PO							
	IV							
	IP							
	IM							
	SC							
	PO							
	IV							
	IP							
	IM							
	SC							
	PO							

CHLORAL HYDRATE

(Notec, Somnos, Lorinal)

mg/kg		Mouse	Rat	Guinea Pig	Rabbit	Cat	Dog	Monkey
Lethal Dose	IV							
Y-LD$_{50}$	IP	Y890 $_{1323}$	500					
Z-MLD	IM							
	SC	825 $_{195}$	Y620 $_{196}$		1000 $_{198}$			
	PO		Y500 $_{197}$		1400 $_{199}$	Z440 $_{201}$	1100 $_{203}$	
Anesthetic	IV					300 $_{1232}$	125	
	IP	400	300 $_{197}$	400 $_{1164}$				
	IM							
	SC						150	
	PO					250	500	
Cardiovascular	IV					25.8 $_{34}$	125	
and	IP							
respiratory	IM							
	SC							
	PO							
Behavioral	IV				30 $_{200}$	30 $_{202}$	40 $_{951}$	
and EEG	IP	64 $_{1155}$						
	IM							
	SC							
	PO	200 $_{935}$			30 $_{200}$			
Increased	IV							
serotonin	IP		300 $_{31}$					
(brain)	IM							
	SC							
	PO							
Loss of	IV							
righting	IP	[a]253 $_{1323}$						
reflex	IM							
[a]ED$_{50}$	SC							
	PO							
	IV							
	IP							
	IM							
	SC							
	PO							
	IV							
	IP							
	IM							
	SC							
	PO							
	IV							
	IP							
	IM							
	SC							
	PO							

α-CHLORALOSE

(Glucochloral, Chloralosane, Somio)

mg/kg		Mouse	Rat	Guinea Pig	Rabbit	Cat	Dog	Monkey	
Lethal Dose	IV						120 [207]		
Y-LD$_{50}$	IP	Y200 [204]				150 [207]			
Z-MLD	IM								
	SC		200		80 [206]				
	PO		400			600 [207]	600 [207]		
Anesthetic	IV				120	75 [208]	100 [209]		
	IP	114 [204]	55 [205]			50			
	IM								
	SC								
	PO								
Increased	IV								
serotonin	IP		100 [31]						
(brain)	IM								
	SC								
	PO								
	IV								
	IP								
	IM								
	SC								
	PO								

IN VITRO

mg %		Cardiac	Vascular	Gut	Uterine	Visceral	Skeletal		

CHLORDIAZEPOXIDE
(A-Poxide, Librium, SK-Lygen)

mg/kg		Mouse	Rat	Guinea Pig	Rabbit	Cat	Dog	Monkey
Lethal Dose $Y\text{-}LD_{50}$ Z-MLD	IV	Y95 210	Y165 115		Y36 845			
	IP	Y268 210						
	IM							
	SC	Y530 210	Y800 210					
	PO	Y720 210	Y2000 115		Y590 1123		Y1000	
Sedative [a]total mg	IV	30 211					[a]10 212	
	IP	50 211						
	IM							100 976
	SC	94 211			25 978			
	PO	224 211	49 211			6 557	7.5 557	1 213
Hypnotic	IV	72 211					80 964	
	IP	210 211						
	IM							
	SC	530 211						
	PO	740 211		50 978			80 213	
Anticonvulsant	IV	6.2 881				1 1117		18
	IP	40 1115						
	IM							
	SC	29 920						
	PO	100 211	12 1072					
Ataxic	IV				17.5 845	10 845		
	IP	40 1115						
	IM							100 976
	SC							
	PO	152 881	6.6 1125			10 1165	10 211	20 211
Behavioral [a]daily	IV						17.8 1527	
	IP	8 1155	15 829			10 1147		
	IM							20 976
	SC							
	PO	50 935	[a]50 1532			10 1108		1 1123
Affect food intake [a]ED_{50}	IV							
	IP		[a]2.8 1528					
	IM							
	SC							
	PO	46 1391	[a]2.5 1528					
Dependence	IV							
	IP							
	IM							
	SC							
	PO		450 1529					
Serotonin release [a]mg %, i. cranial	IV					[a]0.3 1530		
	IP					10 1530		
	IM							
	SC							
	PO							

mg/kg		Mouse	Rat	Guinea Pig	Rabbit	Cat	Dog	Monkey	
Anti-ethanol withdrawal	IV								
	IP		2 [1335]						
	IM								
	SC								
	PO								
Histamine interaction	IV								
	IP								
	IM							10 [1531]	
	SC								
	PO								
Analgesic	IV	[a]8.25 [1533]							
	IP								
	IM								
[a]ED$_{50}$	SC								
	PO								
	IV								
	IP								
	IM								
	SC								
	PO								
	IV								
	IP								
	IM								
	SC								
	PO								
	IV								
	IP								
	IM								
	SC								
	PO								
	IV								
	IP								
	IM								
	SC								
	PO								
	IV								
	IP								
	IM								
	SC								
	PO								
	IV								
	IP								
	IM								
	SC								
	PO								

CHLORIMIPRAMINE

mg/kg		Mouse	Rat	Guinea Pig	Rabbit	Cat	Dog	Monkey	
Lethal Dose	IV								
Y-LD$_{50}$	IP								
Z-MLD	IM								
	SC								
	PO								
Behavioral	IV								
	IP		20 [1466]						
	IM							0.3 [1370]	
	SC								
	PO								
Serotonin	IV								
interaction	IP								
(behavior)	IM								
	SC	7.2 [1536]							
	PO	47.3 [1439]							
Antagonize	IV								
reserpine	IP	3.4 [1371]							
	IM								
	SC								
	PO	10 [1439]							
Cardiac	IV						3.3 [1535]		
	IP		10 [1534]						
	IM								
	SC								
	PO								
Potentiate	IV								
tryptophan	IP	2.6 [1371]							
syndrome	IM								
	SC								
	PO	3.1 [1371]							
	IV								
	IP								
	IM								
	SC								
	PO								
	IV								
	IP								
	IM								
	SC								
	PO								
	IV								
	IP								
	IM								
	SC								
	PO								

CHLORISONDAMINE

(Ecolid, SU-3088)

mg/kg		Mouse	Rat	Guinea Pig	Rabbit	Cat	Dog	Monkey	
Lethal Dose	IV	Y24 [214]	Y28 [215]						
Y-LD$_{50}$	IP								
Z-MLD	IM								
	SC								
	PO	Y401 [214]							
Ganglionic	IV					2 [1538]	0.5		
block	IP								
	IM		5 [867]						
	SC								
	PO						20 [215]		
Cardiovascular	IV		1 [216]		0.32 [216]		2 [1537]	1 [216]	
	IP								
	IM								
	SC		0.11 [916]						
	PO								
Metabolic	IV								
	IP								
	IM								
	SC		5 [884]						
	PO								

IN VITRO

mg %	Cardiac	Vascular	Gut	Uterine	Visceral	Skeletal		
Anticholin.			1 [215]					

p-CHLOROAMPHETAMINE
(PCA)

mg/kg		Mouse	Rat	Guinea Pig	Rabbit	Cat	Dog	Monkey
Lethal Dose	IV							
Y-LD$_{50}$	IP							
Z-MLD	IM							
	SC							
	PO							
Behavioral	IV							
	IP		7.5 1539					
	IM							
	SC							
	PO							
Cardiovascular	IV		3 1540					
	IP							
	IM							
	SC							
	PO							
	IV							
	IP							
	IM							
	SC							
	PO							
	IV							
	IP							
	IM							
	SC							
	PO							
	IV							
	IP							
	IM							
	SC							
	PO							
	IV							
	IP							
	IM							
	SC							
	PO							
	IV							
	IP							
	IM							
	SC							
	PO							
	IV							
	IP							
	IM							
	SC							
	PO							

p-CHLOROPHENYLALANINE
(PCPA)

mg/kg		Mouse	Rat	Guinea Pig	Rabbit	Cat	Dog	Monkey
Lethal Dose	IV							
Y-LD$_{50}$	IP							
Z-MLD	IM							
	SC							
	PO							
Adrenal	IV							
effects	IP		300 $_{1468}$					
	IM							
	SC							
	PO							
Depletion	IV							
of Brain	IP	[a]150 $_{2058}$	310 $_{1188}$					
serotonin and	IM							
histamine	SC							
[a]BID, 3 d	PO							
Gastrointestinal	IV							
	IP							
	IM							
	SC							
	PO						300 $_{1542}$	
Hypersexuality	IV							
	IP		[a]100 $_{1184}$	[a]100 $_{1186}$				
	IM							
[a]daily, 3-5 d	SC							
	PO							
Behavioral	IV							
	IP	[a]300 $_{1890}$	320 $_{1190}$					
	IM							
	SC							
[a]daily, 2 d	PO							
Antagonize	IV							
amantadine	IP	[a]140 $_{1346}$						
tremor	IM							
[a]BID, 2 d	SC							
	PO							
Decrease	IV							
morphine	IP	[a]100 $_{1417}$						
analgesia	IM							
[a]daily, 3 d	SC							
	PO							
Decrease	IV							
L-dopa	IP							
hypoglyemia	IM							
[a]daily, 3 d	SC							
	PO	[a]300 $_{1456}$						

CHLOROTHIAZIDE

(Diuril, Saluric, Salisan)

mg/kg		Mouse	Rat	Guinea Pig	Rabbit	Cat	Dog	Monkey
Lethal Dose	IV	Y1120 [58]					Y1000 [58]	
Y-LD_{50}	IP	1400 [255]	Y1386 [58]					
Z-MLD	IM							
	SC							
	PO	Y8510 [58]	Y10000 [58]					
Diuresis	IV						6 [58]	
	IP		100 [58]					
	IM							
[a]Q12h	SC		2.5 [1285]					
	PO		100 [58]				[a]20-40 [2272]	[a]20-40 [2272]	
Hyperglycemic	IV							
	IP							
	IM							
	SC		50 [1543]					
	PO							
Cardiovascular	IV					25 [1217]		
	IP							
	IM							
	SC							
	PO							
	IV							
	IP							
	IM							
	SC							
	PO							
	IV							
	IP							
	IM							
	SC							
	PO							
	IV							
	IP							
	IM							
	SC							
	PO							
	IV							
	IP							
	IM							
	SC							
	PO							
	IV							
	IP							
	IM							
	SC							
	PO							

CHLORPHENIRAMINE
(Chlor-Trimeton, Noscosed, Teldrin)

mg/kg		Mouse	Rat	Guinea Pig	Rabbit	Cat	Dog	Monkey	
Lethal Dose	IV	39.6 [221]					98 [221]		
Y-LD$_{50}$	IP	76.7 [221]							
Z-MLD	IM								
	SC	104 [221]		101.1 [221]					
	PO	142 [221]		186 [222]					
Antihistaminic	IV			1.16 [221]		0.1 [97]	5		
	IP	1 [1544]							
	IM					0.1 [97]	0.1 [97]		
[a]Q12h	SC			5			5		
	PO			0.13 [222]		[a]1 [2272]	[a]1 [2272]		
CNS	IV								
(stimulant)	IP								
	IM							0.3 [1377]	
	SC								
	PO	12 [222]				12 [222]			
Behavioral	IV								
	IP	25 [1131]	23 [848]						
	IM								
	SC								
	PO								
Cardiac	IV						1 [1545]		
	IP								
	IM								
	SC								
	PO								
Block	IV								
oxotremorine	IP	[a]20.9 [1441]							
hypothermia	IM								
[a]ED$_{50}$	SC								
	PO								

IN VITRO

mg %		Cardiac	Vascular	Gut	Uterine	Visceral	Skeletal	
Antihistamin.				0.0001 [223]				
Guinea Pig			0.00003 [1314]					

CHLORPROMAZINE
(Chlor-PZ, Thorazine, Megaphen)

mg/kg		Mouse	Rat	Guinea Pig	Rabbit	Cat	Dog	Monkey	
Lethal Dose Y-LD$_{50}$ Z-MLD	IV	Y26 [557]	Y29 [115]		Y16 [235]		Y30 [228]		
	IP	Y92 [82]	Y74 [228]						
	IM								
	SC	Y300 [983]	Y542 [82]						
	PO	Y319 [82]	Y493 [82]						
Sedative	IV				10 [236]	2.5 [97]	2.5 [97]	0.3 [248]	
	IP	12.5 [892]	8 [59]					5 [161]	
	IM					5 [557]	4 [557]	0.3 [248]	
	SC	25	20 [88]	50 [978]		1.5 [1232]	4	0.63 [249]	
	PO	96 [1122]		25 [978]		3.3 [97]	3.3 [97]	4.74 [250]	
Behavioral	IV				7 [60]	3 [823]	0.2 [243]		
	IP	6 [224]	4 [229]			2 [926]		5 [185]	
	IM	3 [175]	1 [230]			5 [980]	5 [244]		
	SC	10 [225]	5 [231]	20 [978]	5 [979]		1 [245]	0.3 [977]	
	PO	15.7 [226]	7 [232]	100 [1166]		6 [1108]	20 [246]	10 [977]	
EEG	IV				3 [237]	2 [239]	1 [247]	1 [247]	
	IP		5 [1069]	5 [234]	0.5 [238]	15 [240]			
	IM								
	SC				5 [156]				
	PO					10 [1165]			
Cardiovascular	IV		2.5 [218]		10 [236]	4 [241]	5 [88]		
	IP								
	IM					0.5 [242]			
	SC		2 [986]						
	PO								
Barbiturate sleep potentiation	IV	1	10 [233]						
	IP	4.1 [227]							
	IM								
	SC	50 [142]			25 [142]	2.2 [1232]			
	PO	8 [983]		100 [105]					
Protect from cocaine lethality	IV						12 [1546]		
	IP								
	IM								
	SC								
	PO								
Protect from amphetamine lethality	IV						10 [1375]		
	IP								
	IM								
	SC								
	PO								
Block peripheral norepinephrine	IV								
	IP	1 [1418]							
	IM								
	SC								
	PO								

mg/kg		Mouse	Rat	Guinea Pig	Rabbit	Cat	Dog	Monkey	
Decrease	IV								
methamphetamine	IP								
hyperactivity	IM								
	SC								
[a]MED	PO	[a]10 1372							
Decrease	IV								
brain	IP	12.5 1547							
dopamine	IM								
	SC								
	PO								
Ataxia	IV	0.07 1533							
	IP								
	IM								
	SC								
	PO								
Anticonvulsant	IV								
	IP	20 251	10 982	10 982					
	IM								
	SC	60 252		50 978	5 88	2 110			
	PO	100 142							
Adrenolytic	IV		0.026 253			0.5			
	IP								
	IM						0.5		
	SC				50 88				
	PO						10		
Analgesic	IV	0.07 1533			2 844				
	IP	5 1119							
	IM	0.79 908							
	SC			50 978					
	PO	5 844							
Hypothermic	IV								
	IP	10 985	2 1104	5 984					
	IM		5 1241						
	SC	5 983	25 986						
	PO	12 983							

IN VITRO

mg %	Cardiac	Vascular	Gut	Uterine	Visceral	Skeletal		
Langendorff	1 88							
Anti-5HT			0.01 92					
Rabbit Atria	100 88							

CIMETIDINE

(Tagamet, Gastromet, Tametin)

mg/kg		Mouse	Rat	Guinea Pig	Rabbit	Cat	Dog	Monkey	
Lethal Dose	IV								
Y-LD$_{50}$	IP								
Z-MLD	IM								
	SC								
	PO								
Blocks	IV								
aspirin	IP								
effect on	IM								
Gut	SC								
	PO							2.5 $_{1303}$		
Protects	IV								
from	IP		50 $_{1282}$						
acetaminophen-	IM								
hepatotoxicosis	SC								
	PO								
Gastrointestinal	IV						0.05 $_{1550}$		
(antisecretory)	IP		25 $_{1548}$						
[a]i. gastric	IM								
	SC		0.25 $_{1550}$				[a]2.9 $_{1435}$		
	PO		32 $_{1548}$				3.7 $_{1549}$		
Behavioral	IV								
	IP								
	IM							100 $_{1377}$	
	SC								
	PO								
Histamine	IV								
interaction	IP								
(cardiovascular)	IM							10 $_{1531}$	
	SC								
	PO								
Blocks	IV						0.131 $_{1551}$		
histamine	IP								
secretory	IM								
effects	SC		3.1 $_{1551}$						
	PO					2.5 $_{2272}$	2.37 $_{1551}$		

IN VITRO

mg %	Cardiac	Vascular	Gut	Uterine	Visceral	Skeletal		
Rat	0.252 $_{1552}$							
Guinea Pig	0.252 $_{1394}$							

CINANSERIN

(NSC-125717)

mg/kg		Mouse	Rat	Guinea Pig	Rabbit	Cat	Dog	Monkey	
Lethal Dose	IV								
Y-LD$_{50}$	IP								
Z-MLD	IM								
	SC								
	PO								
Behavioral	IV								
	IP		20 [1553]						
	IM							1 [1554]	
	SC								
	PO								
Peripheral	IV					0.2 [1555]			
nervous	IP								
system	IM								
effects	SC								
(sympathetic)	PO								
	IV								
	IP								
	IM								
	SC								
	PO								
	IV								
	IP								
	IM								
	SC								
	PO								
	IV								
	IP								
	IM								
	SC								
	PO								
	IV								
	IP								
	IM								
	SC								
	PO								
	IV								
	IP								
	IM								
	SC								
	PO								
	IV								
	IP								
	IM								
	SC								
	PO								

CIRAZOLINE

mg/kg		Mouse	Rat	Guinea Pig	Rabbit	Cat	Dog	Monkey	
Lethal Dose $Y-LD_{50}$ $Z-MLD$	IV								
	IP								
	IM								
	SC								
	PO								
Renal effects $^{a}mg/kg/min$	IV		[a]0.04 1556						
	IP								
	IM								
	SC								
	PO								
Cardiac	IV		0.1 1350						
	IP								
	IM								
	SC								
	PO								
Increase blood pressure	IV		0.001 1351						
	IP								
	IM								
	SC								
	PO								
	IV								
	IP								
	IM								
	SC								
	PO								
	IV								
	IP								
	IM								
	SC								
	PO								
	IV								
	IP								
	IM								
	SC								
	PO								
	IV								
	IP								
	IM								
	SC								
	PO								
	IV								
	IP								
	IM								
	SC								
	PO								

CISPLATIN

(Cisplatyl, Neoplatin, Platinex)

mg/kg		Mouse	Rat	Guinea Pig	Rabbit	Cat	Dog	Monkey	
Lethal Dose	IV								
Y-LD$_{50}$	IP								
Z-MLD	IM								
	SC								
	PO								
Nephrotoxic	IV		[5] 1557						
	IP								
	IM								
	SC								
	PO								
Antineoplastic	IV						[a]60 2274		
	IP								
^{a}mg/M^2	IM								
	SC								
	PO								
	IV								
	IP								
	IM								
	SC								
	PO								
	IV								
	IP								
	IM								
	SC								
	PO								
	IV								
	IP								
	IM								
	SC								
	PO								
	IV								
	IP								
	IM								
	SC								
	PO								
	IV								
	IP								
	IM								
	SC								
	PO								
	IV								
	IP								
	IM								
	SC								
	PO								

CLENBUTEROL

(NAB 265, Spiropent, Ventipulmin)

mg/kg		Mouse	Rat	Guinea Pig	Rabbit	Cat	Dog	Monkey	
Lethal Dose Y-LD$_{50}$ Z-MLD	IV								
	IP								
	IM								
	SC								
	PO								
Behavioral	IV								
	IP		0.06 [1558]						
	IM								
	SC								
	PO								
Beta receptor regulation	IV								
	IP		10 [1559]						
	IM								
	SC								
	PO								
	IV								
	IP								
	IM								
	SC								
	PO								
	IV								
	IP								
	IM								
	SC								
	PO								
	IV								
	IP								
	IM								
	SC								
	PO								
	IV								
	IP								
	IM								
	SC								
	PO								
	IV								
	IP								
	IM								
	SC								
	PO								
	IV								
	IP								
	IM								
	SC								
	PO								

CLONIDINE

(Catapres, Isoglaucon, Dixarit)

mg/kg		Mouse	Rat	Guinea Pig	Rabbit	Cat	Dog	Monkey
Lethal Dose	IV							
Y-LD_{50}	IP	[a]100 1562						
Z-MLD	IM							
[a]LD 100	SC							
	PO							
Inhibit	IV							
aggression	IP	0.15 1561						
sedation	IM	0.25 1440						
	SC	0.05 1560						
	PO							
Behavioral	IV							
	IP	10 1562	0.16 1575					
	IM							0.3 1576
	SC							
	PO							
Convulsive	IV							
	IP	50 1562						
	IM							
	SC							
	PO							
Cardiovascular	IV		0.003 1563		0.03 1564		0.02 1565	
[a]daily [b]ICV	IP		[e]0.3 1574					
[c]total μg ICV	IM		[a]0.01 1566					
[d]IA	SC		d 0.004 1572			d 0.002 1573		
[e]total μg IT	PO		b 0.005 1570			[c]1 1571	b 0.001 1568	
Analgesic	IV		0.0125 1577		0.0125 1577			
	IP							
	IM							
	SC	0.1 1578						
	PO							
Antagonize	IV							
cardiotoxic	IP		0.5 1579					
effect of	IM							
ouabain	SC							
	PO							
CNS	IV							
	IP		0.01 1580	0.0017 1581				
	IM							
	SC		0.5 1591					
	PO							
Gastrointestinal	IV		[a]0.02 1582					
[a]ICV	IP		0.625 1582					
[b]i. duodenal	IM							
	SC		0.01 1590					
	PO		b 0.042					

mg/kg		Mouse	Rat	Guinea Pig	Rabbit	Cat	Dog	Monkey	
Anticholinergic	IV		0.1 [1589]						
	IP								
	IM								
	SC	1 [1584]							
	PO								
Hyperglycemia	IV		0.1 [1585]				0.03 [1586]		
	IP		0.1 [1585]						
	IM								
	SC								
	PO		0.1 [1585]						
Diuretic	IV		0.0017 [1587]						
	IP								
	IM								
	SC		0.05 [1588]						
	PO								
Dependence	IV								
	IP								
	IM								
	SC								
[a]daily	PO		[a]0.6 [1592]						
Adrenal effects	IV		0.003 [1593]						
	IP								
	IM								
	SC								
	PO								
Thermoregulatory	IV								
	IP								
	IM								
	SC		0.05 [1337]						
	PO								
Tolerance	IV								
	IP								
	IM								
[a]daily	SC								
	PO		[a]1 [1594]						

IN VITRO

mg %		Cardiac	Vascular	Gut	Uterine	Visceral	Skeletal	
Dog			0.01 [1567]					
Monkey			0.009 [1569]					
Rat				0.23 [1583]				

CLOZAPINE

(Clozaril, Leponex, Lepotex)

mg/kg		Mouse	Rat	Guinea Pig	Rabbit	Cat	Dog	Monkey	
Lethal Dose	IV								
Y-LD$_{50}$	IP								
Z-MLD	IM								
	SC								
	PO								
Behavioral	IV								
	IP		3 $_{1595}$						
	IM							0.1 $_{1377}$	
	SC								
	PO								
Reverse	IV		10 $_{1380}$						
amphetamine	IP								
effect on	IM								
dopamine	SC								
neurons	PO								
	IV								
	IP								
	IM								
	SC								
	PO								
	IV								
	IP								
	IM								
	SC								
	PO								
	IV								
	IP								
	IM								
	SC								
	PO								
	IV								
	IP								
	IM								
	SC								
	PO								
	IV								
	IP								
	IM								
	SC								
	PO								
	IV								
	IP								
	IM								
	SC								
	PO								

COCAINE

mg/kg		Mouse	Rat	Guinea Pig	Rabbit	Cat	Dog	Monkey
Lethal Dose Y-LD$_{50}$ Z-MLD	IV	Z30 [256]	Y17.5 [258]	Z20 [67]	Y17 [259]	Z14.6 [63]	Y22 [1546]	
	IP	Y95 [1598]	Y70 [259]	Z60 [67]				
	IM							
	SC	100 [257]	Y250 [259]	Z50 [67]	Z126	Z31.9 [63]	Z35 [63]	
	PO	Z100 [1596]						
Cardiovascular	IV			1	1 [262]	5	2 [262]	
	IP		20					
	IM						10 [263]	
	SC				1.5 [7]	20	20	
	PO							
CNS Stimulant	IV		0.06 [1604]		1.3 [262]	1.3 [262]		
	IP	55 [251]						
	IM	10 [175]						
	SC	20 [176]		10 [978]	10 [978]			
	PO							
Convulsant	IV		10.5 [260]					
	IP					50 [948]		
	IM							
	SC				80			
	PO							
Counteract bulbocapnine catatonia	IV							
	IP							
	IM							
	SC							5 [170]
	PO							
Decreased norepinephrine in heart, spleen, and adrenals	IV					5 [91]		
	IP							
	IM							
	SC							
	PO							
Reverse effects of α-methyl tyrosine	IV							
	IP	40 [1597]						
	IM							
	SC							
	PO							
Potentiate Straub tail reaction	IV							
	IP	40 [1598]						
	IM							
	SC							
	PO							
Tolerance [a] daily infusion	IV							
	IP	[a]25 [1601]	20 [1602]					
	IM							
	SC							
	PO							

COCAINE (continued)

mg/kg		Mouse	Rat	Guinea Pig	Rabbit	Cat	Dog	Monkey	
Hepatotoxic	IV								
	IP	60 1603							
	IM								
	SC								
	PO								
Self administration	IV		0.1 1605				0.1 1606	0.01 1607	
	IP								
	IM								
	SC								
	PO								
Potentiate morphine	IV								
	IP	40 1608	40 1608						
	IM								
	SC								
	PO								
Reserpine antagonist	IV				6.8 988				
	IP	40 264							
	IM								
	SC								
	PO								
Hyperthermic	IV								
	IP								
	IM				25				
	SC								
	PO								
Behavioral	IV								
	IP	25 987	21 1501						
	IM						0.03 1599	0.09 1600	
	SC	16 1101	10 988						
	PO								
Diuretic	IV								
	IP								
	IM								
	SC						10 854		
	PO								

IN VITRO

mg %	Cardiac	Vascular	Gut	Uterine	Visceral	Skeletal		
Poten. epi	0.05 265	0.01	0.14 1157		1			
Antidopamine	[a]0.008 266							
Anti-5HT			10 92					
Rat	0.303 1609							
[a] total mg								

103

CODEINE

(Methylmorphine, Codicept)

mg/kg		Mouse	Rat	Guinea Pig	Rabbit	Cat	Dog	Monkey	
Lethal Dose Y-LD50 Z-MLD	IV	Y68 267	Y55 267		Y60 990				
	IP	Y130 17	Y102 268						
	IM								
	SC	Y183 267	Y332 267		Y32 270		150 989		
	PO	Y395 267	Y542 267	Z120 109	100 109		200 109		
Analgesic	IV	25.5 267	6.2 267		10 191				
	IP	40	63						
	IM		14.8 267					3 1612	
	SC	5.6 908	17 908	28 991			5		
	PO	97 267	22.5 267		10 271		31 1114		
Antitussive	IV		10 269			2.3 989			
	IP			2 948					
	IM								
	SC		50 269				2.2 24		
	PO			42 1124			2.2 24		
Behavioral	IV	10 191							
	IP	100 989				50 948			
	IM								
	SC								
	PO								
Emetic	IV								
	IP								
	IM								
	SC						6.5 267		
	PO						5 267		
Depress spinal reflexes	IV					12 990	5 894		
	IP								
	IM								
	SC								
	PO						20 894		
Self administration	IV							2.5 1497	
	IP								
	IM								
	SC								
a IG	PO							a0.5 1611	
Thermoregulatory	IV								
	IP								
	IM								
	SC	40 1613							
	PO								
Gastrointestinal	IV		1.18 1614						
	IP								
	IM								
	SC								
	PO								

mg/kg		Monkey	Rat	Guniea Pig	Rabbit	Cat	Dog	Monkey	
	IV								
	IP								
	IM								
	SC								
	PO								
	IV								
	IP								
	IM								
	SC								
	PO								
	IV								
	IP								
	IM								
	SC								
	PO								
	IV								
	IP								
	IM								
	SC								
	PO								

IN VITRO

mg %	Cardiac	Vascular	Gut	Uterine	Visceral	Skeletal		
Guinea Pig			0.2395_{1610}					

COLCHICINE

mg/kg		Mouse	Rat	Guinea Pig	Rabbit	Cat	Dog	Monkey	
Lethal Dose	IV		Y1.7 [275]		Z5.5 [277]	Y0.25 [279]			
Y-LD$_{50}$	IP	Y3.5 [272]	4 [275]						
Z-MLD	IM								
	SC	Y3.1 [273]	Y4 [276]		Z7.5 [277]	0.8 [109]	0.57 [109]		
	PO	66.6 [272]				0.13 [109]	0.13 [109]		
Cardiovascular	IV					5 [275]			
	IP								
	IM								
	SC				15 [278]				
	PO								
Arrest mitotic division	IV								
	IP								
	IM								
	SC	2 [274]							
	PO								
	IV								
	IP								
	IM								
	SC								
	PO								

IN VITRO

mg %	Cardiac	Vascular	Gut	Uterine	Visceral	Skeletal		

CORTICOSTERONE

mg/kg		Mouse	Rat	Guinea Pig	Rabbit	Cat	Dog	Monkey
Lethal Dose	IV							
Y-LD$_{50}$	IP							
Z-MLD	IM							
	SC							
	PO							
Increase	IV							
spontaneous	IP							
motor	IM							
activity	SC	3 $_{1619}$						
	PO							
Increase	IV							
antagonistic	IP	10 $_{1620}$						
potency of	IM							
naloxone	SC							
	PO							
	IV							
	IP							
	IM							
	SC							
	PO							
	IV							
	IP							
	IM							
	SC							
	PO							
	IV							
	IP							
	IM							
	SC							
	PO							
	IV							
	IP							
	IM							
	SC							
	PO							
	IV							
	IP							
	IM							
	SC							
	PO							
	IV							
	IP							
	IM							
	SC							
	PO							

CORTICOSTERONE ACETATE

mg/kg		Mouse	Rat	Guinea Pig	Rabbit	Cat	Dog	Monkey
Lethal Dose $Y-LD_{50}$ $Z-MLD$	IV							
	IP							
	IM							
	SC							
	PO							
Attenuate hypotension of ganglionic block	IV			7.5 [1615]				
	IP							
	IM							
	SC							
	PO							
Improve pneumonia model [a]twice weekly	IV							
	IP							
	IM							
	SC	[a]100 [1618]						
	PO							
Effects on hemopoietic system	IV							
	IP	1 [1617]						
	IM							
	SC							
	PO							
Teratogenic [a]cleft palate ED_{61}	IV							
	IP	[a]100 [1618]						
	IM							
	SC							
	PO							
	IV							
	IP							
	IM							
	SC							
	PO							
	IV							
	IP							
	IM							
	SC							
	PO							
	IV							
	IP							
	IM							
	SC							
	PO							
	IV							
	IP							
	IM							
	SC							
	PO							

CORTISONE

(Cortone, Incortin, Corlin)

mg/kg		Mouse	Rat	Guinea Pig	Rabbit	Cat	Dog	Monkey
Lethal Dose	IV							
Y-LD$_{50}$	IP							
Z-MLD	IM							
	SC							
	PO							
Anti-	IV							
inflammatory	IP							
^{a}ED$_{50}$	IM		^{b}0.25 $_{2275}$	^{b}5-10 $_{2275}$	^{b}5 $_{2274}$			
^{b}total mg	SC		^{b}0.25 $_{2275}$					
	PO	^{a}78 $_{1526}$	^{a}45 $_{1526}$	^{b}5-10 $_{2275}$	^{b}5 $_{2275}$	^{b}5-15 $_{2275}$	^{b}25-75 $_{2275}$	
Replacement	IV							
therapy	IP							
	IM							
	SC							
	PO						0.1-1.2 *	
	IV							
	IP							
	IM							
	SC							
	PO							
	IV							
	IP							
	IM							
	SC							
	PO							
	IV							
	IP							
	IM							
	SC							
	PO							
	IV							
	IP							
	IM							
	SC							
	PO							
	IV							
	IP							
	IM							
	SC							
	PO							
	IV							
	IP							
	IM							
	SC							
	PO							

*2275

CYCLAZOCINE
(WIN 20740, NSC 107429)

mg/kg		Mouse	Rat	Guinea Pig	Rabbit	Cat	Dog	Monkey	
Lethal Dose	IV								
Y-LD$_{50}$	IP								
Z-MLD	IM								
	SC								
	PO								
Suppress	IV								
ACh writhing	IP								
	IM								
	SC	0.098 $_{1296}$							
	PO								
Behavioral	IV							11 $_{1624}$	
	IP		30 $_{1621}$						
	IM							0.03 $_{1625}$	
	SC		0.3 $_{1622}$						
	PO		0.3 $_{1623}$						
Analgesia	IV								
	IP								
	IM								
^{a}ED$_{50}$	SC	^{a}0.05 $_{1489}$							
	PO								
Antitussive	IV					1.57 $_{1626}$			
	IP								
	IM								
	SC								
	PO								
Thermoregulatory	IV								
	IP								
	IM								
	SC	2.5 $_{1495}$	0.1 $_{1496}$						
	PO								
	IV								
	IP								
	IM								
	SC								
	PO								
	IV								
	IP								
	IM								
	SC								
	PO								
	IV								
	IP								
	IM								
	SC								
	PO								

CYCLOPHOSPHAMIDE

(Cytoxan, Neosar)

mg/kg		Mouse	Rat	Guinea Pig	Rabbit	Cat	Dog	Monkey
Lethal Dose Y-LD$_{50}$ Z-MLD	IV							
	IP							
	IM							
	SC							
	PO							
Stimulate cell-mediated immunity	IV							
	IP							
	IM							
	SC							
	PO	10 1446						
Decrease subepidermal and glomerular Ig cells [a]daily	IV							
	IP	[a]15 1627						
	IM							
	SC							
	PO							
Inhibit lung and HeLa tumor growth	IV							
	IP	180 1628						
	IM							
	SC							
	PO							
Increased survival in spontaneous systemic lupus [a]monthly	IV							
	IP							
	IM							
	SC							
	PO	[a]240 1629						
Reduce bone marrow derived lymphocyte	IV							
	IP	400 1630						
	IM							
	SC							
	PO							
	IV							
	IP							
	IM							
	SC							
	PO							
	IV							
	IP							
	IM							
	SC							
	PO							
	IV							
	IP							
	IM							
	SC							
	PO							

CYCLORPHAN

mg/kg		Mouse	Rat	Guinea Pig	Rabbit	Cat	Dog	Monkey
Lethal Dose	IV							
Y-LD$_{50}$	IP							
Z-MLD	IM							
	SC							
	PO							
Analgesic	IV							
	IP							
	IM							
^{a}ED$_{50}$	SC	^{a}0.037 $_{1482}$		^{a}0.021 $_{1482}$				
	PO							
	IV							
	IP							
	IM							
	SC							
	PO							
	IV							
	IP							
	IM							
	SC							
	PO							
	IV							
	IP							
	IM							
	SC							
	PO							
	IV							
	IP							
	IM							
	SC							
	PO							
	IV							
	IP							
	IM							
	SC							
	PO							
	IV							
	IP							
	IM							
	SC							
	PO							
	IV							
	IP							
	IM							
	SC							
	PO							

CYCLOSPORINE

(Cyclosporin A, Sandimmune)

mg/kg		Mouse	Rat	Guinea Pig	Rabbit	Cat	Dog	Monkey
Lethal Dose	IV							
Y-LD$_{50}$	IP							
Z-MLD	IM							
	SC							
	PO							
Nephrotoxic	IV							
	IP							
	IM							
[a]daily, 4-10d	SC		[a]100 1631					
	PO							
Immuno-	IV							
suppressive	IP	[a]3 1632						
	IM							
	SC							
[a]daily	PO							
Stimulate	IV							
renin-AT	IP							
system	IM							
[a]daily, 4-5d	SC							
	PO		[a]25 1633					
	IV							
	IP							
	IM							
	SC							
	PO							
	IV							
	IP							
	IM							
	SC							
	PO							
	IV							
	IP							
	IM							
	SC							
	PO							
	IV							
	IP							
	IM							
	SC							
	PO							
	IV							
	IP							
	IM							
	SC							
	PO							

CYPROHEPTADINE
(Periactin, Anarexol, Peritol)

mg/kg		Mouse	Rat	Guinea Pig	Rabbit	Cat	Dog	Monkey
Lethal Dose	IV	Y23 [58]			4 [58]			
Y-LD$_{50}$	IP	Y55 [58]	Y52 [58]					
Z-MLD	IM							
	SC	Y107 [58]						
	PO	Y125 [58]	Y295 [58]				50 [58]	
Antiserotonin	IV						0.1 [58]	
	IP							
	IM							
	SC		0.05 [58]					
	PO		0.08 [58]					
Antihistaminic	IV						0.05 [82]	
	IP			0.25 [58]				
	IM							
	SC							
	PO							
Affect	IV						0.01 [1635]	
coronary	IP							
artery	IM							
flow	SC							
	PO							
Behavioral	IV							
	IP							
	IM							0.1 [1554]
	SC							
	PO							
Gastrointestinal	IV						0.2 [1542]	
	IP							
	IM							
	SC							
	PO							
	IV							
	IP							
	IM							
	SC							
	PO							
	IV							
	IP							
	IM							
	SC							
	PO							
	IV							
	IP							
	IM							
	SC							
	PO							

CYPROHEPTADINE (continued)

mg/kg		Mouse	Rat	Guinea Pig	Rabbit	Cat	Dog	Monkey
Block 5-HTP- and L-dopa-induced hypoglycemia	IV							
	IP							
	IM							
	SC	0.1 1456						
	PO							
Block 5HT- induced twitching	IV							
	IP	1 1636						
	IM							
	SC							
	PO							
Reverse oxotremorine- induced hypothermia [a]ED$_{50}$	IV							
	IP	[a]10 1441						
	IM							
	SC							
	PO							
	IV							
	IP							
	IM							
	SC							
	PO							

IN VITRO

mg %	Cardiac	Vascular	Gut	Uterine	Visceral	Skeletal		
Anti-5HT Rat				4×10^{-5}*				
	0.0112 1634		0.017 1157					

*58

115

DANTROLENE

(Dantrium, F-440, Dantamacrin)

mg/kg		Mouse	Rat	Guinea Pig	Rabbit	Cat	Dog	Monkey
Lethal Dose	IV							
Y-LD$_{50}$	IP							
Z-MLD	IM							
	SC							
	PO							
Relax	IV							
urethral	IP							
sphincter	IM							
^{a}Q8h	SC							
^{b}Q12h	PO						^{b}0.5-2$_{2272}$	^{a}1-5$_{2272}$	
	IV							
	IP							
	IM							
	SC							
	PO							
	IV							
	IP							
	IM							
	SC							
	PO							

IN VITRO

mg %	Cardiac	Vascular	Gut	Uterine	Visceral	Skeletal	Renal
Rat	1.103$_{1640}$						0.974$_{1639}$
Dog	0.277$_{1641}$						

DECAMETHONIUM
(Syncurine, C-10)

mg/kg		Mouse	Rat	Guinea Pig	Rabbit	Cat	Dog	Monkey	
Lethal Dose	IV	Y0.75 280			Y0.2 281				
Y-LD$_{50}$	IP								
Z-MLD	IM								
	SC								
	PO								
Neuromuscular	IV	0.17 280			0.1 281	0.015	0.2 282	0.1 283	
block	IP								
	IM								
	SC								
	PO								
Behavioral	IV								
	IP		0.8 61						
	IM								
	SC								
	PO								
	IV								
	IP								
	IM								
	SC								
	PO								

IN VITRO

mg %	Cardiac	Vascular	Gut	Uterine	Visceral	Skeletal		
Rat						1.5 1157		

4-DEOXYPYRIDOXINE

mg/kg		Mouse	Rat	Guinea Pig	Rabbit	Cat	Dog	Monkey	
Lethal Dose	IV								
Y-LD$_{50}$	IP	$^a 1.7\ _{1354}$							
Z-MLD	IM								
	SC								
^{a}mMol/Kg	PO								
Seizures	IV								
	IP	$^a 1.1\ _{1354}$						$^a 0.53\ _{1354}$	
	IM								
^{a}mMol/Kg	SC								
	PO								
	IV								
	IP								
	IM								
	SC								
	PO								
	IV								
	IP								
	IM								
	SC								
	PO								
	IV								
	IP								
	IM								
	SC								
	PO								
	IV								
	IP								
	IM								
	SC								
	PO								
	IV								
	IP								
	IM								
	SC								
	PO								
	IV								
	IP								
	IM								
	SC								
	PO								
	IV								
	IP								
	IM								
	SC								
	PO								

DESIPRAMINE

(Desmethylimipramine, Norpramin, Pertofrane)

mg/kg		Mouse	Rat	Guinea Pig	Rabbit	Cat	Dog	Monkey	
Lethal Dose	IV								
Y-LD$_{50}$	IP								
Z-MLD	IM								
	SC								
	PO								
Antagonize	IV								
reserpine	IP	0.8 1371							
	IM								
	SC								
	PO	10 1439							
Suppress	IV								
ACh	IP								
writhing	IM								
	SC	2.2 1296							
	PO								
Potentiate	IV								
norepinephrine	IP	2.5 1418	20 1642						
	IM								
	SC								
	PO								
CNS	IV								
	IP	30 1393	[b]10						
[a]daily	IM								
[b]BID	SC		[a]5 1366						
	PO								
Behavioral	IV								
	IP		20 1643						
	IM							1 1370	
	SC								
	PO	185 1372							
Cardiovascular	IV						2.4 1535	5 1646	
	IP		10 1644						
	IM								
	SC								
	PO		45 1645						
Block	IV								
oxotremorine	IP								
	IM								
	SC	32 1439							
	PO								
Mydriatic	IV								
	IP								
	IM								
	SC	3.2 1439							
	PO								

DESOXYCORTICOSTERONE ACETATE
(DOCA Acetate, Dorcostrin, Percorten Acetate)

mg/kg		Mouse	Rat	Guinea Pig	Rabbit	Cat	Dog	Monkey	
Lethal Dose	IV								
Y-LD$_{50}$	IP								
Z-MLD	IM								
	SC								
	PO								
Renal	IV								
effects	IP								
	IM						[a]10 $_{1648}$		
[a]total mg	SC								
	PO								
Affect on	IV								
salt intake	IP								
	IM								
[a]total mg daily	SC		[a]2.5 $_{1518}$						
	PO								
Mineralo-	IV								
corticoid	IP								
replacement	IM					[a]0.5-1 $_{2273}$	[a]1-5 $_{2273}$		
	SC								
[a]total mg	PO						[a]0.5		
	IV								
	IP								
	IM								
	SC								
	PO								
	IV								
	IP								
	IM								
	SC								
	PO								
	IV								
	IP								
	IM								
	SC								
	PO								
	IV								
	IP								
	IM								
	SC								
	PO								
	IV								
	IP								
	IM								
	SC								
	PO								

DEXAMETHASONE

(Azium, Decadron, Gammacorten, Maxidex)

mg/kg		Mouse	Rat	Guinea Pig	Rabbit	Cat	Dog	Monkey
Lethal Dose Y-LD$_{50}$ Z-MLD	IV							
	IP							
	IM							
	SC							
	PO							
Antileukemia	IV							
	IP	[a]0.002 [1649]						
[a]total mg, 3 times weekly	IM							
	SC							
	PO							
Tumorigenesis	IV							
	IP	1 [1650]						
	IM							
	SC							
	PO							
Inhibit bone marrow	IV							
	IP	1 [1651]						
	IM							
	SC							
	PO							
Protect against gastric damage	IV							
	IP							
	IM							
	SC		2 [1652]					
	PO							
Protect against anaphylaxis	IV	2 [1653]				5 [2273]	5 [2273]	
	IP							
	IM							
	SC							
	PO							
Anti-inflammatory	IV					[a]0.25 [2272]	0.07-0.15*	
	IP							
[a]total mg	IM					[a]0.25 [2272]	0.07-0.15*	
	SC							
	PO					[a]0.125 [2273]	0.07-0.15*	
Immune suppression	IV							
	IP							
	IM						0.3-0.6*	
	SC							
	PO							
	IV							
	IP							
	IM							
	SC							
	PO							

*2273

DEXOXADROL
(CL-911C, U-22559A)

mg/kg		Mouse	Rat	Guinea Pig	Rabbit	Cat	Dog	Monkey	
Lethal Dose	IV								
Y-LD$_{50}$	IP								
Z-MLD	IM								
	SC								
	PO								
Behavioral	IV							0.32 [1654]	
	IP								
	IM							1 [1477]	
	SC							0.32 [1655]	
	PO								
	IV								
	IP								
	IM								
	SC								
	PO								
	IV								
	IP								
	IM								
	SC								
	PO								

IN VITRO

mg %	Cardiac	Vascular	Gut	Uterine	Visceral	Skeletal		

DEXTROAMPHETAMINE
(Dexampex, Dexedrine, Amphetasul)

mg/kg		Mouse	Rat	Guinea Pig	Rabbit	Cat	Dog	Monkey
Lethal Dose $Y-LD_{50}$ $Z-MLD$	IV	Y14.3						
	IP	Y72.2 [284]						
	IM							
	SC	Y84 [285]	Y200					
	PO	Y37 [82]	Y80 [82]				Z6.4 [82]	Z32 [82]
Cardiovascular	IV	0.4	0.4	0.4	0.4	0.35	0.4	
	IP							
	IM							
	SC							
	PO							
CNS stimulant	IV				0.5 [108]	1 [184]	2.5	
	IP	10 [286]				3 [993]		
	IM					0.5-2 [2275]	0.5-2 [2275]	
	SC		3 [180]			0.5-2 [2275]	2.5	
	PO		1 [232]				0.2-1.3*	
Behavioral	IV				5 [288]		1 [945]	
	IP	2 [992]	2 [287]					0.2 [185]
	IM							0.5 [289]
	SC	5 [933]						
	PO	20 [935]	1 [232]					
Antagonize adrenolytic action of bretylium	IV					0.35 [153]		
	IP							
	IM							
	SC							
	PO							
Analeptic	IV					10	20	
	IP							
	IM							
	SC							
	PO							
EEG (desynchro- nization)	IV							
	IP							
	IM							
	SC	10 [109]						
	PO							
Reverse adrenergic action of guanethidine	IV					0.48 [285]		
	IP							
	IM							
	SC							
	PO							
	IV							
	IP							
	IM							
	SC							
	PO							

*2272

DEXTROAMPHETAMINE (continued)

mg/kg		Mouse	Rat	Guinea Pig	Rabbit	Cat	Dog	Monkey	
	IV								
	IP								
	IM								
	SC								
	PO								
	IV								
	IP								
	IM								
	SC								
	PO								
	IV								
	IP								
	IM								
	SC								
	PO								
	IV								
	IP								
	IM								
	SC								
	PO								

IN VITRO

mg %	Cardiac	Vascular	Gut	Uterine	Visceral	Skeletal		
Rabbit		[a]0.004	0.1					
[a] total mg								

124

DEXTROMETHORPHAN

(Benylin, Dormethan, Methorate)

mg/kg		Mouse	Rat	Guinea Pig	Rabbit	Cat	Dog	Monkey	
Lethal Dose	IV								
Y-LD$_{50}$	IP								
Z-MLD	IM								
	SC								
	PO								
Gastrointestinal	IV		50 1656						
	IP								
	IM								
	SC								
	PO		10 1656						
Antitussive	IV					0.77 1657			
[a]Q6h	IP					[b]0.07 1657			
[b]IA	IM								
[c]Total mg, chimp	SC								
	PO					[a]1-2 2272	[a]1-2 2272	[c]15-30*	
	IV								
	IP								
	IM								
	SC								
	PO								

*2275

IN VITRO

mg %		Cardiac	Vascular	Gut	Uterine	Visceral	Skeletal		
Guinea Pig				0.402 1610					

125

DEXTRORPHAN

(D-Levorphanol, Ro 1-6794)

mg/kg		Mouse	Rat	Guinea Pig	Rabbit	Cat	Dog	Monkey	
Lethal Dose	IV								
Y-LD$_{50}$	IP								
Z-MLD	IM								
	SC								
	PO								
Thermoregulatory	IV								
	IP								
	IM								
	SC		[1] 1496						
	PO								
Behavioral	IV							[a][1] 1654	
	IP								
	IM								
[a]Self	SC								
administration	PO								
	IV								
	IP								
	IM								
	SC								
	PO								

IN VITRO

mg %	Cardiac	Vascular	Gut	Uterine	Visceral	Skeletal	CNS	
Mouse							0.380 1658	

DIACETYLMORPHINE
(Diamorphine, Heroin)

mg/kg		Mouse	Rat	Guinea Pig	Rabbit	Cat	Dog	Monkey
Lethal Dose	IV							
Y-LD$_{50}$	IP							
Z-MLD	IM							
	SC							
	PO							
Thermoregulatory	IV							
	IP							
	IM							
	SC		0.1 [1496]					
	PO							
Behavioral	IV							[a]0.01 [1677]
	IP							
	IM							
[a]Self	SC							
administration	PO							
	IV							
	IP							
	IM							
	SC							
	PO							
	IV							
	IP							
	IM							
	SC							
	PO							
	IV							
	IP							
	IM							
	SC							
	PO							
	IV							
	IP							
	IM							
	SC							
	PO							
	IV							
	IP							
	IM							
	SC							
	PO							
	IV							
	IP							
	IM							
	SC							
	PO							

DIAZEPAM
(Valium, Valrelease, Tranimul)

mg/kg		Mouse	Rat	Guinea Pig	Rabbit	Cat	Dog	Monkey
Lethal Dose Y-LD_{50} Z-MLD	IV				Y8.8 [845]			
	IP	Y220 [1145]						
	IM							
	SC							
	PO	Y970 [1145]						
Skeletal muscle relaxant [a]total mg	IV				6.6 [845]	3 [845]	[a]2.5-20*	
	IP							
	IM				5-10 [2275]	0.66-1.1*	0.66-1.1*	1.2-2.2**
	SC							
	PO	25 [977]						1.2-2.2**
CNS	IV		0.31 [1664]		2 [1223]	10 [843]		
	IP		5 [1069]					
	IM							1 [1195]
	SC							
	PO							
Behavioral	IV					5 [1148]	1 [1107]	10 [1660]
	IP	6 [1115]	10 [977]			4 [1147]		
	IM							
	SC		1 [1129]					
	PO	13 [1372]	152 [977]			6 [1108]	1 [977]	
Cardiovascular	IV					0.1 [875]	0.3 [1107]	
	IP		2 [1243]					
	IM							
	SC							
	PO							
Ataxic	IV							
	IP							
	IM							
	SC							
	PO	57 [881]						
Anticonvulsant [a]ED_{50}	IV	[a]0.28 [1659]				0.25 [1117]	1 [2272]	
	IP	10 [1148]				0.6 [1149]		
	IM	[a]1.5 [1349]			5-10 [2275]	0.5 [1662]		1.2-2.2**
	SC							
	PO	2.5 [2275]						1.2-2.2**
Methadone interaction	IV		0.5 [1663]					
	IP	1 [2042]						
	IM							
	SC		20 [1661]					
	PO							
Antagonize anorexia, Taste aversion	IV							
	IP		3 [1528]					
	IM							
	SC							
	PO	21 [1391]	3.7 [1528]					

*2273   **2275

128

mg/kg		Mouse	Rat	Guinea Pig	Rabbit	Cat	Dog	Monkey
Thermoregulatory	IV				5 1405			
	IP							
	IM							
	SC							
	PO							
Analgesia	IV							
	IP							
	IM							0.5 1612
	SC							
	PO							
Dependency	IV							
	IP		60 1668					
	IM							
[a]daily	SC							
	PO	1000 1665					[a]24 1666	
Sensitization and tolerance	IV							
	IP							
	IM							
	SC							
	PO		100 1667					
Peripheral nervous system effects [a]Sympathetic	IV					[a]0.3 1469		
	IP							
	IM							
	SC							
	PO							
Effect on micturition reflex	IV		0.2 1467					
	IP							
	IM							
	SC							
	PO							
Anxiolytic	IV							
	IP							
	IM							
	SC							
[a]Q8h	PO					[a]0.25 2272	[a]0.25 2272	
	IV							
	IP							
	IM							
	SC							
	PO							
	IV							
	IP							
	IM							
	SC							
	PO							

N-(2-CHLOROETHYL)DIBENZYLAMINE
(Dibenamine)

mg/kg		Mouse	Rat	Guinea Pig	Rabbit	Cat	Dog	Monkey	
Lethal Dose	IV								
Y-LD$_{50}$	IP								
Z-MLD	IM								
	SC	Y800 [217]							
	PO								
Adrenolytic	IV		20 [218]		50 [220]	30 [220]	15 [220]		
	IP		10 [219]						
	IM								
	SC								
	PO								
Inhibit analeptic effect of amphetamine	IV				15				
	IP								
	IM								
	SC								
	PO								
Cardiovascular	IV					20 [821]	10 [1177]		
	IP								
	IM								
	SC								
	PO								

IN VITRO

mg %	Cardiac	Vascular	Gut	Uterine	Visceral	Skeletal		
Anti-5HT			0.03 [92]					
[a]Total mg								

DIBOZANE
(McN-181)

mg/kg		Mouse	Rat	Guinea Pig	Rabbit	Cat	Dog	Monkey	
Lethal Dose	IV				Y43 [293]		60 [293]		
Y-LD	IP	Y260 [293]							
Z-MLD	IM								
	SC								
	PO								
Adrenolytic	IV						2 [294]		
	IP								
	IM								
	SC								
	PO						1 [293]		
Sympatholytic	IV						3 [295]		
	IP								
	IM								
	SC								
	PO								
	IV								
	IP								
	IM								
	SC								
	PO								

IN VITRO

mg %	Cardiac	Vascular	Gut	Uterine	Visceral	Skeletal		
Adrenolytic					0.003			

DICHLOROISOPROTERENOL
(DCI)

mg/kg		Mouse	Rat	Guinea Pig	Rabbit	Cat	Dog	Monkey
Lethal Dose	IV	Y48 [296]						
Y-LD$_{50}$	IP	Y132 [296]						
Z-MLD	IM							
	SC							
	PO							
Cardiovascular	IV				10	10 [296]	10 [299]	
	IP							
	IM							
	SC							
	PO							
Adrenolytic	IV		0.1 [297]		4 [298]	4 [298]	2 [300]	
(ß-Block)	IP							
	IM							
	SC							
	PO							
CNS	IV				4 [995]	7 [994]		
	IP	10 [1670]						
	IM							
	SC							
	PO							

IN VITRO

mg %	Cardiac	Vascular	Gut	Uterine	Visceral	Skeletal	
Adrenolytic	0.04 [301]			1 [296]			
Sympathomimetic	0.65 [302]						

DICUMAROL

(Bishydroxycoumarin, Dicoumarol, Melitoxin)

mg/kg		Mouse	Rat	Guinea Pig	Rabbit	Cat	Dog	Monkey	
Lethal Dose	IV	Y64 [146]	Y52 [146]	Y59 [146]			40		
Y-LD$_{50}$	IP	Y350							
Z-MLD	IM								
	SC								
	PO	Y233 [146]	Y542 [146]						
Anticoagulant	IV						10 [7]		
	IP								
	IM								
	SC								
	PO		8 [147]				20		
	IV								
	IP								
	IM								
	SC								
	PO								
	IV								
	IP								
	IM								
	SC								
	PO								

IN VITRO

mg %	Cardiac	Vascular	Gut	Uterine	Visceral	Skeletal		

DIGITOXIN

(Cardidigin, Crystodigin, Digisidin)

mg/kg		Mouse	Rat	Guinea Pig	Rabbit	Cat	Dog	Monkey	
Lethal Dose	IV		12.2 74	Z1.2 922	3 303	0.35 303	Z0.65 897		
Y-LD$_{50}$	IP								
Z-MLD	IM								
	SC	Y22.2 922	Y16.4 922			0.35 303	0.5 303		
	PO	Y32.7 922	Y23.8 922	Y>100 922	100 303	0.25			
Cardiovascular	IV						0.15		
	IP								
	IM					0.02 2275	0.01 2275		
	SC						0.15		
	PO		4 1671			0.02 2275	0.03 2272		
	IV								
	IP								
	IM								
	SC								
	PO								
	IV								
	IP								
	IM								
	SC								
	PO								

IN VITRO

mg %	Cardiac	Vascular	Gut	Uterine	Visceral	Skeletal		
Guinea Pig	0.2142 1672							

DIGOXIN

(Lanoxin, Lanacordin, Digacin)

mg/kg		Mouse	Rat	Guinea Pig	Rabbit	Cat	Dog	Monkey	
Lethal Dose	IV	20 [149]		[a]0.5 [1674]	3.56 [149]	0.35 [149]	0.3 [149]		
Y-LD$_{50}$	IP		>10 [149]						
Z-MLD	IM			0.6 [149]					
[a]followed with	SC			0.45 [149]					
0.05 mg/kg/min	PO			1.8 [149]			0.3 [149]		
Cardiac	IV					0.15 [149]	0.2 [149]		
arrhythmia	IP								
	IM								
	SC								
[a]mg/M^2	PO					0.01 [2272]	[a]0.22 [2272]		
Tolerance	IV					[a]0.001 [1675]			
	IP								
	IM								
[a]mg/kg/min	SC								
	PO								
Sympathetic	IV					[a]0.02 [1676]			
neuroexcitatory	IP								
	IM								
	SC								
[a]Q15min	PO								

IN VITRO

mg %	Cardiac	Vascular	Gut	Uterine	Visceral	Skeletal		
Guinea Pig	0.1406 [1673]							

DIHYDROERGOTAMINE

(D H E-45)

mg/kg		Mouse	Rat	Guinea Pig	Rabbit	Cat	Dog	Monkey	
Lethal Dose	IV	Y118 [304]	Y110 [304]		Y25 [304]				
Y-LD$_{50}$	IP								
Z-MLD	IM								
	SC					Y68 [304]			
	PO								
Adrenolytic	IV		0.5 [218]		1 [305]		10		
	IP								
	IM								
	SC	3.16 [1212]							
	PO								
Sympathomimetic	IV						0.1 [306]		
	IP								
	IM								
	SC								
	PO								
Antiarrhythmic	IV						0.1 [1181]		
	IP								
	IM								
	SC								
	PO								

IN VITRO

mg %	Cardiac	Vascular	Gut	Uterine	Visceral	Skeletal		
Adrenolytic					0.02			

DIISOPROPYL FLUOROPHOSPHATE
(DFP, Floropryl, Diflupyl)

mg/kg		Mouse	Rat	Guinea Pig	Rabbit	Cat	Dog	Monkey	
Lethal Dose	IV				Y0.34 [311]	Y1.63 [311]	Y3.43 [311]	Y0.25 [311]	
Y-LD$_{50}$	IP								
Z-MLD	IM		Y1.82 [311]						
	SC	Y3.71 [311]	Y3 [311]		Y1 [311]		Y3 [311]		
	PO	Y36.8 [311]	Y6 [311]		Y9.78 [311]				
Anticholin-esterase	IV								
	IP								
	IM		1 [312]				1 [312]	0.2 [312]	
	SC								
	PO							0.5 [312]	
Sedative	IV								
	IP								
	IM		1 [312]				2 [312]		
	SC	2.5 [996]							
	PO								
Behavioral	IV								
	IP								
	IM								
	SC		1 [1140]						
	PO								

IN VITRO

mg %	Cardiac	Vascular	Gut	Uterine	Visceral	Skeletal		

DILTIAZEM
(Cardizem, Anginyl, Dilzem)

mg/kg		Mouse	Rat	Guinea Pig	Rabbit	Cat	Dog	Monkey
Lethal Dose	IV							
Y-LD$_{50}$	IP							
Z-MLD	IM							
	SC							
	PO							
Cardiovascular	IV		3 [1678]				0.09 [1459]	
[a]IA	IP				[c]9.119 [1687]	[a]5 [1686]	[b]0.01 [1679]	
[b]mg/kg/min IA	IM							
[c]Total mg IA	SC							
	PO		10 [1683]					
Pulmonary	IV							
antihyper-	IP			10 [1680]				
sensitivity	IM							
	SC							
	PO							
Decrease	IV		2 [1685]					
uterine	IP							
contractions	IM							
	SC							
	PO							

IN VITRO

mg %	Cardiac	Vascular	Gut	Uterine	Visceral	Skeletal	Kidney
Rat	0.916 [1299]	0.004 [1634]					2.487 [1639]
Rabbit	0.1244 [1681]	0.0207 [1682]				2.6114 [1684]	
Guinea Pig	0.0415 [1320]						

DIMAPRIT

mg/kg		Mouse	Rat	Guinea Pig	Rabbit	Cat	Dog	Monkey
Lethal Dose	IV							
Y-LD$_{50}$	IP							
Z-MLD	IM							
	SC							
	PO							
Gastric	IV		150 1637					
ulceragenic	IP							
	IM							
	SC							
	PO							
Stimulate GI	IV					[a]0.4 1435		
secretions	IP							
[a]mg/min,	IM							
follows SC dose	SC					0.2 1435		
	PO							
	IV							
	IP							
	IM							
	SC							
	PO							
	IV							
	IP							
	IM							
	SC							
	PO							
	IV							
	IP							
	IM							
	SC							
	PO							
	IV							
	IP							
	IM							
	SC							
	PO							
	IV							
	IP							
	IM							
	SC							
	PO							
	IV							
	IP							
	IM							
	SC							
	PO							

DIMETHINDENE

(Forhistal, Fenistil, Fenostil)

mg/kg		Mouse	Rat	Guinea Pig	Rabbit	Cat	Dog	Monkey	
Lethal Dose	IV		Y26.8 93				Y45 93		
Y-LD$_{50}$	IP								
Z-MLD	IM								
	SC								
	PO		Y618.2 93	Y888 93					
Antihistaminic	IV								
	IP								
	IM								
	SC								
	PO			0.06 93					
Cardiovascular	IV						9 93		
	IP								
	IM								
	SC								
	PO								
	IV								
	IP								
	IM								
	SC								
	PO								

IN VITRO

mg %	Cardiac	Vascular	Gut	Uterine	Visceral	Skeletal		
Antihistaminic			0.0007 93					
Anticholinergic			0.4 93					

DIMETHYL PHENYLPIPERAZINIUM
(DMPP)

mg/kg		Mouse	Rat	Guinea Pig	Rabbit	Cat	Dog	Monkey	
Lethal Dose	IV				1 [314]		20 [313]		
Y-LD$_{50}$	IP	Y40 [313]							
Z-MLD	IM	Y27.5 [314]							
	SC								
	PO	Y365 [314]	Y2000 [313]						
Inhibit	IV		0.099 [1521]	0.1 [1419]					
GI	IP								
activity	IM								
	SC								
	PO								
Cardiovascular	IV				20 [313]	0.25 [313]	2 [313]		
	IP								
	IM								
	SC								
	PO								
Ganglionic	IV					0.2 [314]	0.15 [314]		
stimulant	IP								
	IM		0.5 [1167]						
	SC								
	PO								

IN VITRO

mg %	Cardiac	Vascular	Gut	Uterine	Visceral	Skeletal		
Langendorff	[a]0.025 [314]							
Guinea Pig			0.4 [314]					
[a]total mg								

DIMETHYL SULFOXIDE

(DMSO, Domoso, Demasorb)

mg/kg		Mouse	Rat	Guinea Pig	Rabbit	Cat	Dog	Monkey	
Lethal Dose	IV								
Y-LD$_{50}$	IP	Y14,700[1688]							
Z-MLD	IM								
	SC								
	PO								
Prevents	IV								
alloxan-	IP	7,500[1689]							
induced	IM								
diabetes	SC								
	PO								
Suppress	IV								
cholesterol-	IP								
induced athero-	IM								
slerosis [a]% in	SC								
drinking water	PO				[a]4[1690]				
Anti-	IV								
inflammatory	IP								
	IM								
[a]total ml,	SC						[a]<24[2273]		
topical	PO								
	IV								
	IP								
	IM								
	SC								
	PO								
	IV								
	IP								
	IM								
	SC								
	PO								
	IV								
	IP								
	IM								
	SC								
	PO								
	IV								
	IP								
	IM								
	SC								
	PO								
	IV								
	IP								
	IM								
	SC								
	PO								

2,4-DINITROPHENOL

(α-Dinitrophenol, Aldifen)

mg %		Mouse	Rat	Guinea Pig	Rabbit	Cat	Dog	Monkey	
Lethal Dose	IV						Y30 315		
Y-LD$_{50}$	IP				100 318				
Z-MLD	IM						Y20 315		
	SC		Y25 315		30 315		Y22 315		
	PO		Y30 316		Y200 318		Y25 315		
Hyperthermic	IV						5 319		
	IP				10 120				
	IM						5 319		
	SC		10 317		20 319		5 319		
	PO						5 319		
Respiratory	IV						20 319		
	IP								
	IM				20 319				
	SC				20 311				
	PO								
	IV								
	IP								
	IM								
	SC								
	PO								

IN VITRO

mg %	Cardiac	Vascular	Gut	Uterine	Visceral	Skeletal		

DINOPROST

(Prostin F_2 Alpha, Enzaprost F, Prostarmon F, $PGF_{2\alpha}$)

mg/kg		Mouse	Rat	Guinea Pig	Rabbit	Cat	Dog	Monkey	
Lethal Dose	IV								
Y-LD$_{50}$	IP								
Z-MLD	IM								
	SC								
	PO								
Pulmonary	IV								
circulation	IP						[a]0.1 1897		
	IM								
[a]μg/kg/min	SC								
	PO								
Inhibit	IV						[a]0.003 2168		
broncho-	IP								
constriction	IM								
[a]aerosol	SC								
	PO								
Natriuretic	IV						[a]0.3 2169		
and	IP								
diuretic	IM								
	SC								
[a]μg/kg/min IA	PO								

IN VITRO

mg %	Cardiac	Vascular	Gut	Uterine	Visceral	Skeletal		
Monkey		3.5×10^{-5}*						

*2162

DINOPROSTONE

(Prostin E$_2$, ProstarmonE, PGE$_2$)

mg/kg		Mouse	Rat	Guinea Pig	Rabbit	Cat	Dog	Monkey
Lethal Dose	IV							
Y-LD$_{50}$	IP							
Z-MLD	IM							
	SC							
	PO							
Cardiovascular	IV			[a]0.01 $_{2166}$				
[a]total µg IC	IP						[b]0.01 $_{1897}$	
[b]µg/kg/min	IM							
	SC							
	PO							
Gastrointestinal	IV		[a]0.05 $_{1816}$			0.0005$_{1799}$		
	IP							
	IM							
[a]total µg	SC							
	PO							
Anticonvulsant	IV	[a]45.7$_{2122}$						
(total µg ICV)	IP	[b]6.29$_{2122}$						
[a] vs strychnine	IM							
[b] vs picrotoxin	SC							
	PO							
Erythropoietic	IV						[a]0.5 $_{2167}$	
	IP							
	IM							
[a]µg/min IA	SC	0.1 $_{2167}$						
	PO							
Renal	IV						[a]4×10^{-6}*	
neurotrans-	IP							
mission	IM							
	SC							
[a]mg/kg/min IA	PO							
	IV							
	IP							
	IM							
	SC							
	PO							
	IV							
	IP							
	IM							
	SC							
	PO							
	IV							
	IP							
	IM							
	SC							
	PO							

*2157

DIPHENHYDRAMINE
(Benadryl, Amidryl, Benylan)

mg/kg		Mouse	Rat	Guinea Pig	Rabbit	Cat	Dog	Monkey
Lethal Dose Y-LD$_{50}$ Z-MLD	IV	Y31	Y42 $_{321}$		Y10 $_{321}$		Y24 $_{321}$	
	IP	Y84 $_{320}$	Y82 $_{324}$	Y75 $_{324}$				
	IM							
	SC	Y127 $_{321}$	Y475 $_{321}$	40.2 $_{221}$				
	PO	Y164 $_{321}$	Y500 $_{325}$	284 $_{221}$				
Antihistaminic	IV			23 $_{221}$		1.8 $_{97}$	1.8 $_{97}$	
	IP	50 $_{1458}$		12.5				
	IM					1.8 $_{97}$	1.8 $_{97}$	1 $_{1531}$
	SC		10 $_{997}$	5				
	PO					4 $_{2272}$	2.2 $_{97}$	
Anticonvulsant	IV							
	IP	30 $_{251}$	2 $_{930}$					
	IM	15.7 $_{140}$						
	SC							
	PO	30 $_{322}$	25 $_{326}$					
CNS	IV				15 $_{108}$	1.5 $_{1206}$		
	IP							
	IM							
	SC							
	PO							
Behavioral	IV							
	IP	40 $_{323}$						
	IM						0.3 $_{1377}$	
	SC							
	PO	50 $_{935}$						
Anticholinergic	IV				8 $_{839}$		1 $_{1545}$	
	IP							
	IM							
	SC	22 $_{839}$						
	PO							
	IV							
	IP							
	IM							
	SC							
	PO							
	IV							
	IP							
	IM							
	SC							
	PO							
	IV							
	IP							
	IM							
	SC							
	PO							

DIPHENOXYLATE

(Lomotil, Diarsed, Reasec)

mg/kg		Mouse	Rat	Guinea Pig	Rabbit	Cat	Dog	Monkey	
Lethal Dose	IV								
Y-LD$_{50}$	IP								
Z-MLD	IM								
	SC								
	PO								
Decrease	IV		0.065 $_{1614}$						
GI motility	IP								
	IM								
	SC								
[a]IG	PO	[a]9.4 $_{1691}$				0.063 $_{2272}$	0.063 $_{2272}$		
Analgesic	IV		1.68 $_{1614}$						
	IP								
	IM								
	SC								
	PO								
	IV								
	IP								
	IM								
	SC								
	PO								

IN VITRO

mg %	Cardiac	Vascular	Gut	Uterine	Visceral	Skeletal	CNS	
Guinea Pig							0.0453	

*1692

DIPRENORPHINE

(Nororipavine, Cyprenorphine, M50-50, Revivon)

mg/kg		Mouse	Rat	Guinea Pig	Rabbit	Cat	Dog	Monkey	
Lethal Dose	IV								
Y-LD$_{50}$	IP								
Z-MLD	IM								
	SC								
	PO								
Behavioral	IV								
	IP								
	IM							0.1 $_{1494}$	
	SC								
	PO								
Thermoregulatory	IV								
	IP								
	IM								
	SC	0.1 $_{1495}$							
	PO								
Antagonize	IV						0.03 $_{2275}$		
etorphine	IP								
	IM								
	SC								
	PO								
	IV								
	IP								
	IM								
	SC								
	PO								
	IV								
	IP								
	IM								
	SC								
	PO								
	IV								
	IP								
	IM								
	SC								
	PO								
	IV								
	IP								
	IM								
	SC								
	PO								
	IV								
	IP								
	IM								
	SC								
	PO								

DIPYRIDAMOLE

(Persantine, Cardoxin, Peridamol)

mg/kg		Mouse	Rat	Guinea Pig	Rabbit	Cat	Dog	Monkey	
Lethal Dose	IV								
Y-LD$_{50}$	IP								
Z-MLD	IM								
	SC								
	PO								
Thrombosis	IV						0.2 [1307]		
	IP								
	IM								
	SC								
	PO								
	IV								
	IP								
	IM								
	SC								
	PO								
	IV								
	IP								
	IM								
	SC								
	PO								

IN VITRO

mg %	Cardiac	Vascular	Gut	Uterine	Visceral	Skeletal		
Guinea Pig	0.0252 [1694]							
Dog	0.0252 [1694]		0.0504 [1693]					

DISULFIRAM

(TTD, Abstensil, Antabuse)

mg/kg		Mouse	Rat	Guinea Pig	Rabbit	Cat	Dog	Monkey	
Lethal Dose	IV								
Y-LD$_{50}$	IP								
Z-MLD	IM								
	SC								
	PO								
Restore dopamine	IV								
after L-dopa	IP	[a]37.5 $_{1292}$							
[a]ED$_{50}$,	IM								
reserpinized	SC								
	PO								
Decrease	IV								
motor	IP	45 $_{1416}$							
activity	IM								
	SC								
	PO								
Decrease	IV								
aggression	IP	95 $_{1416}$							
(isolation-	IM								
induced)	SC								
	PO								
Enhance	IV								
respiratory O$_2$	IP		200 $_{1695}$						
toxicosis	IM								
	SC								
	PO								
	IV								
	IP								
	IM								
	SC								
	PO								
	IV								
	IP								
	IM								
	SC								
	PO								
	IV								
	IP								
	IM								
	SC								
	PO								
	IV								
	IP								
	IM								
	SC								
	PO								

DOBUTAMINE

(Dobutrex, LY 174008)

mg/kg		Mouse	Rat	Guinea Pig	Rabbit	Cat	Dog	Monkey
Lethal Dose	IV							
Y-LD$_{50}$	IP							
Z-MLD	IM							
	SC							
	PO							
Cardiovascular	IV		0.001_{1696}		$^a0.011_{1697}$	$^a0.012_{1367}$	0.015_{1698}	
^{a}mg/kg/min	IP							
	IM							
	SC							
	PO							
	IV							
	IP							
	IM							
	SC							
	PO							
	IV							
	IP							
	IM							
	SC							
	PO							
	IV							
	IP							
	IM							
	SC							
	PO							
	IV							
	IP							
	IM							
	SC							
	PO							
	IV							
	IP							
	IM							
	SC							
	PO							
	IV							
	IP							
	IM							
	SC							
	PO							
	IV							
	IP							
	IM							
	SC							
	PO							

DOMPERIDONE

(Motilium, R 33812)

mg/kg		Mouse	Rat	Guinea Pig	Rabbit	Cat	Dog	Monkey
Lethal Dose Y-LD$_{50}$ Z-MLD	IV							
	IP							
	IM							
	SC							
	PO							
Cardiovascular	IV		2.5 1699		0.02 1700			
	IP							
	IM							
	SC							
	PO							
Gastrointestinal	IV							
	IP							
	IM		5 1423					
	SC							
	PO							
	IV							
	IP							
	IM							
	SC							
	PO							
	IV							
	IP							
	IM							
	SC							
	PO							
	IV							
	IP							
	IM							
	SC							
	PO							
	IV							
	IP							
	IM							
	SC							
	PO							
	IV							
	IP							
	IM							
	SC							
	PO							
	IV							
	IP							
	IM							
	SC							
	PO							

DOPAMINE

(3-hydroxytyramine, Dopastat, Intropin)

mg/kg		Mouse	Rat	Guinea Pig	Rabbit	Cat	Dog	Monkey	
Lethal Dose	IV								
Y-LD$_{50}$	IP								
Z-MLD	IM								
	SC								
	PO								
Cardiovascular	IV		0.088 $_{1709}$	[a]0.08 $_{350}$	[a]0.8 $_{330}$	[a]0.16 $_{330}$	0.15 $_{330}$		
	IP								
[a]total mg	IM						[b]0.002 $_{171}$		
[b]mg/kg/min IA	SC								
	PO								
EEG	IV				15 $_{331}$				
	IP								
(desynchroni-	IM								
zation)	SC								
	PO								
Neuromuscular	IV					5 $_{1132}$			
block	IP								
	IM								
	SC								
	PO								
CNS	IV						0.3 $_{1225}$		
	IP								
	IM								
	SC								
	PO								
Decrease	IV								
adrenal	IP								
ascorbic	IM								
acid	SC		10 $_{857}$						
	PO								
Gastrointestinal	IV		0.005 $_{1423}$						
	IP								
	IM								
	SC								
	PO								
Thermoregulatory	IV								
	IP								
[a]total mg ICV	IM		[a]0.1 $_{1408}$						
	SC								
	PO								
Increase	IV								
gestation	IP								
	IM								
[a]BID	SC		[a]150 $_{1703}$						
	PO								

DOPAMINE (continued)

mg/kg		Mouse	Rat	Guinea Pig	Rabbit	Cat	Dog	Monkey
	IV							
	IP							
	IM							
	SC							
	PO							
	IV							
	IP							
	IM							
	SC							
	PO							
	IV							
	IP							
	IM							
	SC							
	PO							
	IV							
	IP							
	IM							
	SC							
	PO							

IN VITRO

mg %	Cardiac	Vascular	Gut	Uterine	Visceral	Skeletal		
Rabbit	0.16 266	100 330	0.024 266					
Cat	[a]5 266		0.164 266	0.26 266				
Guinea Pig			0.00015*					
[a]total mg								

*1710

154

DOXORUBICIN

(Adriblastina, Adriamycin, Adriacin)

mg/kg		Mouse	Rat	Guinea Pig	Rabbit	Cat	Dog	Monkey
Lethal Dose	IV							
Y-LD$_{50}$	IP							
Z-MLD	IM							
	SC							
	PO							
Antineoplastic	IV						[a]30 2273	
	IP							
[a]mg/M^2, Q3wks	IM							
	SC							
	PO							
Inhibit	IV							
leukemia	IP	10 1712						
cell	IM							
proliferation	SC							
	PO							
Cardiac	IV		[a]1 1713		[b]1 1697			
toxicosis	IP							
[a]daily, 5 d	IM							
[b]BID, 8 wks	SC							
	PO							
	IV							
	IP							
	IM							
	SC							
	PO							
	IV							
	IP							
	IM							
	SC							
	PO							
	IV							
	IP							
	IM							
	SC							
	PO							
	IV							
	IP							
	IM							
	SC							
	PO							
	IV							
	IP							
	IM							
	SC							
	PO							

DYNORPHIN

mg/kg		Mouse	Rat	Guinea Pig	Rabbit	Cat	Dog	Monkey	
Lethal Dose	IV								
Y-LD$_{50}$	IP								
Z-MLD	IM								
	SC								
	PO								
Anterior	IV							0.03_{1714}	
pituitary	IP								
effects	IM								
	SC								
	PO								
Cardiovascular	IV								
	IP								
	IM								
$^a\mu$Mol/kg	SC		$^a0.3_{1715}$						
	PO								
Anticonvulsive	IV		$^a1_{1716}$						
	IP								
	IP								
^{a}total nMol,	SC								
i. cranial	PO								

IN VITRO

mg %	Cardiac	Vascular	Gut	Uterine	Visceral	Skeletal	Ocular	
Rat			$^a1.26 \times 10^{-7}$*					
Rabbit							1×10^{-7}**	
^{a}molar solution								

*1717　　**1718

EDETATE, CALCIUM DISODIUM
(Calcium Disodium Versenate, Versene CA)

mg/kg		Mouse	Rat	Guinea Pig	Rabbit	Cat	Dog	Monkey
Lethal Dose	IV							
Y-LD$_{50}$	IP							
Z-MLD	IM							
	SC							
	PO							
Mobilization and	IV					[a]25 2272	[a]25 2272	
redistribution	IP		75 1509					
of lead	IM							
[a]Q6h	SC							
	PO							
Cardiac	IV		[a]15 1508					
	IP							
	IM							
[a]total mg/hr	SC							
	PO							
	IV							
	IP							
	IM							
	SC							
	PO							
	IV							
	IP							
	IM							
	SC							
	PO							
	IV							
	IP							
	IM							
	SC							
	PO							
	IV							
	IP							
	IM							
	SC							
	PO							
	IV							
	IP							
	IM							
	SC							
	PO							
	IV							
	IP							
	IM							
	SC							
	PO							

EDROPHONIUM

(Enlon, Tensilon, Antirex)

mg/kg		Mouse	Rat	Guinea Pig	Rabbit	Cat	Dog	Monkey	
Lethal Dose	IV	Y9 210			Y28.5 210		Y15 250		
Y-LD$_{50}$	IP	Y37 210							
Z-MLD	IM								
	SC	Y130 210							
	PO	Y600 210							
Curare	IV					0.4	0.4		
antagonist	IP								
	IM								
	SC		2.5						
	PO								
Muscle	IV					0.5	0.5		
relaxant	IP								
	IM								
	SC								
	PO								
Cholinergic	IV						0.11-0.22*		
	IP								
	IM								
	SC								
	PO								

*2273

IN VITRO

mg %		Cardiac	Vascular	Gut	Uterine	Visceral	Skeletal		

ß-ENDORPHIN

(ß-Lipotropin)

mg/kg		Mouse	Rat	Guinea Pig	Rabbit	Cat	Dog	Monkey	
Lethal Dose	IV								
Y-LD$_{50}$	IP								
Z-MLD	IM								
	SC								
	PO								
Analgesia	IV								
	IP								
^{a}IT	IM		^{a}0.19 1719						
^{b}Total μg ICV	SC		^{b}0.8 1719						
	PO								
	IV								
	IP								
	IM								
	SC								
	PO								
	IV								
	IP								
	IM								
	SC								
	PO								

IN VITRO

mg %	Cardiac	Vascular	Gut	Uterine	Visceral	Skeletal		
Dog			0.1 1720					

ENKEPHALIN

mg/kg		Mouse	Rat	Guinea Pig	Rabbit	Cat	Dog	Monkey
Lethal Dose	IV							
Y-LD$_{50}$	IP							
Z-MLD	IM							
	SC							
	PO							
Cardiovascular	IV				0.001 [261]			
	IP							
	IM							
$^a\mu$Mol/kg	SC		^{a}0.45 [1715]					
^{b}IA	PO				^{b}0.003 [1721]			
Analgesic	IV							
	IP	5 [1722]						
^{a}Total mg ICV	IM	^{a}0.04 [1722]						
^{b}IT	SC		^{b}0.12 [1719]					
	PO							
Anticonvulsive	IV							
	IP							
	IM							
^{a}total nMol,	SC							
i. cranial	PO	^{a}35 [1716]						
Respiratory	IV						0.006 [1723]	
effects	IP							
	IM							
	SC							
	PO							
Affect	IV						0.01 [1724]	
catecholamine	IP							
concentrations	IM							
	SC							
^{a}Total μg ICV	PO	^{a}0.5 [1725]						
	IV							
	IP							
	IM							
	SC							
	PO							
	IV							
	IP							
	IM							
	SC							
	PO							
	IV							
	IP							
	IM							
	SC							
	PO							

ENPROSTIL

(RS-84135)

mg/kg		Mouse	Rat	Guinea Pig	Rabbit	Cat	Dog	Monkey
Lethal Dose	IV							
Y-LD$_{50}$	IP							
Z-MLD	IM							
	SC							
	PO							
Antisecretory	IV							
(GI)	IP							
	IM							
	SC							
[a]IG	PO		0.0099_{1435}			[a]0.001_{1435}	[a]0.0066*	
Antiulcer	IV							
(GI)	IP							
	IM							
	SC		0.022_{1435}					
	PO		0.0061_{1435}					
Increase	IV							
blood	IP							
pressure	IM							
	SC							
[a]IG	PO					[a]0.005_{1435}		
	IV							
	IP							
	IM							
	SC							
	PO							
	IV							
	IP							
	IM							
	SC							
	PO							
	IV							
	IP							
	IM							
	SC							
	PO							
	IV							
	IP							
	IM							
	SC							
	PO							
	IV							
	IP							
	IM							
	SC							
	PO							

*1435

EPHEDRINE

(Ephedral, Sanedrine, Biophedrin)

mg/kg		Mouse	Rat	Guinea Pig	Rabbit	Cat	Dog	Monkey	
Lethal Dose Y-LD$_{50}$ Z-MLD	IV	200 [6]	Z137 [334]		Z60 [6]	Z60 [6]	Z72.5 [333]		
	IP	Z400 [332]	800 [335]		Z335 [334]				
	IM				Z340 [333]				
	SC	500 [333]	Y650	400 [6]	Z360 [333]		Z220 [333]		
	PO	Y1550 [960]	Z160 [335]		Z590 [334]				
Behavioral	IV							15	
	IP	1.25 [177]	29 [1501]						
	IM								
	SC	10 [940]							
	PO	100 [960]	100 [336]				0.06 [337]		
Cardiovascular	IV		1	1	1	1	0.5		
	IP								
	IM								
	SC								
	PO								
CNS stimulant [a]total mg	IV						2.5		
	IP						3.3 [97]		
	IM								
	SC						2.5		
	PO						"20 [97]		
Antagonize adrenolytic action of bretylium	IV					0.35 [153]			
	IP								
	IM								
	SC								
	PO								
Antagonize reserpine	IV								
	IP	20 [78]							
	IM								
	SC								
	PO						2 [1168]		
Increase rate of catecholamine disappearance	IV								
	IP	50 [338]							
	IM								
	SC								
	PO								
Hyperthermic	IV								
	IP								
	IM								
	SC		60 [259]						
	PO								
Bronchodilation	IV					[a]5 [2275]	1.5-3 [2275]		
	IP					[a]5 [2275]	1.5-3 [2275]		
	IM					[a]5 [2275]	1.5-3 [2275]		
	SC					[a]5 [2275]	1.5-3 [2275]		
[a]Total mg	PO					[a]5 [2275]	[a]5 15 [2272]		

EPHEDRINE (continued)

mg/kg		Mouse	Rat	Guinea Pig	Rabbit	Cat	Dog	Monkey
	IV							
	IP							
	IM							
	SC							
	PO							
	IV							
	IP							
	IM							
	SC							
	PO							
	IV							
	IP							
	IM							
	SC							
	PO							
	IV							
	IP							
	IM							
	SC							
	PO							

IN VITRO

mg %	Cardiac	Vascular	Gut	Uterine	Visceral	Skeletal	
Rabbit			2 [1157]				
Rat			0.8 [92]	0.2 [1157]			
Guinea Pig			0.3 [92]				
Rabbit Ear		[a]0.016 [339]					
[a]total mg							

EPINEPHRINE
(Adrenalin, Epifrin, Glaucon)

mg/kg		Mouse	Rat	Guinea Pig	Rabbit	Cat	Dog	Monkey
Lethal Dose Y-LD$_{50}$ Z-MLD	IV	Y0.5 896	Y0.98	0.15 341	0.2 341	0.7 341	0.15 341	
	IP	Y4 340	10 343					
	IM		Y3.5 7					
	SC	Y1.47 341	Y5 341	1.5 341	15 341	20 341	5.5 341	
	PO	Y50	30 341		30 341			
Cardiovascular [a] mg/kg/min [b] mg/kg/min IA [c] total mg	IV	0.002 1197	0.002 855	0.003	0.003	0.003	[a]0.005 1727	0.001 1079
	IP						[b]0.001 1728	
	IM					0.01 2272	0.01 2272	
	SC		1 862			[c]0.1-0.5 *	0.05	
	PO							
Behavioral	IV						0.05 99	
	IP	2.5 177	1 334					
	IM							
	SC	2 940						
	PO							
CNS	IV				0.01 345	0.15 998		
	IP							
	IM							
	SC		0.1 1730					
	PO							
Barbiturate sleep potentiation	IV							
	IP	2 342						
	IM	0.4 7						
	SC							
	PO							
Antagonize reserpine ptosis	IV							
	IP	1 78						
	IM							
	SC							
	PO							
Diuretic	IV							
	IP							
	IM							
	SC		0.5 151				1 885	
	PO							
EEG	IV				0.004 827	0.004 827		
	IP							
	IM							
	SC							
	PO							
Metabolic	IV						0.022 865	
	IP		0.05 1082					
	IM							
	SC	0.1 1200	0.2 864		0.15 863			
	PO							

*2275

mg/kg		Mouse	Rat	Guinea Pig	Rabbit	Cat	Dog	Monkey
Bronchiole dilatation	IV							
	IP							
	IM							
	SC			0.05_{1081}				
	PO							
	IV							
	IP							
	IM							
	SC							
	PO							
	IV							
	IP							
	IM							
	SC							
	PO							
	IV							
	IP							
	IM							
	SC							
	PO							

IN VITRO

mg %	Cardiac	Vascular	Gut	Uterine	Visceral	Trachea	CNS	
Sympathomimetic	0.01	0.0183_{1726}	0.01	0.02	0.01	0.006_{1157}		
Dog		0.00018_{1729}						
Anti-5HT			0.002_{92}					
Rat							0.00018*	

*1730

EPININE
(N-Methyl Dopamine)

mg/kg		Mouse	Rat	Guinea Pig	Rabbit	Cat	Dog	Monkey
Lethal Dose	IV							
Y-LD$_{50}$	IP							
Z-MLD	IM							
	SC							
	PO							
Cardiovascular	IV		0.0032_{1709}			0.003_{1731}		
	IP							
	IM							
[a]IA, perfused	SC							
lung	PO						[a]0.004_{1732}	
	IV							
	IP							
	IM							
	SC							
	PO							
	IV							
	IP							
	IM							
	SC							
	PO							

IN VITRO

mg %	Cardiac	Vascular	Gut	Uterine	Visceral	Skeletal		

EPOPROSTENOL

(Cyclo-Prostin, Flolan, Prostacyclin, PGI_2)

mg/kg		Mouse	Rat	Guinea Pig	Rabbit	Cat	Dog	Monkey	
Lethal Dose	IV								
Y-LD_{50}	IP								
Z-MLD	IM								
	SC								
	PO								
Cardiovascular	IV						[a]0.01 1515		
[a]mg/kg/min	IP						[b]0.25 2155		
[b]Total μg, IA	IM								
	SC								
	PO								
Renal	IV		[a]0.5 2156						
[a]mg/kg/min	IP		[b]0.25 2156				[b]4×10^{-6}*		
[b]mg/kg/min IA	IM								
	SC								
	PO								
Effects	IV						[a]25×10^{-6}**		
on blood	IP	0.1 2158							
	IM								
	SC								
[a]mg/kg/min	PO								

*2157   **1356

IN VITRO

mg %	Cardiac	Vascular	Gut	Uterine	Visceral	Skeletal		

ERGONOVINE

(Ergotrate, Ergobasine, Ergometrine)

mg/kg		Mouse	Rat	Guinea Pig	Rabbit	Cat	Dog	Monkey	
Lethal Dose	IV	145 $_{346}$		80 $_{346}$	27.5				
Y-LD$_{50}$	IP								
Z-MLD	IM								
	SC		0.5 $_{346}$						
	PO								
Oxytocic	IV						^{a}0.35 $_{97}$		
	IP								
^{a}total mg	IM					^{a}0.07-0-.2*	^{a}0.35 $_{97}$		
	SC		500 $_{257}$						
	PO					^{a}0.1 $_{2275}$	^{a}0.2-1$_{2275}$		
Antagonize	IV		0.085						
epinephrine	IP								
toxicosis	IM								
	SC								
	PO								
Behavioral	IV								
	IP		0.063 $_{1403}$						
	IM								
	SC								
	PO								

*2273

IN VITRO

mg %	Cardiac	Vascular	Gut	Uterine	Visceral	Skeletal		
Oxytocic				50 $_{347}$				

168

ERGOTAMINE

(Gynergen, Cafergot, Ergomar)

mg/kg		Mouse	Rat	Guinea Pig	Rabbit	Cat	Dog	Monkey
Lethal Dose	IV	Y52 [348]	Y62 [304]	36 [351]	Y3.55 [352]			
Y-LD$_{50}$	IP							
Z-MLD	IM							
	SC		Z125 [349]			Y11 [352]		
	PO							
Adrenolytic	IV				0.15 [352]	1	8 [354]	
	IP							
	IM							
	SC							
	PO							
CNS	IV					0.1 [353]		
	IP							
	IM							
	SC	5 [350]						
	PO							
Oxytocic	IV							
	IP							
[a]total mg	IM						[a]0.2-0.5*	
	SC						[a]0.2-0.5*	
	PO						[a]0.5-1 [2275]	

*2275

IN VITRO

mg %	Cardiac	Vascular	Gut	Uterine	Visceral	Skeletal		
Rabbit				0.5 [352]				
Guinea Pig				0.002 [352]				

ESTRADIOL

(Dihydrofolliculin, Dihydroxyestrin)

mg/kg		Mouse	Rat	Guinea Pig	Rabbit	Cat	Dog	Monkey	
Lethal Dose	IV								
Y-LD$_{50}$	IP								
Z-MLD	IM								
	SC								
	PO								
Endothelium	IV								
responses	IP								
	IM				0.033 $_{1733}$				
	SC								
	PO								
CNS	IV								
drug	IP								
binding	IM								
modulation	SC		0.007 $_{1734}$						
	PO								
Estrogenic	IV								
	IP								
	IM					[a]0.2-0.5*	[a]0.2-2*		
[a]total mg	SC								
	PO								
	IV								
	IP								
	IM								
	SC								
	PO								
	IV								
	IP								
	IM								
	SC								
	PO								
	IV								
	IP								
	IM								
	SC								
	PO								
	IV								
	IP								
	IM								
	SC								
	PO								
	IV								
	IP								
	IM								
	SC								
	PO								

*2275

ETHACRYNIC ACID
(Edecrin, Endecril)

mg/kg		Mouse	Rat	Guinea Pig	Rabbit	Cat	Dog	Monkey	
Lethal Dose	IV								
Y-LD$_{50}$	IP								
Z-MLD	IM								
	SC								
	PO								
Renal	IV	50 1736					[1] 1735		
	IP								
	IM								
	SC								
	PO								
	IV								
	IP								
	IM								
	SC								
	PO								
	IV								
	IP								
	IM								
	SC								
	PO								
	IV								
	IP								
	IM								
	SC								
	PO								
	IV								
	IP								
	IM								
	SC								
	PO								
	IV								
	IP								
	IM								
	SC								
	PO								
	IV								
	IP								
	IM								
	SC								
	PO								
	IV								
	IP								
	IM								
	SC								
	PO								

ETHOSUXIMIDE

(Zarontin, Suxilep, Suximal)

mg/kg		Mouse	Rat	Guinea Pig	Rabbit	Cat	Dog	Monkey
Lethal Dose	IV							
Y-LD$_{50}$	IP							
Z-MLD	IM							
	SC							
	PO							
Anticonvulsant	IV							
	IP	150 1737						
	IM							
	SC							
	PO							
Neurotoxic	IV							
	IP	400 1737						
	IM							
	SC							
	PO							
Behavioral	IV							
toxicosis	IP							
	IM							[a]45 1738
	SC							
[a]daily	PO							
CNS	IV		12.5 1664					
	IP							
	IM							
	SC							
	PO							
Inhibit	IV					200 1739		
spinal	IP							
neurotrans-	IM							
mission	SC							
	PO							
	IV							
	IP							
	IM							
	SC							
	PO							
	IV							
	IP							
	IM							
	SC							
	PO							
	IV							
	IP							
	IM							
	SC							
	PO							

ETHYLKETOCYCLAZOCINE

(Ethylketazocine)

mg/kg		Mouse	Rat	Guinea Pig	Rabbit	Cat	Dog	Monkey	
Lethal Dose	IV								
Y-LD$_{50}$	IP								
Z-MLD	IM								
	SC								
	PO								
Analgesic	IV								
	IP								
[a]ED$_{50}$	IM								
	SC	[a]0.08 $_{1482}$	[a]0.14 $_{1482}$	[a]0.046$_{1482}$			0.02 $_{1479}$		
	PO								
Sedative	IV								
	IP								
	IM								
	SC	1.59 $_{1482}$						0.0056*	
	PO								
Increase	IV				0.2 $_{1481}$				
spinal	IP								
reflexes	IM								
	SC								
	PO								
Diuretic	IV								
	IP								
	IM								
	SC		1.25 $_{1478}$					0.0001*	
	PO								
Behavioral	IV								
	IP								
	IM							0.01$_{1741}$	
	SC	32 $_{1740}$							
	PO								
Cardiovascular	IV						[a]0.01$_{1742}$		
	IP								
	IM								
[a]total mg,	SC								
i. cerebral	PO								
Decrease	IV								
respiratory	IP								
rate	IM							0.1 $_{1477}$	
	SC								
	PO								
Inhibit	IV		[a]10 $_{1743}$						
urinary	IP								
bladder	IM								
[a]total nMol ICV	SC								
	PO								

*1479

173

mg/kg		Mouse	Rat	Guinea Pig	Rabbit	Cat	Dog	Monkey	
	IV								
	IP								
	IM								
	SC								
	PO								
	IV								
	IP								
	IM								
	SC								
	PO								
	IV								
	IP								
	IM								
	SC								
	PO								
	IV								
	IP								
	IM								
	SC								
	PO								

IN VITRO

mg %	Cardiac	Vascular	Gut	Uterine	Visceral	Skeletal		
Rat			$^a 5\times10^{-8}$*					
^{a}molar solution								

*1717

ETHYLNOREPINEPHRINE

(Protocatechuyl Alcohol, Ethylnoradrenaline, Ethylnorsuprarenin)

mg/kg		Mouse	Rat	Guinea Pig	Rabbit	Cat	Dog	Monkey	
Lethal Dose	IV	Y117 [47]							
Y-LD$_{50}$	IP								
Z-MLD	IM								
	SC								
	PO								
Bronchiolar	IV					1 [48]	1 [47]		
dilatation	IP			500 [47]					
	IM								
	SC		80 [47]						
	PO								
Hyperglycemic	IV								
	IP								
	IM								
	SC				10 [47]				
	PO								
	IV								
	IP								
	IM								
	SC								
	PO								

IN VITRO

mg %		Cardiac	Vascular	Gut	Uterine	Visceral	Skeletal		

ETORPHINE

(M-99, Oripavine)

mg/kg		Mouse	Rat	Guinea Pig	Rabbit	Cat	Dog	Monkey	
Lethal Dose Y-LD_{50} Z-MLD	IV								
	IP								
	IM								
	SC								
	PO								
Analgesic [a]ED_{50} [b]total mg to immobilize	IV								
	IP								
	IM						[b]0.0075*		
	SC	[a]0.6 1744							
	PO								
Thermoregulatory	IV								
	IP								
	IM								
	SC	0.0005 1613	0.0001 1496						
	PO								
Behavioral	IV								
	IP								
	IM							0.007 1494	
	SC								
	PO								
Increase corticoids	IV								
	IP		0.05 1745						
	IM								
	SC								
	PO								
Inhibit urinary bladder [a]total ug ICV	IV		[a]0.165 1743						
	IP								
	IM								
	SC								
	PO								
	IV								
	IP								
	IM								
	SC								
	PO								
	IV								
	IP								
	IM								
	SC								
	PO								
	IV								
	IP								
	IM								
	SC								
	PO								

*2275

FAMOTIDINE

(MK-208)

mg/kg		Mouse	Rat	Guinea Pig	Rabbit	Cat	Dog	Monkey
Lethal Dose	IV							
Y-LD$_{50}$	IP							
Z-MLD	IM							
	SC							
	PO							
Inhibit	IV							
gastric	IP							
acid	IM							
secretion	SC							
[a]ED$_{50}$	PO		[a]0.8 $_{1637}$					
Anti-ulcer	IV							
(GI)	IP							
	IM							
	SC							
	PO		3 $_{1637}$					
	IV							
	IP							
	IM							
	SC							
	PO							
	IV							
	IP							
	IM							
	SC							
	PO							
	IV							
	IP							
	IM							
	SC							
	PO							
	IV							
	IP							
	IM							
	SC							
	PO							
	IV							
	IP							
	IM							
	SC							
	PO							
	IV							
	IP							
	IM							
	SC							
	PO							

FENGABINE

(SK-79.229-00)

mg/kg		Mouse	Rat	Guinea Pig	Rabbit	Cat	Dog	Monkey	
Lethal Dose	IV								
Y-LD$_{50}$	IP								
Z-MLD	IM								
	SC								
	PO								
Behavioral	IV								
	IP		25 $_{1466}$						
	IM								
	SC								
	PO								
GABA	IV								
receptor	IP		^{a}50 $_{1366}$						
regulation	IM								
	SC								
^{a}daily	PO								
	IV								
	IP								
	IM								
	SC								
	PO								
	IV								
	IP								
	IM								
	SC								
	PO								
	IV								
	IP								
	IM								
	SC								
	PO								
	IV								
	IP								
	IM								
	SC								
	PO								
	IV								
	IP								
	IM								
	SC								
	PO								
	IV								
	IP								
	IM								
	SC								
	PO								

FENOLDOPAM

(SKF-82526-J)

mg/kg		Mouse	Rat	Guinea Pig	Rabbit	Cat	Dog	Monkey	
Lethal Dose	IV								
Y-LD$_{50}$	IP								
Z-MLD	IM								
	SC								
	PO								
Cardiovascular	IV		1_{1747}		0.001_{1700}	0.3_{1746}	$^a0.01_{1748}$		
	IP								
	IM								
^{a}mg/kg/min	SC								
	PO								
	IV								
	IP								
	IM								
	SC								
	PO								
	IV								
	IP								
	IM								
	SC								
	PO								

IN VITRO

mg %	Cardiac	Vascular	Gut	Uterine	Visceral	Skeletal		

179

FENTANYL
(Leptanal, Sublimaze, Pentanyl)

mg/kg		Mouse	Rat	Guinea Pig	Rabbit	Cat	Dog	Monkey
Lethal Dose	IV							
Y-LD$_{50}$	IP							
Z-MLD	IM							
.	SC							
	PO							
Decrease	IV				0.1 [1481]			
spinal	IP							
reflexes	IM							
	SC							
	PO							
Analgesic	IV					0.02-0.04*	0.02-0.04*	
	IP		[b]0.0016 [1752]					
	IM					0.02-0.04*	0.02-0.04*	
[a]ED$_{50}$	SC	[a]0.004 [1482]	[a]0.003 [1482]	[a]0.004 [1482]		0.02-0.04*	0.02-0.04*	
[b]total mg IT	PO							
Sedative	IV					0.02-0.04*	0.02-0.04*	
	IP							
	IM					0.02-0.04*	0.02-0.04*	
[a]Rotorod test	SC	[a]0.81 [1482]				0.02-0.04*	0.02-0.04*	
	PO							
Respiratory	IV		0.002 [1749]					
depression	IP							
	IM							
	SC							
	PO							
Urinary	IV		0.0008 [1750]					
system	IP							
effect	IM							
	SC		0.025 [1492]					
	PO							
Behavioral	IV		[a]0.0025 [1387]					
	IP							
	IM							
[a]Self	SC	0.03 [1483]	0.04 [1751]					
administration	PO							
Cardiovascular	IV		0.0077 [1753]					
	IP						[a]0.005 [1742]	
	IM							
[a]total mg	SC							
i. cerebral	PO							
Thermoregulatory	IV							
	IP							
	IM							
	SC	0.125 [1613]	0.025 [1496]					
	PO							

*2273

180

FENTANYL (continued)

mg/kg		Mouse	Rat	Guinea Pig	Rabbit	Cat	Dog	Monkey	
	IV								
	IP								
	IM								
	SC								
	PO								
	IV								
	IP								
	IM								
	SC								
	PO								
	IV								
	IP								
	IM								
	SC								
	PO								
	IV								
	IP								
	IM								
	SC								
	PO								

IN VITRO

mg %	Cardiac	Vascular	Gut	Uterine	Visceral	Skeletal		
Cat	3.365 1754							

FLUMAZENIL

(Flumazepil, Ro 15-1788/000)

mg/kg		Mouse	Rat	Guinea Pig	Rabbit	Cat	Dog	Monkey	
Lethal Dose	IV								
$Y-LD_{50}$	IP								
Z-MLD	IM								
	SC								
	PO								
Induce	IV								
Diazepam	IP								
withdrawal	IM								
syndrome	SC								
	PO						[2] 1666		
	IV								
	IP								
	IM								
	SC								
	PO								
	IV								
	IP								
	IM								
	SC								
	PO								

IN VITRO

mg %	Cardiac	Vascular	Gut	Uterine	Visceral	Skeletal	CNS	
Rat							[a]1×10^{-5}*	
[a]molar								
solution								

*1755

FLUNIXIN

(Banamine, Finadyne)

mg/kg		Mouse	Rat	Guinea Pig	Rabbit	Cat	Dog	Monkey	
Lethal Dose Y-LD$_{50}$ Z-MLD	IV								
	IP								
	IM								
	SC								
	PO								
Analgesic	IV								
	IP								
	IM							10 [1901]	
	SC	2.3 [1901]	2.4 [1901]						
	PO		4.8 [1901]						
Anti- inflammatory	IV						0.5-1 [2272]		
	IP								
	IM						0.3 [2273]		
	SC								
	PO								
	IV								
	IP								
	IM								
	SC								
	PO								
	IV								
	IP								
	IM								
	SC								
	PO								
	IV								
	IP								
	IM								
	SC								
	PO								
	IV								
	IP								
	IM								
	SC								
	PO								
	IV								
	IP								
	IM								
	SC								
	PO								
	IV								
	IP								
	IM								
	SC								
	PO								

FLUOROACETIC ACID
(Fluoroacetate, 1080, Fratol)

mg/kg		Mouse	Rat	Guinea Pig	Rabbit	Cat	Dog	Monkey	
Lethal Dose	IV				Y0.25 [346]	Y0.2 [346]	Y0.06 [346]	Y4 [346]	
Y-LD$_{50}$	IP	Y10 [346]	Y0.4 [346]	Y0.35 [346]					
Z-MLD	IM		Y5 [346]						
	SC	Y16 [346]	Y2.5 [346]	0.25 [346]	0.75 [346]				
	PO	Y8 [346]	Y2.5 [346]						
Decreased	IV						1 [355]		
mitotic	IP								
index of	IM								
mucosal	SC								
epithelium	PO								
	IV								
	IP								
	IM								
	SC								
	PO								
	IV								
	IP								
	IM								
	SC								
	PO								

IN VITRO

mg %	Cardiac	Vascular	Gut	Uterine	Visceral	Skeletal		
Rabbit			0.004 [356]					

FLUOROURACIL

(Adrucil, Efudex, Fluoroplex)

mg/kg		Mouse	Rat	Guinea Pig	Rabbit	Cat	Dog	Monkey	
Lethal Dose	IV								
Y-LD$_{50}$	IP								
Z-MLD	IM								
	SC								
	PO								
Antileukemic	IV								
(L1210 cells)	IP	[a]20 1756							
	IM								
	SC								
[a]days 1,5,9	PO								
Teratogenesis;	IV								
Embryo	IP	40 1757							
lethality	IM								
	SC								
	PO								
Antineoplastic	IV						5 2273		
	IP	50 1628							
	IM								
	SC								
	PO								
Block	IV								
humoral	IP	50 1758							
(not cell)-	IM								
mediated	SC								
immunity	PO								
Regression	IV								
of antigen-	IP	80 1759							
dependent	IM								
tumor	SC								
	PO								
	IV								
	IP								
	IM								
	SC								
	PO								
	IV								
	IP								
	IM								
	SC								
	PO								
	IV								
	IP								
	IM								
	SC								
	PO								

FLUOXETINE

(Prozac)

mg/kg		Mouse	Rat	Guinea Pig	Rabbit	Cat	Dog	Monkey
Lethal Dose	IV							
Y-LD$_{50}$	IP							
Z-MLD	IM							
	SC							
	PO							
Anticonvulsant	IV							
	IP	[a]13 $_{1760}$						
	IM							
[a]ED$_{50}$	SC							
	PO							
Behavioral	IV							
	IP							
	IM							
	SC	0.44 $_{1365}$	12.7 $_{1365}$					
	PO	9.9 $_{1439}$						
Mydriatic	IV							
	IP							
	IM							
	SC	32 $_{1439}$						
	PO							
GABA	IV							
binding	IP		[a]10 $_{1366}$					
regulation	IM							
	SC							
[a]daily	PO							
Block	IV		3 $_{1540}$					
PCA-induced	IP							
hemodynamic	IM							
effects	SC							
	PO							
	IV							
	IP							
	IM							
	SC							
	PO							
	IV							
	IP							
	IM							
	SC							
	PO							
	IV							
	IP							
	IM							
	SC							
	PO							

ß-FUNALTREXAMINE

(ß-FNA)

mg/kg		Mouse	Rat	Guinea Pig	Rabbit	Cat	Dog	Monkey	
Lethal Dose	IV								
Y-LD$_{50}$	IP								
Z-MLD	IM								
	SC								
	PO								
Antagonize	IV	[a]0.15 [1761]	[b]10 [1480]						
opioids	IP								
[a]ICV	IM								
[b]total nMol ICV	SC	80 [1489]	20 [1478]					1 [1762]	
	PO								
Behavioral	IV		[a]0.005 [1764]					[b]0.003 [*]	
	IP								
[a]ICV	IM								
[b]Total mg ICV	SC							10 [1763]	
	PO								
	IV								
Muscle	IP								
relaxation	IM								
and stupor	SC							10 [1763]	
	PO								
	IV								
	IP								
	IM								
	SC								
	PO								
	IV								
	IP								
	IM								
	SC								
	PO								
	IV								
	IP								
	IM								
	SC								
	PO								
	IV								
	IP								
	IM								
	SC								
	PO								
	IV								
	IP								
	IM								
	SC								
	PO								

*1763

FUROSEMIDE

(Frusemide, Furose, Lasix)

mg/kg		Mouse	Rat	Guinea Pig	Rabbit	Cat	Dog	Monkey
Lethal Dose Y-LD$_{50}$ Z-MLD	IV							
	IP							
	IM							
	SC							
	PO							
Hyperglycemic	IV	200 1736						
	IP	200 1765						
	IM							
	SC							
	PO							
Renal	IV	200 1736	0.1 1766		5 1767	0.2 1768	1 1648	
	IP	25 1765	5 1769			[a]0.001 1768		
	IM					2.5-5 2273	2.5-5 2273	
[a]mg/kg/min	SC		0.5 1285					
	PO					2-4 2272	2.5-5 2273	
Renal toxicosis [a]Follow with 0.26 mg/kg/min	IV						[a]5 1770	
	IP							
	IM							
	SC							
	PO							
Increase antibiotic excretion	IV							
	IP							
	IM				1 1771			
	SC							
	PO							
Decrease growth [a]mg/M^2/d	IV							
	IP		[a]100 1772					
	IM							
	SC							
	PO							
Decrease pulmonary artery pressure	IV						2 1773	
	IP							
	IM							
	SC							
	PO							
	IV							
	IP							
	IM							
	SC							
	PO							
	IV							
	IP							
	IM							
	SC							
	PO							

FUROSEMIDE (continued)

mg/kg		Mouse	Rat	Guinea Pig	Rabbit	Cat	Dog	Monkey
	IV							
	IP							
	IM							
	SC							
	PO							
	IV							
	IP							
	IM							
	SC							
	PO							
	IV							
	IP							
	IM							
	SC							
	PO							
	IV							
	IP							
	IM							
	SC							
	PO							

IN VITRO

mg %	Cardiac	Vascular	Gut	Uterine	Visceral	Skeletal	Hepatic	
Rat							0.331_{1774}	

GALLAMINE

(Flaxedil, Relaxan, Tricuran)

mg/kg		Mouse	Rat	Guinea Pig	Rabbit	Cat	Dog	Monkey
Lethal Dose	IV	Y4.3	Y5.5 [361]		Y0.65 [361]		Y0.8 [361]	
Y-LD$_{50}$	IP	Y9.6 [1143]						
Z-MLD	IM				Y2.5 [361]			
	SC	Y17.4 [360]	Y25 [361]		Y3 [361]			
	PO	Y425 [361]			Y100 [361]			
Neuromuscular	IV		0.01 [1143]		4 [1485]	5 [362]	2 [1775]	
block	IP							
	IM				0.75 [361]		0.25 [2275]	
	SC				1.5 [361]		0.25 [2275]	
	PO							
CNS	IV		2 [1000]			1 [1000]		
	IP							
	IM							
	SC							
	PO							
Ganglionic	IV					2 [1538]		
effects	IP							
	IM							
	SC							
	PO							

IN VITRO

mg %	Cardiac	Vascular	Gut	Uterine	Visceral	Skeletal	
Rat						0.25 [1157]	

GENTAMICIN

(Bristagen, Garasin, Gentacidin, U-Gencin)

mg/kg		Mouse	Rat	Guinea Pig	Rabbit	Cat	Dog	Monkey	
Lethal Dose	IV								
Y-LD$_{50}$	IP								
Z-MLD	IM								
	SC								
	PO								
Nephrotoxic	IV		100 1776						
	IP								
	IM								
[a]Daily	SC		[a]40 1777						
	PO								
	IV								
	IP								
	IM								
	SC								
	PO								
	IV								
	IP								
	IM								
	SC								
	PO								

IN VITRO

mg %	Cardiac	Vascular	Gut	Uterine	Visceral	Skeletal	Renal	
Rat							20 1776	

GLUCAGON

(Hyperglycemic-glycogenolytic Factor, HGF)

mg/kg		Mouse	Rat	Guinea Pig	Rabbit	Cat	Dog	Monkey	
Lethal Dose	IV								
Y-LD$_{50}$	IP								
Z-MLD	IM								
	SC								
	PO								
Cardiac	IV		1 1508				0.004 1778		
	IP								
	IM								
	SC								
	PO								
Tolerance	IV						0.03 2272		
test	IP								
	IM								
	SC								
	PO								
	IV								
	IP								
	IM								
	SC								
	PO								

IN VITRO

mg %	Cardiac	Vascular	Gut	Uterine	Visceral	Skeletal		

GUANABENZ

(Wytensin, Rexitene)

mg/kg		Mouse	Rat	Guinea Pig	Rabbit	Cat	Dog	Monkey
Lethal Dose	IV							
Y-LD$_{50}$	IP							
Z-MLD	IM							
	SC							
	PO							
Hyperglycemic	IV		0.1 $_{1585}$					
	IP							
	IM							
	SC							
	PO							
Renal	IV						^{a}0.001 $_{1779}$	
effects	IP							
	IM							
^{a}mg/kg/min	SC							
	PO							
Cardiovascular	IV		0.01 $_{1780}$					
	IP							
	IM							
	SC							
	PO							
	IV							
	IP							
	IM							
	SC							
	PO							
	IV							
	IP							
	IM							
	SC							
	PO							
	IV							
	IP							
	IM							
	SC							
	PO							
	IV							
	IP							
	IM							
	SC							
	PO							
	IV							
	IP							
	IM							
	SC							
	PO							

GUANETHIDINE
(Ismelin, Utensol, Dopom)

mg/kg		Mouse	Rat	Guinea Pig	Rabbit	Cat	Dog	Monkey
Lethal Dose Y-LD$_{50}$ Z-MLD	IV	Y22 93	Y23 363		50	50		
	IP							
	IM							
	SC							
	PO		Y1000 363					
Autonomic effects	IV				3	15 363	15	3 1646
	IP	2.5 1243	50 1782	100 1219		15 367		
	IM							
	SC			3.75 1781		7.5 171		
	PO					15 171	35 93	
Catecholamine depletion	IV		5 150		12.5 366	15 91		
	IP	10 861	8 364					
	IM		25 150					
	SC		15 365			15 366		
	PO							
Neurocytotoxic	IV							
	IP		[a]15 1783					
	IM							
[a]daily	SC							
	PO							

IN VITRO

mg %	Cardiac	Vascular	Gut	Uterine	Visceral	Skeletal	
Finkleman 812			0.4 365				

HALOPERIDOL

(Haldol, Aloperidine, Brotopon)

mg/kg		Mouse	Rat	Guinea Pig	Rabbit	Cat	Dog	Monkey
Lethal Dose Y-LD$_{50}$ Z-MLD	IV	Y13 1784						
	IP							
	IM							
	SC	Y54 1784						
	PO	Y144 1784						
Antagonize amphetamine effects	IV						1 1375	
	IP	0.5 1392	1 1381					
	IM							
	SC							
	PO	0.25 1372						
Alter brain neurotrans- mitters (ACh, NE, DA)	IV		0.1 1380					
	IP	4 1785						
	IM							1 1791
	SC		4 1786		1 1411			
	PO							
Block peripheral effects of norepinephrine	IV							
	IP	5 1418						
	IM							
	SC							
	PO							
Tranquilize [a]ED$_{50}$	IV							
	IP							
	IM							
	SC							
	PO	[a]8.3 1372						
Increase morphine analgesia	IV							
	IP	2.5 1417						
	IM							
	SC							
	PO							
Behavioral	IV				0.25 1790			
	IP		0.08 1789					
	IM							
	SC							
	PO							
Thermoregulatory	IV				0.05 1405			
	IP	0.12 1414						
	IM							
	SC							
	PO							
Gastrointestinal [a]antiemetic	IV							
	IP							
	IM		5 1423				[a]0.02 2272	
	SC							
	PO						[a]0.02 2272	

mg/kg		Mouse	Rat	Guinea Pig	Rabbit	Cat	Dog	Monkey
Decrease	IV		[a]1 1788					
locomotor	IP		0.001 1787					
activity	IM							
[a]BID, 15 d	SC							
i. cisternal	PO							
Ocular	IV							
	IP		0.4 1384					
	IM							
	SC							
	PO							
Increase	IV							
endorphins	IP		[a]0.1 1792					
	IM							
[a]chronic	SC							
	PO							
	IV							
	IP							
	IM							
	SC							
	PO							
	IV							
	IP							
	IM							
	SC							
	PO							
	IV							
	IP							
	IM							
	SC							
	PO							
	IV							
	IP							
	IM							
	SC							
	PO							
	IV							
	IP							
	IM							
	SC							
	PO							
	IV							
	IP							
	IM							
	SC							
	PO							

HARMALINE

(3,4-Dihydroharmine, Harmidine, Harmalol methyl ether)

mg/kg		Mouse	Rat	Guinea Pig	Rabbit	Cat	Dog	Monkey
Lethal Dose	IV				20 1105			
Y-LD50	IP							
Z-MLD	IM							
	SC	Y120 115	Z120 368	Z100 368	Z100 368	Z100 368	33.3 368	
	PO							
Cardiovascular	IV				10 371	1 368	5	
and	IP							
uterine	IM							
	SC							
	PO							
Behavioral	IV							
	IP	8 992	5 370					
	IM							
	SC		2.5					
	PO							
Ataxic	IV				5 1105			
	IP	15 369	10					
	IM							
	SC			10 368				
	PO							
Spinal reflex	IV					5 372		
depressant	IP							
	IM							
	SC							
	PO							
Tremor	IV				3 1105	5 1244		
	IP		15 1105					
	IM							
	SC							
	PO							
	IV							
	IP							
	IM							
	SC							
	PO							
	IV							
	IP							
	IM							
	SC							
	PO							
	IV							
	IP							
	IM							
	SC							
	PO							

HARMINE
(Banisterine, Yageine, Telepathine)

mg/kg		Mouse	Rat	Guinea Pig	Rabbit	Cat	Dog	Monkey	
Lethal Dose Y-LD$_{50}$ Z-MLD	IV				60 [1105]				
	IP								
	IM								
	SC	300 [373]	Z200 [374]	100 [375]	200 [375]	Z200 [373]		Z30 [373]	
	PO								
Cardiovascular	IV				10 [374]	4 [374]	5		
	IP								
	IM								
	SC								
	PO								
Tremor ^{a}ED$_{50}$	IV				3 [1105]				
	IP	15 [369]	15 [1105]						
	IM	10 [175]							
	SC	^{a}3.3 [1793]							
	PO								
Behavioral	IV								
	IP								
	IM	1 [175]							
	SC								
	PO								
Ganglionic block	IV					25 [376]	15 [376]		
	IP								
	IM								
	SC								
	PO								
EEG	IV					5 [842]			
	IP								
	IM								
	SC								
	PO								
	IV								
	IP								
	IM								
	SC								
	PO								
	IV								
	IP								
	IM								
	SC								
	PO								
	IV								
	IP								
	IM								
	SC								
	PO								

mg/kg		Mouse	Rat	Guinea Pig	Rabbit	Cat	Dog	Monkey	
Lethal Dose	IV				1.2 [1110]	1 [378]	2.5 [1110]		
Y-LD_{50}	IP	Y0.064 [377]	Y0.45 [1110]	0.75 [1110]					
Z-MLD	IM								
	SC								
	PO								
Parasympatho-lytic	IV				5.9 [377]	10 [1444]	0.013 [377]		
	IP								
	IM								
	SC								
	PO								
CNS	IV		[a]0.001 [1794]			3.5 [379]	10 [1078]		
	IP								
	IM								
[a]total mg ICV	SC								
	PO								
Neuromuscular block	IV				1.8 [872]				
	IP								
	IM								
	SC								
	PO								

IN VITRO

mg %	Cardiac	Vascular	Gut	Uterine	Visceral	Skeletal		
Guinea Pig						20 [100]		
Rat						20		
Rabbit	4 [100]			2.4 [100]				
Cat	50 [100]							

HEPARIN

(Calciparin, Hep-Lock, Lipo-Hepin)

mg/kg		Mouse	Rat	Guinea Pig	Rabbit	Cat	Dog	Monkey
Lethal Dose Y-LD$_{50}$ Z-MLD	IV	Y1780 380						
	IP							
	IM							
	SC							
	PO							
Anticoagulant [a]units/kg	IV		10 381		5 383	5 385	8 209	2
	IP							
	IM							
	SC					[a]250 2272	[a]500 2272	
	PO							
Increased lipoproteinase activity	IV		6 382		1.5 384			
	IP							
	IM							
	SC							
	PO							
Shock protection [a]units/kg	IV						[a]250 1795	
	IP							
	IM							
	SC							
	PO							

IN VITRO

mg %	Cardiac	Vascular	Gut	Uterine	Visceral	Skeletal		

HEXAMETHONIUM
(Bistrium, C-6, Hexameton)

mg/kg		Mouse	Rat	Guinea Pig	Rabbit	Cat	Dog	Monkey
Lethal Dose	IV	Y21 [214]						
Y-LD$_{50}$	IP	Y42 [214]						
Z-MLD	IM							
	SC							
	PO	Y484 [214]						
Ganglionic	IV		20 [386]	5	10-15 [2275]	10	40 [1398]	
block	IP		2.8 [387]	10 [1219]				
	IM							
	SC							
	PO		100 [387]					
CNS	IV							
	IP	5 [350]						
	IM							
	SC		2 [350]					
	PO							
Behavioral	IV							
	IP		5 [1109]					
	IM							
	SC		10 [1092]					
	PO	40 [935]						
Gastrointestinal	IV		11.13 [1521]			10 [1444]		
	IP							
	IM							
	SC			3 [1781]				
	PO							
Cardiac	IV						10 [1545]	
	IP							
	IM							
	SC							
	PO							
Decrease	IV		25.2 [1310]					
bladder	IP							
contraction	IM							
	SC							
	PO							
Suppress	IV							
ACh	IP							
writhing	IM							
	SC	[a]12.2 [1296]						
[a]ED$_{50}$	PO							
	IV							
	IP							
	IM							
	SC							
	PO							

mg/kg		Mouse	Rat	Guinea Pig	Rabbit	Cat	Dog	Monkey	
	IV								
	IP								
	IM								
	SC								
	PO								
	IV								
	IP								
	IM								
	SC								
	PO								
	IV								
	IP								
	IM								
	SC								
	PO								
	IV								
	IP								
	IM								
	SC								
	PO								

IN VITRO

mg %	Cardiac	Vascular	Gut	Uterine	Visceral	Skeletal		
Rat			0.24 388			1.5 1157		
Rabbit	10		5					
Guinea Pig			2 1157					

HEXOBARBITAL

(Evipal, Sombulex, Cyclonal)

mg/kg		Mouse	Rat	Guinea Pig	Rabbit	Cat	Dog	Monkey	
Lethal Dose	IV	190 389			Y80 66	100 66	100 66		
Y-LD50	IP	Y340 390	Y280 393	100 66	Z225 393				
Z-MLD	IM								
	SC	250 66	404 66						
	PO	Y468 391	Y468		Z1200 394	400 66			
Anesthetic	IV	47 392	25 1076		25	25 66	30 66		
	IP	75	75 393		40 395	40 395			
	IM								
	SC	150 66	90 66						
	PO	150 66				100 66			
Increased	IV								
brain	IP		100 31						
serotonin	IM								
	SC								
	PO								
Behavioral	IV								
	IP	26 204						20 1230	
	IM								
	SC								
	PO								
Decreased	IV					20 396			
hippocampal	IP								
seizure	IM								
	SC								
	PO								
Decreased	IV		5 1000			5 1000			
spinal	IP								
reflexes	IM								
	SC								
	PO								
	IV								
	IP								
	IM								
	SC								
	PO								
	IV								
	IP								
	IM								
	SC								
	PO								
	IV								
	IP								
	IM								
	SC								
	PO								

HEXOCYCLIUM
(Tral, Tralin)

mg/kg		Mouse	Rat	Guinea Pig	Rabbit	Cat	Dog	Monkey	
Lethal Dose	IV	Y10.5 [111]							
Y-LD$_{50}$	IP	Y55 [111]							
Z-MLD	IM								
	SC	Y360 [111]							
	PO	Y600 [111]							
Anticholinergic	IV					4 [111]	5 [111]		
	IP								
	IM								
	SC								
	PO								
Antispasmodic	IV						0.04 [111]		
	IP								
	IM								
	SC								
	PO								
	IV								
	IP								
	IM								
	SC								
	PO								

IN VITRO

mg %	Cardiac	Vascular	Gut	Uterine	Visceral	Skeletal		

HISTAMINE

(Imido, Ergamine, Peremine)

mg/kg		Mouse	Rat	Guinea Pig	Rabbit	Cat	Dog	Monkey	
Lethal Dose	IV			Y0.18 [398]	0.1 [109]		30	50 [109]	
Y-LD$_{50}$	IP	2000 [1322]		33 [399]					
Z-MLD	IM								
	SC	2500 [195]		7 [399]	13.5 [399]				
	PO				300 [400]				
Cardiovascular	IV		0.01 [855]	0.1	0.15	0.0005 [1796]	0.0001 [1797]		
	IP								
	IM								
	SC						1.0		
	PO								
Increase	IV		[a]0.05 [1798]			[b]0.1 [1462]			
gastric	IP								
HCl	IM								
[a]mg/kg/min	SC		40 [1435]				0.064 [1433]		
[b]mg/kg/h	PO		25 [397]				0.5 [397]		
Behavioral	IV							0.03 [1531]	
	IP								
	IM								
	SC	10 [935]							
	PO								
Broncho-	IV			0.003 [1295]					
constriction	IP								
	IM								
	SC								
	PO								
Increased	IV						0.001 [1799]		
gastric blood	IP								
flow	IM								
	SC								
	PO								
Increased	IV						[a]0.01 [1802]		
renal blood	IP								
flow	IM								
	SC								
[a]total mg/min	PO								

IN VITRO

mg %	Cardiac	Vascular	Gut	Uterine	Visceral	Trachea	Lung	
Guinea Pig		0.111 [1314]	0.005	0.005		0.06 [1157]	0.0111 [1801]	
Rabbit	0.1	0.003 [1157]		0.5				
Rat			0.3 [1157]	3 [1157]				
Dog			0.111 [1693]			0.0111 [1800]		

205

HOMATROPINE

(Homapin, Malcotran, Mesopin, Novatropine)

mg/kg		Mouse	Rat	Guinea Pig	Rabbit	Cat	Dog	Monkey
Lethal Dose	IV							
$Y-LD_{50}$	IP	Y60 [101]	Y82 [101]	Y120 [101]				
Z-MLD	IM							
	SC	Y650 [101]	Y 800 [101]					
	PO	Y1400 [101]	Y1200 [101]	Y1000 [101]				
Anticholinergic	IV							
	IP							
	IM				0.16 [101]			
	SC	0.13 [101]	27 [101]					
	PO	12 [101]	18 [101]					
Ganglionic	IV					1 [101]		
block	IP							
	IM							
	SC							
	PO							
	IV							
	IP							
	IM							
	SC							
	PO							

IN VITRO

mg %	Cardiac	Vascular	Gut	Uterine	Visceral	Skeletal		
Rabbit			0.01					

HORDENINE

(Anhaline, Eremursine, Peyocactine)

mg/kg		Mouse	Rat	Guinea Pig	Rabbit	Cat	Dog	Monkey	
Lethal Dose	IV			300 [401]	275 [109]		275 [109]		
Y-LD$_{50}$	IP								
Z-MLD	IM								
	SC		1000 [401]	2000 [401]					
	PO						2000 [109]		
Cardiovascular	IV					^{a}2 [402]			
^{a}total mg	IP								
	IM								
	SC								
	PO								
Block	IV								
diarrhea	IP								
	IM								
	SC						35 [274]		
	PO								
	IV								
	IP								
	IM								
	SC								
	PO								

IN VITRO

mg %	Cardiac	Vascular	Gut	Uterine	Visceral	Skeletal	Trachea	
Stimulation			0.8 [402]	0.8 [402]				

HYDRALAZINE

(Apresoline, Vasodur, Hypophthalin)

mg/kg		Mouse	Rat	Guinea Pig	Rabbit	Cat	Dog	Monkey
Lethal Dose	IV		34 [403]				64 [817]	
Y-LD$_{50}$	IP	Y83 [817]						
Z-MLD	IM							
	SC							
	PO		173 [93]					
Cardiovascular	IV		10 [1803]	1 [403]	0.3 [1804]	1 [403]	1 [1805]	
	IP		2.6 [404]				b1 [1177]	
a IV	IM		a1 [403]					
b IV; Reflex	SC		0.57 [916]					
	PO		5 [1683]				0.5 [1806]	
Adrenolytic	IV					1 [405]	8 [817]	
	IP							
	IM							
	SC							
	PO							
Increased	IV							
renal blood	IP							
flow	IM							
	SC							
	PO		5 [1683]				1 [1806]	

IN VITRO

mg %	Cardiac	Vascular	Gut	Uterine	Visceral	Skeletal	Vas Deferens
Guinea Pig		0.016 [1320]					
Rabbit		4.645 [1807]					
Rat						12.49 [1807]	
Spasmogenic		10 [403]					

HYDROCHLOROTHIAZIDE

(Esidrex, Hydro-Diuril, Oretic, Thiuretic)

mg/kg		Mouse	Rat	Guinea Pig	Rabbit	Cat	Dog	Monkey	
Lethal Dose	IV	Y884 58			Y461 58		Y250 58		
Y-LD50	IP	Y578 58	Y234 58						
Z-MLD	IM								
	SC	Y1470 58	Y1270 58						
	PO	Y3080 58	Y6190 58						
Diuretic	IV						0.5 58		
	IP		15 58						
	IM						10 1077		
	SC								
	PO		15 58			2-4 2272	0.25 58	1 1809	
	IV								
	IP								
	IM								
	SC								
	PO								
	IV								
	IP								
	IM								
	SC								
	PO								

IN VITRO

mg %	Cardiac	Vascular	Gut	Uterine	Visceral	Skeletal		
Rabbit			2.977 1808					

HYDROMORPHONE

(Dihydromorphinone, Dilaudid, Laudicon, Hymorphan)

mg/kg		Mouse	Rat	Guinea Pig	Rabbit	Cat	Dog	Monkey
Lethal Dose Y-LD$_{50}$ Z-MLD	IV	Y88 307						
	IP							
	IM							
	SC	Y84 308						
	PO							
Anesthetic	IV						3.5 557	
	IP							
	IM							
	SC						7.5 557	
	PO							
Analgesic	IV		1.32 269					
	IP	0.25 309	1.7 269	3.1 309				
	IM					0.26 310		
	SC		0.9 269				2	
	PO		18 269					
Behavioral [a]Self administration	IV						10	[a]0.02 1677
	IP		7.1 310					
	IM							
	SC							
	PO							
Catatonic	IV							
	IP		4 269					
	IM							
	SC							
	PO							
	IV							
	IP							
	IM							
	SC							
	PO							
	IV							
	IP							
	IM							
	SC							
	PO							
	IV							
	IP							
	IM							
	SC							
	PO							
	IV							
	IP							
	IM							
	SC							
	PO							

6-HYDROXYDOPA

mg/kg		Mouse	Rat	Guinea Pig	Rabbit	Cat	Dog	Monkey	
Lethal Dose $Y-LD_{50}$ $Z-MLD$	IV								
	IP								
	IM								
	SC								
	PO								
Decrease brain norepinephrine	IV	100 1393							
	IP								
	IM								
	SC								
	PO								
Block amphetamine activity	IV	100 1810							
	IP								
	IM								
	SC								
	PO								
	IV								
	IP								
	IM								
	SC								
	PO								
	IV								
	IP								
	IM								
	SC								
	PO								
	IV								
	IP								
	IM								
	SC								
	PO								
	IV								
	IP								
	IM								
	SC								
	PO								
	IV								
	IP								
	IM								
	SC								
	PO								
	IV								
	IP								
	IM								
	SC								
	PO								

6-HYDROXYDOPAMINE

mg/kg		Mouse	Rat	Guinea Pig	Rabbit	Cat	Dog	Monkey
Lethal Dose	IV							
Y-LD$_{50}$	IP							
Z-MLD	IM							
	SC							
	PO							
Cardiovascular	IV							
	IP							
	IM							
	SC		100 1811					
	PO							
Lesion	IV		50 1812			25 1813		
catecholamine	IP		[a]0.2 1815					
pathways	IM							
[a]total mg	SC		150 1814					
i.cisternal	PO							
Gastrointestinal	IV		50 1816					
	IP							
	IM							
	SC							
	PO			250 1781				
Deplete	IV							
brain	IP		[a]0.2 1817					
dopamine	IM							
[a]total mg ICV	SC							
	PO							
Behavioral	IV							
	IP		[a]0.2 1818					
	IM							
[a]total mg	SC							
i.cisternal	PO							
Suppress	IV							
capsaicin-	IP							
induced	IM							
corneal	SC	30 1512						
lesions	PO							
	IV							
	IP							
	IM							
	SC							
	PO							
	IV							
	IP							
	IM							
	SC							
	PO							

mg/kg		Mouse	Rat	Guinea Pig	Rabbit	Cat	Dog	Monkey
Effects	IV			100 1820				
on vas	IP							
deferens	IM							
smooth	SC							
muscle	PO							
	IV							
	IP							
	IM							
	SC							
	PO							
	IV							
	IP							
	IM							
	SC							
	PO							
	IV							
	IP							
	IM							
	SC							
	PO							

IN VITRO

mg %	Cardiac	Vascular	Gut	Uterine	Visceral	Skeletal		
Dog		2.056 1819						

5-HYDROXYTRYPTOPHAN
(5-HTP)

mg/kg		Mouse	Rat	Guinea Pig	Rabbit	Cat	Dog	Monkey
Lethal Dose	IV							
Y-LD$_{50}$	IP							
Z-MLD	IM							
	SC							
	PO							
Behavioral	IV	25 286	25 411					
	IP	100 204	25 1528					
	IM							
	SC	10 1001	40 286					
	PO							
CNS	IV				65 410	100 412	50 410	
	IP	45 410	75 410					
	IM							
	SC							
	PO							
Gastrointestinal stimulant	IV					60 410	60 410	
	IP	60 410	60 410					
	IM							
	SC							
	PO							
Cardiovascular	IV				87.5 410		30 413	
	IP							
	IM							
	SC							
	PO							
Anticonvulsant	IV							
	IP	100 1821						
	IM							
	SC		30 414					
	PO							
Induce hypoglycemia	IV	4 1456						
	IP							
	IM							
	SC							
	PO							
Motor activity	IV					50 410	30 413	
	IP	150 1536						
	IM							
	SC							
	PO							
Hypothermia	IV							
	IP	300 1822						
	IM							
	SC							
	PO							

mg/kg		Mouse	Rat	Guinea Pig	Rabbit	Cat	Dog	Monkey
EEG	IV				0.03 827	0.03 827		
	IP							
	IM							
	SC							
	PO							
Decrease catecholamines	IV							
	IP	5 861						
	IM							
	SC							
	PO							
Increase morphine analgesia and naloxone blockade of morphine	IV							
	IP	25 1417						
	IM							
	SC							
	PO							
	IV							
	IP							
	IM							
	SC							
	PO							
	IV							
	IP							
	IM							
	SC							
	PO							
	IV							
	IP							
	IM							
	SC							
	PO							
	IV							
	IP							
	IM							
	SC							
	PO							
	IV							
	IP							
	IM							
	SC							
	PO							
	IV							
	IP							
	IM							
	SC							
	PO							

215

HYDROXYZINE

(Atarax, Durrax, Orgatrax, Quiess, Vistaril)

mg/kg		Mouse	Rat	Guinea Pig	Rabbit	Cat	Dog	Monkey	
Lethal Dose $Y-LD_{50}$ $Z-MLD$	IV	137 [117]	Y45 [986]						
	IP	137 [117]	137 [117]						
	IM								
	SC								
	PO	515 [226]	Y1000 [986]						
Behavioral	IV							10 [418]	
	IP	70 [137]	20 [416]				0.1 [417]		
	IM	250 [175]							
	SC	100 [415]	25 [1002]						
	PO	50 [1002]	250 [1002]						
Tolerated	IV							12.5 [117]	
	IP								
	IM								
	SC								
	PO	490 [226]					20 [117]	87.5 [117]	
Barbiturate sleep potentiation	IV								
	IP								
	IM								
	SC	50 [142]		50 [142]	50 [142]				
	PO		50 [986]						
Analgesic	IV								
	IP	89 [1119]							
	IM								
	SC			50 [142]					
	PO			100 [142]					
EEG (synchronization)	IV				6 [108]				
	IP								
	IM								
	SC								
	PO								
Cardiovascular	IV				1 [1002]	2 [1002]	7.5 [419]		
	IP								
	IM								
	SC		10 [986]						
	PO								
Increased EEG arousal threshold	IV				16 [831]				
	IP								
	IM								
	SC								
	PO								
Antidiuretic	IV						5 [420]		
	IP								
	IM								
	SC								
	PO								

IBOPAMINE

(SB 7505)

mg/kg		Mouse	Rat	Guinea Pig	Rabbit	Cat	Dog	Monkey	
Lethal Dose Y-LD$_{50}$ Z-MLD	IV								
	IP								
	IM								
	SC								
	PO								
Cardiovascular	IV		0.035 [1709]						
	IP								
	IM								
	SC								
	PO								
Pulmonary pressor effect [a]IA (perfused lung)	IV						[a]0.016 [1732]		
	IP								
	IM								
	SC								
	PO								
	IV								
	IP								
	IM								
	SC								
	PO								

IN VITRO

mg %	Cardiac	Vascular	Gut	Uterine	Visceral	Skeletal	Vas Deferens	

IBUPROFEN

(Advil, Medipren, Motrin, Nuprin)

mg/kg		Mouse	Rat	Guinea Pig	Rabbit	Cat	Dog	Monkey	
Lethal Dose	IV								
Y-LD$_{50}$	IP								
Z-MLD	IM								
	SC								
	PO								
Analgesic	IV								
	IP								
	IM								
	SC								
	PO	100 [1578]							
Suppress	IV								
ACh	IP								
writing	IM								
[a]ED$_{50}$	SC	[a]800 [1296]							
	PO								
Anti-	IV				2.7 [1823]				
inflammatory	IP								
	IM								
	SC								
	PO		136 [1283]						
Cardiovascular	IV						10 [1824]		
	IP								
	IM								
	SC								
	PO						75 [1825]		
Renal	IV						20 [1826]		
	IP						[a]0.1 [1824]		
[a]total mg IA	IM								
(renal)	SC								
	PO								
Shock	IV		1 [1827]						
protection	IP								
	IM								
	SC								
	PO								

IN VITRO

mg %	Cardiac	Vascular	Gut	Uterine	Visceral	Skeletal	Hepatic	
Rabbit	5 [1828]							
Rat							7.22 [1829]	

IDAZOXAN

mg/kg		Mouse	Rat	Guinea Pig	Rabbit	Cat	Dog	Monkey
Lethal Dose	IV							
Y-LD$_{50}$	IP							
Z-MLD	IM							
	SC							
	PO							
Cardiovascular	IV		0.3 1830				0.3 1832	
	IP							
	IM							
	SC							
	PO							
Noradrenergic	IV		[a]0.2 1580					
receptor	IP		20 1831					
regulation	IM							
[a]total mg ICV	SC							
	PO							
	IV							
	IP							
	IM							
	SC							
	PO							
	IV							
	IP							
	IM							
	SC							
	PO							
	IV							
	IP							
	IM							
	SC							
	PO							
	IV							
	IP							
	IM							
	SC							
	PO							
	IV							
	IP							
	IM							
	SC							
	PO							
	IV							
	IP							
	IM							
	SC							
	PO							

IMIPRAMINE

(Imavate, Janimine, Preamine, SK-Pramine, Tofranil)

mg/kg		Mouse	Rat	Guinea Pig	Rabbit	Cat	Dog	Monkey
Lethal Dose	IV	Y35 235	Y22 235		Y18 235			
Y-LD$_{50}$	IP	Y115 59	Y79					
Z-MLD	IM							
	SC	Y189	Y250					
	PO	Y400 235	Y625 235					
Barbiturate	IV						5 425	
sleep	IP	50 978						
potentiation	IM							
	SC	50 423			50 142			
	PO			25 105				
CNS	IV	14 838			10 235	8 1005		
	IP	32 949	20 59			4 1004		
	IM							
	SC	50 235	50 235	50 978		20 235		
	PO							
Antagonize	IV				15 988			
reserpine	IP	75 264	15 810					
	IM							
	SC							
	PO	100 79	5.8 1833					
Cardiovascular	IV					1 235	4 426	
	IP		35.05 1373					
	IM							
	SC							
	PO							
Decreased	IV							
motor activity	IP		40 1003	30 978				
	IM							
	SC	50 105				10 424		
	PO							
Potentiate	IV							
peripheral	IP	2.5 1418						
action of	IM							
norepinephrine	SC							
	PO							
Potentiate	IV							
5-hydroxy-	IP	20 1371						
tryptophan	IM							
syndrome	SC							
	PO	31 1371						
Antidepressant	IV							
	IP	1.15 1365						
	IM							
	SC							
	PO		10.9 1365					

mg/kg		Mouse	Rat	Guinea Pig	Rabbit	Cat	Dog	Monkey
Corneal lesions	IV							
	IP							
	IM							
	SC							
	PO		13.9_{1374}					
Suppress ACh writhing	IV							
	IP							
	IM							
	SC	5.5_{1296}						
	PO							
Increase GABA binding	IV							
	IP	7.5_{1647}						
	IM							
	SC							
	PO							
EEG	IV				4.5_{831}	3_{1102}		7_{949}
	IP							
	IM						10_{1006}	
	SC			20_{837}				
	PO							
Decreased catecholamine uptake	IV							
	IP	20_{910}				20_{91}		
	IM							
	SC							
	PO							
Serotonin and catecholamine potentiation	IV					2.4_{427}		
	IP							
	IM							
	SC	31_{1536}						
	PO							
Behavioral	IV					5_{850}		3.5_{949}
	IP	20_{874}	8_{848}			10_{1149}		
	IM							0.3_{1370}
	SC							
	PO	100_{935}	160_{949}					20_{949}

IN VITRO

mg %	Cardiac	Vascular	Gut	Uterine	Visceral	Skeletal	Trachea
Anticholin.			[a]0.16_{235}				
Antihistaminic		[a]0.006_{235}					
Anti-BaCl$_2$			[a]0.3_{235}				
Anti-5HT			[a]0.004_{235}				
[a]total mg							

INDOMETHACIN

(Indocin, Indomed, Inacid)

mg/kg		Mouse	Rat	Guinea Pig	Rabbit	Cat	Dog	Monkey
Lethal Dose Y-LD$_{50}$ Z-MLD	IV	40 1844						
	IP	28 1844						
	IM							
	SC							
	PO	50 1844						
Anti-inflammatory	IV		3.5 1310					
	IP	2 1305	10 1834					
	IM							
	SC							
	PO		2 1835				1.2 1311	
Analgesic	IV							
	IP							
	IM							
	SC	1 1578						
	PO	1 1578	2.45 1284					
Cardiovascular [a]IA [b]mg/min IA	IV						5 1515	
	IP						[b]1 1837	
	IM		[a]5 1836					
	SC							
	PO							
Gastrointestinal	IV						10 1838	
	IP							
	IM							
	SC		10 1302					
	PO		30 1302					
Urinary system effects [a]total mg IA (renal)	IV		0.36 1310		10 1841			8 1648
	IP						[a]0.25 1824	
	IM							
	SC		2.5 1839					
	PO		10 1840					
Antagonize furosemide	IV		5 1842				5 1773	
	IP							
	IM							
	SC							
	PO							
Inhibit ascites tumor [a]BID IG	IV							
	IP							
	IM							
	SC							
	PO	[a]5 1843						
Suppress ACh writhing	IV							
	IP							
	IM							
	SC	200 1296						
	PO							

INDOMETHACIN (continued)

mg/kg		Mouse	Rat	Guinea Pig	Rabbit	Cat	Dog	Monkey
	IV							
	IP							
	IM							
	SC							
	PO							
	IV							
	IP							
	IM							
	SC							
	PO							
	IV							
	IP							
	IM							
	SC							
	PO							
	IV							
	IP							
	IM							
	SC							
	PO							

IN VITRO

mg %	Cardiac	Vascular	Gut	Uterine	Visceral	Skeletal	Hepatic
Rat	1_{1313}		3.578_{1845}			2.147_{1829}	
Guinea Pig		0.358_{1314}					
Rabbit		0.358_{1315}					

223

IPRINDOLE

(Tertran, Prondol, Galatur)

mg/kg		Mouse	Rat	Guinea Pig	Rabbit	Cat	Dog	Monkey	
Lethal Dose	IV								
Y-LD$_{50}$	IP								
Z-MLD	IM								
	SC								
	PO								
Behavioral	IV								
	IP		30 $_{1846}$						
	IM								
	SC								
	PO								
Effects on	IV								
dopaminergic	IP		10 $_{1847}$						
and serotonergic	IM								
systems	SC								
	PO								
Potentiate	IV								
adrenergic	IP		10 $_{1534}$						
nerve	IM								
stimulation	SC								
(atria)	PO								
	IV								
	IP								
	IM								
	SC								
	PO								
	IV								
	IP								
	IM								
	SC								
	PO								
	IV								
	IP								
	IM								
	SC								
	PO								
	IV								
	IP								
	IM								
	SC								
	PO								
	IV								
	IP								
	IM								
	SC								
	PO								

IPRONIAZID

(Euphozid, Marsilid)

mg/kg		Mouse	Rat	Guinea Pig	Rabbit	Cat	Dog	Monkey
Lethal Dose Y-LD$_{50}$ Z-MLD	IV	Y725 [428]			Y150 [428]		140 [429]	
	IP	Y690 [428]						
	IM	Y683 [428]						
	SC	Y750 [428]						
	PO	Y968 [428]	Y383 [428]		Y150 [428]		140 [428]	640 [429]
Monoamine oxidase inhibition	IV	100 [430]			100 [430]		65 [372]	
	IP	25 [429]	50 [429]					
	IM							
	SC	100 [430]	12 [868]		100 [430]	100 [430]		
	PO		100 [433]					
Increased brain 5HT and norepinephrine	IV							
	IP	300 [431]	100 [148]					
	IM							
	SC		100 [434]		100			
	PO							
Barbiturate sleep potentiation	IV							
	IP	100 [411]						
	IM							
	SC	50 [142]		50 [142]	50 [142]			
	PO							
Cardiovascular	IV					8 [428]	163 [372]	
	IP							
	IM							
	SC							
	PO							
Behavioral	IV							
	IP	200 [874]	155 [848]					
	IM							
	SC	100 [432]	100 [370]				129 [955]	
	PO					2 [1007]		
Analgesic	IV							
	IP							
	IM							
	SC	100 [1008]		50 [142]				
	PO							
Ganglionic block	IV					100 [376]		
	IP							
	IM							
	SC							
	PO							
Decreased motor activity	IV							
	IP	200 [204]						
	IM							
	SC	100 [1008]						
	PO							

mg/kg		Mouse	Rat	Guinea Pig	Rabbit	Cat	Dog	Monkey	
Affect	IV								
brain	IP		150 1706						
dopamine	IM								
concentrations	SC								
	PO								
	IV								
	IP								
	IM								
	SC								
	PO								
	IV								
	IP								
	IM								
	SC								
	PO								
	IV								
	IP								
	IM								
	SC								
	PO								

IN VITRO

mg %	Cardiac	Vascular	Gut	Uterine	Visceral	Skeletal		
Cat	10 429							

ISOCARBOXAZID

(Marplan)

mg/kg		Mouse	Rat	Guinea Pig	Rabbit	Cat	Dog	Monkey	
Lethal Dose	IV								
Y-LD$_{50}$	IP	Y110 $_{210}$	Y199 $_{210}$						
Z-MLD	IM								
	SC								
	PO	Y173 $_{210}$	Y280 $_{115}$				40 $_{429}$	160 $_{429}$	
Monoamine	IV								
oxidase	IP	0.75 $_{429}$	2 $_{429}$	[a]5 $_{1169}$				20 $_{1170}$	
inhibition	IM								
[a] 6 d	SC								
	PO								
Reserpine	IV								
antagonist	IP	5 $_{455}$							
	IM								
	SC								
	PO	15 $_{455}$							
Barbiturate	IV								
sleep	IP								
potentiation	IM								
	SC	25 $_{142}$							
	PO			50 $_{142}$					
Behavioral	IV								
	IP								
	IM								
	SC		1.2 $_{456}$						
	PO								
CNS	IV					5 $_{1009}$			
	IP		3 $_{1201}$						
	IM								
	SC								
	PO								
	IV								
	IP								
	IM								
	SC								
	PO								
	IV								
	IP								
	IM								
	SC								
	PO								
	IV								
	IP								
	IM								
	SC								
	PO								

ISOMAZOLE
(LY 175326)

mg/kg		Mouse	Rat	Guinea Pig	Rabbit	Cat	Dog	Monkey
Lethal Dose	IV							
Y-LD$_{50}$	IP							
Z-MLD	IM							
	SC							
	PO							
Inotropic	IV						0.1 $_{1848}$	
	IP							
	IM							
	SC							
	PO							
	IV							
	IP							
	IM							
	SC							
	PO							
	IV							
	IP							
	IM							
	SC							
	PO							

IN VITRO

mg %	Cardiac	Vascular	Gut	Uterine	Visceral	Skeletal	Trachea	
Cat	$^a 3 \times 10^{-4}$ *							
^{a}molar								
solution								

*1848

ISONIAZID

(Cotinazin, Dinacrin, INH, Nidrazid)

mg/kg		Mouse	Rat	Guinea Pig	Rabbit	Cat	Dog	Monkey
Lethal Dose	IV	Y153 428			Y94 428		100 428	
Y-LD$_{50}$	IP	Y132 428						
Z-MLD	IM	Y140 428						
	SC	Y160 428						
	PO	Y142 428	Y650 115		250 428		100 428	
Cardiovascular	IV					8 428		
	IP							
	IM							
	SC							
	PO							
Behavioral	IV							
	IP							
	IM							
	SC		100 1010					
	PO							
Diamine	IV							
oxidase	IP	78 1849						
inhibition	IM							
	SC							
	PO							

IN VITRO

mg %	Cardiac	Vascular	Gut	Uterine	Visceral	Skeletal	Trachea	

ISOPROTERENOL

(Isuprel, Norisodrine, Aludrin)

mg/kg		Mouse	Rat	Guinea Pig	Rabbit	Cat	Dog	Monkey
Lethal Dose	IV	Y128 1084					Y50 1084	
Y-LD$_{50}$	IP	Y300 111						
Z-MLD	IM							
	SC			Y0.32 1084				
	PO	Y450 111		Y270 1084				
Sympathomimetic	IV		0.0005 1352		0.002 298	0.0005	0.0005	
(CV, respir.)	IP		0.17 1644		b 0.0001*		0.2 1851	
a ug/min IA	IM						a 0.03 1728	
b total mg IA	SC	5 1850	0.1 862	0.06 1084				
	PO			17 1084				
EEG	IV				0.005 298	0.005 298	0.005 298	
(Desynchro-	IP							
nization)	IM							
	SC							
	PO							
Metabolic	IV						0.022 865	
	IP		0.05 1082					
	IM							
	SC		0.02 864		25 863			
	PO							
Tolerance	IV							
a mg/kg/h	IP							
	IM							
	SC		a 0.4 1852					
	PO							
Hyperthermic	IV							
	IP		0.5 1853					
	IM							
	SC							
	PO							
Cardiotoxic	IV							
	IP							
	IM							
	SC		250 1854					
	PO							
Endorphin	IV							
release	IP							
	IM							
	SC		0.2 1730					
	PO							
Erythropoietic	IV							
	IP							
	IM							
	SC	0.05 1855						
	PO							

*1687

ISOPROTERENOL (continued)

mg/kg		Mouse	Rat	Guinea Pig	Rabbit	Cat	Dog	Monkey	
Renin	IV								
release	IP								
	IM						$^a0.03_{1858}$		
$^a\mu$g/kg/min	SC								
IA (renal)	PO								
	IV								
	IP								
	IM								
	SC								
	PO								
	IV								
	IP								
	IM								
	SC								
	PO								
	IV								
	IP								
	IM								
	SC								
	PO								

IN VITRO

mg %	Cardiac	Vascular	Gut	Uterine	Visceral	Skeletal	Trachea	CNS
Rat	0.0019_{1856}		0.0021_{1583}	0.0003_{1157}				0.0002^*
Guinea Pig						0.01	0.002^{**}	
Rabbit	0.025	0.01_{1157}	0.01		$2\times10^{-5***}$			
Dog	0.1056_{1857}		0.003_{1157}					

^{*1730} $^{**}1358$ $^{***}1859$

KAINIC ACID
(Digenin, Helminal)

mg/kg		Mouse	Rat	Guinea Pig	Rabbit	Cat	Dog	Monkey
Lethal Dose	IV							
Y-LD$_{50}$	IP							
Z-MLD	IM							
	SC							
	PO							
Convulsions	IV							
and hypothalamic	IP							
destruction	IM							
(immature animal)	SC	4 1860						
	PO	4 1860						
Convulsions	IV							
and hypothalamic	IP							
destruction	IM							
(mature animal)	SC	100 1860						
	PO	100 1860						
Limbic	IV							
seizures	IP		[a]0.2 1448					
	IM							
[a]total μg ICV	SC							
	PO							

IN VITRO

mg %	Cardiac	Vascular	Gut	Uterine	Visceral	Skeletal	Trachea	CNS

KETAMINE

(Ketaset, Ketaject, Ketalar, Ketavet, Vetalar)

mg/kg		Mouse	Rat	Guinea Pig	Rabbit	Cat	Dog	Monkey	
Lethal Dose	IV								
Y-LD$_{50}$	IP	Y360.6*							
Z-MLD	IM								
	SC								
	PO								
Ataxia	IV								
	IP	[a]15.27*							
	IM								
[a]ED$_{50}$	SC								
	PO								
Analgesia	IV								
and catatonia	IP		45 1863						
	IM								
	SC								
	PO								
Behavioral	IV		[b]2.5 1866				[a]0.375 1864	[a]0.125**	
[a]Self	IP							[c]1 1654	
administration	IM								
[b]mg/kg/h	SC							1 1655	
[c]IV	PO							14.5 1389	
Restraint and	IV					2-4 2272			
anesthesia	IP								
	IM		100 2267			11-33 2272			
	SC								
	PO								
	IV								
	IP								
	IM								
	SC								
	PO								

*1861   **1865

IN VITRO

mg %	Cardiac	Vascular	Gut	Uterine	Visceral	Skeletal		
Guinea Pig			2.74 1862					

KETANSERIN

(R-41,468)

mg/kg		Mouse	Rat	Guinea Pig	Rabbit	Cat	Dog	Monkey	
Lethal Dose	IV								
$Y-LD_{50}$	IP								
$Z-MLD$	IM								
	SC								
	PO								
Cardiovascular	IV		1_{1867}		0.03_{1869}	0.05_{1868}	0.01_{1635}		
	IP								
	IM								
	SC								
	PO								
Gastrointestinal	IV						0.033_{1870}		
	IP								
	IM								
	SC								
	PO								
Behavioral	IV								
	IP		1.25_{1871}						
	IM							0.3_{1554}	
	SC								
	PO								

IN VITRO

mg %		Cardiac	Vascular	Gut	Uterine	Visceral	Skeletal		
Rat			$a_{10}{}^{-10}{}_{*}$						
a_{molar}									
solution									

*1872

KETAZOCINE

(WIN 34,276)

mg/kg		Mouse	Rat	Guinea Pig	Rabbit	Cat	Dog	Monkey	
Lethal Dose	IV								
Y-LD$_{50}$	IP								
Z-MLD	IM								
	SC								
	PO								
Analgesic	IV								
	IP								
	IM								
[a]ED$_{25}$	SC	[a]0.29 1482	[a]0.37 1482						
	PO								
	IV								
	IP								
	IM								
	SC								
	PO								
	IV								
	IP								
	IM								
	SC								
	PO								

IN VITRO

mg %	Cardiac	Vascular	Gut	Uterine	Visceral	Skeletal		

LABETALOL

(Normodyne, Trandate, Ibidomide)

mg/kg		Mouse	Rat	Guinea Pig	Rabbit	Cat	Dog	Monkey	
Lethal Dose	IV								
Y-LD$_{50}$	IP								
Z-MLD	IM								
	SC								
	PO								
Cardiovascular	IV								
	IP								
	IM								
	SC								
	PO		30 1873						
	IV								
	IP								
	IM								
	SC								
	PO								
	IV								
	IP								
	IM								
	SC								
	PO								

IN VITRO

mg %	Cardiac	Vascular	Gut	Uterine	Visceral	Skeletal		
Rat		0.0033 1874						

LEUKOTRIENE D$_4$
(LTD$_4$)

mg/kg		Mouse	Rat	Guinea Pig	Rabbit	Cat	Dog	Monkey	
Lethal Dose	IV								
Y-LD$_{50}$	IP								
Z-MLD	IM								
	SC								
	PO								
Cardiovascular	IV		0.02 $_{1397}$				0.0001$_{1875}$		
	IP								
[a]IA	IM		[a]0.001$_{1836}$				[b]0.003$_{1876}$		
[b]Total mg IA	SC								
	PO								
	IV								
	IP								
	IM								
	SC								
	PO								
	IV								
	IP								
	IM								
	SC								
	PO								

IN VITRO

mg %	Cardiac	Vascular	Gut	Uterine	Visceral	Skeletal		
Guinea Pig	[a]2×10^{-10}*							
[a]molar								
solution								

*1877

LEVALLORPHAN

(Lorfan)

mg/kg		Mouse	Rat	Guinea Pig	Rabbit	Cat	Dog	Monkey
Lethal Dose $Y-LD_{50}$ $Z-MLD$	IV							
	IP	Y184 210	Y185 210					
	IM							
	SC							
	PO	Y949 1878	Y949 210					
Morphine antagonist	IV				0.45 1011		0.2	
	IP							
	IM							
	SC	0.3 908						
	PO							
EEG (desynchroni- zation)	IV				10 157	10 184		
	IP							
	IM							
	SC							
	PO							
Cardiovascular and respiratory	IV				10 157			
	IP							
	IM							
	SC		125 908					
	PO							
Behavioral	IV							
	IP	6 989						
	IM							
	SC							
	PO							
Analgesic	IV							
	IP							
	IM							
	SC	2.4 908						
	PO							
	IV							
	IP							
	IM							
	SC							
	PO							
	IV							
	IP							
	IM							
	SC							
	PO							
	IV							
	IP							
	IM							
	SC							
	PO							

LEVODOPA
(L-Dopa, 3-Hydroxy-L-tyrosine)

mg/kg		Mouse	Rat	Guinea Pig	Rabbit	Cat	Dog	Monkey
Lethal Dose	IV							
Y-LD$_{50}$	IP		^{a}10 328					
Z-MLD	IM							
	SC							
^{a}total mg	PO							
Behavioral	IV	200 1561				25 14		
	IP	750 327	20 329					
	IM							
	SC		200 942					
	PO							
Cardiovascular	IV		12 328			30 1702	20 1701	
	IP		12 328				^{a}3 1573	
	IM							
^{a}IA	SC							
	PO							
CNS	IV		50 1226		50 1102	20 1098	1.3 1225	
	IP							
	IM							
	SC							
	PO							
Anorexic	IV							
	IP							
	IM							
	SC		50 1383					
	PO							
Increase	IV							
gestation	IP							
	IM							
^{a}BID+Carbidopa,	SC		^{a}200 1703					
20 BID	PO							
Antagonize	IV							
drug-induced	IP	25 1704						
hypothermia	IM							
	SC							
	PO	185 1292						
Increase	IV							
brain	IP	25 1705	250 1706					
dopamine	IM							
	SC							
	PO							
Counteract	IV							
reserpine	IP	^{a}259 1292						
	IM							
^{a}ED$_{50}$	SC							
	PO	^{a}400 1707						

LEVODOPA (continued)

mg/kg		Mouse	Rat	Guinea Pig	Rabbit	Cat	Dog	Monkey	
Antagonize	IV								
morphine	IP	200 1708							
analgesia	IM								
	SC	100 1709							
	PO								
	IV								
	IP								
	IM								
	SC								
	PO								
	IV								
	IP								
	IM								
	SC								
	PO								
	IV								
	IP								
	IM								
	SC								
	PO								

IN VITRO

mg %		Cardiac	Vascular	Gut	Uterine	Visceral	Skeletal		

LEVORPHANOL

(Levo-Dromoran)

mg/kg		Mouse	Rat	Guinea Pig	Rabbit	Cat	Dog	Monkey	
Lethal Dose	IV	Y41.5 [210]			Y 20 [210]				
Y-LD$_{50}$	IP	Y73 [1879]							
Z-MLD	IM								
	SC	Y187 [210]	Y110 [210]						
	PO	Y285 [210]	Y150 [210]						
Analgesic	IV								
	IP								
	IM								
	SC		2 [435]				2		
	PO								
Respiratory	IV				0.5 [435]				
	IP								
	IM							0.03 [1880]	
	SC	0.3 [1881]							
	PO								
Antitussive	IV						2 [435]		
	IP								
	IM								
	SC								
	PO								
Induce locomotor activity	IV								
	IP	20 [1879]							
	IM								
	SC								
	PO								
Thermoregulatory	IV								
	IP								
	IM								
	SC	10 [1613]	0.5 [1496]						
	PO								
Tolerance	IV		0.5 [1883]						
	IP								
	IM								
	SC	12 [1882]							
	PO								
Ocular	IV					0.5 [1884]			
	IP								
	IM								
	SC								
	PO								
	IV								
	IP								
	IM								
	SC								
	PO								

mg/kg		Mouse	Rat	Guinea Pig	Rabbit	Cat	Dog	Monkey	
	IV								
	IP								
	IM								
	SC								
	PO								
	IV								
	IP								
	IM								
	SC								
	PO								
	IV								
	IP								
	IM								
	SC								
	PO								
	IV								
	IP								
	IM								
	SC								
	PO								

IN VITRO

mg %	Cardiac	Vascular	Gut	Uterine	Visceral	Skeletal	Neurons	
Mouse							1.03 1658	

LIDOCAINE

(Anestacon, Dalcaine)

mg/kg		Mouse	Rat	Guinea Pig	Rabbit	Cat	Dog	Monkey	
Lethal Dose	IV	Y31.5 $_{436}$							
Y-LD$_{50}$	IP								
Z-MLD	IM								
	SC	Y400 $_{437}$							
	PO	Y457 $_{1012}$							
Anticonvulsant	IV					2.5 $_{440}$		3 $_{442}$	
	IP	75 $_{925}$							
	IM								
	SC	4.9 $_{252}$							
	PO	13 $_{1012}$			25 $_{1012}$				
Convulsant	IV	a18.6 $_{1349}$			10 $_{438}$	20 $_{440}$			
	IP	a76 $_{1821}$		>60 $_{991}$					
	IM								
aED$_{50}$	SC								
	PO								
EEG	IV				5 $_{439}$	16 $_{1214}$			
and	IP								
ECP	IM								
	SC								
	PO				30 $_{1012}$				
Block	IV						20 $_{441}$		
afferent	IP								
nerve	IM								
discharge	SC								
	PO								
Cardiovascular	IV						3 $_{1234}$		
	IP								
	IM								
	SC								
	PO								
Antiarrhythmic	IV						a 0.8$_{1727}$		
	IP						b 2 $_{1368}$		
	IM								
a mg/kg/min	SC								
b IV	PO								
Attenuate	IV						10 $_{1887}$		
myocardial	IP								
acidosis	IM								
	SC								
	PO								
	IV								
	IP								
	IM								
	SC								
	PO								

mg/kg		Mouse	Rat	Guinea Pig	Rabbit	Cat	Dog	Monkey	
	IV								
	IP								
	IM								
	SC								
	PO								
	IV								
	IP								
	IM								
	SC								
	PO								
	IV								
	IP								
	IM								
	SC								
	PO								
	IV								
	IP								
	IM								
	SC								
	PO								

IN VITRO

mg %	Cardiac	Vascular	Gut	Uterine	Visceral	Skeletal	Trachea	
Rat						5 1157		
Guinea Pig	2.34 1886		0.3 1157					
Dog	1 1228							
Dog	0.4 1885							

LISURIDE

(Methylergolcarbamide, Lysuride)

mg/kg		Mouse	Rat	Guinea Pig	Rabbit	Cat	Dog	Monkey
Lethal Dose	IV							
Y-LD$_{50}$	IP							
Z-MLD	IM							
	SC							
	PO							
Hypothermia	IV							
	IP	0.1 $_{1888}$						
	IM							
	SC							
	PO							
Production of	IV							
stereotypy	IP	^{a}1.5 $_{1888}$						
	IM							
^{a}ED$_{50}$	SC							
	PO	^{a}5.8 $_{1888}$						
	IV							
	IP							
	IM							
	SC							
	PO							
	IV							
	IP							
	IM							
	SC							
	PO							
	IV							
	IP							
	IM							
	SC							
	PO							
	IV							
	IP							
	IM							
	SC							
	PO							
	IV							
	IP							
	IM							
	SC							
	PO							
	IV							
	IP							
	IM							
	SC							
	PO							

LITHIUM

(Eskalith, Lithane, Lithobid)

mg/kg		Mouse	Rat	Guinea Pig	Rabbit	Cat	Dog	Monkey	
Lethal Dose	IV								
Y-LD$_{50}$	IP								
Z-MLD	IM								
	SC								
	PO								
Taste	IV								
aversion	IP		30 $_{1528}$						
	IM								
	SC								
	PO								
Behavioral	IV								
	IP	100 $_{1890}$							
	IM								
	SC								
^{a}g/kg diet	PO		^{a}1.7 $_{1404}$						
Increase	IV								
brain	IP		211.97$_{1891}$						
substance P	IM								
	SC								
	PO								

IN VITRO

mg %	Cardiac	Vascular	Gut	Uterine	Visceral	Skeletal	Neurons	
Dog							0.212$_{1889}$	

LOPERAMIDE

(Imodium, Lopemid, Loperyl)

mg/kg		Mouse	Rat	Guinea Pig	Rabbit	Cat	Dog	Monkey	
Lethal Dose	IV		Y5.92*						
Y-LD$_{50}$	IP								
Z-MLD	IM								
	SC								
	PO								
Antidiarrheal	IV		0.02 $_{1614}$						
	IP								
	IM								
[a]Total mg	SC								
	PO			1 $_{1692}$			[a]2-4 $_{2273}$		
Behavioral	IV								
	IP								
	IM								
	SC	4.5 $_{1483}$							
	PO								
Analgesia	IV		2.83 $_{1614}$						
	IP								
	IM								
	SC								
	PO								

*1614

IN VITRO

mg %	Cardiac	Vascular	Gut	Uterine	Visceral	Skeletal	Brain	
Guinea Pig			0.382 $_{1610}$			0.477 $_{1692}$		

LORAZEPAM

(Ativan, Lorax, Lorsilan)

mg/kg		Mouse	Rat	Guinea Pig	Rabbit	Cat	Dog	Monkey	
Lethal Dose	IV								
Y-LD$_{50}$	IP								
Z-MLD	IM								
	SC								
	PO								
Antagonize	IV								
taste	IP		0.7 1528						
aversion	IM								
	SC								
	PO		1.5 1528						
Behavioral	IV								
	IP								
	IM							0.03 1892	
	SC								
	PO								
Dependence	IV								
	IP								
	IM								
	SC								
^{a}daily	PO						^{a}100 1893		
	IV								
	IP								
	IM								
	SC								
	PO								
	IV								
	IP								
	IM								
	SC								
	PO								
	IV								
	IP								
	IM								
	SC								
	PO								
	IV								
	IP								
	IM								
	SC								
	PO								
	IV								
	IP								
	IM								
	SC								
	PO								

LYSERGIDE

(Lysergic acid diethylamide, LSD)

mg/kg		Mouse	Rat	Guinea Pig	Rabbit	Cat	Dog	Monkey	
Lethal Dose	IV	Y54 $_{443}$			2 $_{92}$				
Y-LD$_{50}$	IP								
Z-MLD	IM								
	SC								
	PO								
Behavioral	IV				0.5 $_{446}$	0.4	0.5 $_{446}$	0.01$_{452}$	
	IP	4 $_{369}$	2 $_{833}$	10 $_{833}$	0.0003$_{1895}$	0.02 $_{447}$		0.1$_{185}$	
	IM	1 $_{175}$				0.1 $_{448}$		0.025$_{289}$	
	SC	2.5 $_{940}$						0.06$_{1894}$	
	PO	5 $_{935}$							
Hyperthermic	IV				0.05 $_{443}$				
	IP		4 $_{444}$						
	IM								
	SC				0.06				
	PO								
EEG	IV				0.04	0.1 $_{184}$	0.1 $_{451}$		
and	IP		2 $_{833}$	10 $_{833}$			0.004 $_{1196}$		
ECP	IM								
	SC								
	PO								
Pentobarbital	IV				0.14 $_{159}$				
antagonist	IP					50 $_{449}$			
	IM								
	SC								
	PO								
Metabolic	IV					0.3 $_{450}$			
	IP		1.3 $_{1239}$						
	IM								
	SC		0.625 $_{445}$						
	PO								
Anti-5HT	IV		0.025 $_{386}$			0.05 $_{453}$			
	IP								
	IM								
	SC	0.03 $_{1014}$		0.013 $_{917}$					
	PO		1 $_{997}$						
Ataxic	IV								
	IP								
	IM							0.1 $_{161}$	
	SC								
	PO								
Catatonic	IV								
	IP								
	IM							1 $_{161}$	
	SC								
	PO								

mg/kg		Mouse	Rat	Guinea Pig	Rabbit	Cat	Dog	Monkey
Fetal damage	IV							
	IP							
	IM							
	SC		0.005_{1094}					
	PO		0.02_{1094}					
	IV							
	IP							
	IM							
	SC							
	PO							
	IV							
	IP							
	IM							
	SC							
	PO							
	IV							
	IP							
	IM							
	SC							
	PO							

IN VITRO

mg %	Cardiac	Vascular	Gut	Uterine	Visceral	Skeletal	Trachea	
Anti-5HT				0.002_{443}				

MAGNESIUM SULFATE

(Epsom Salts)

mg/kg		Mouse	Rat	Guinea Pig	Rabbit	Cat	Dog	Monkey	
Lethal Dose	IV	1100 [97]	1100 [97]	1100 [97]	1100 [97]	1100 [97]	750	1100 [97]	
Y-LD$_{50}$	IP						1600 [109]		
Z-MLD	IM								
	SC			Z1800 [454]	Z1750 [454]	Z1000 [454]	1750 [109]		
	PO								
CNS	IV								
depressant	IP								
	IM								
	SC								
	PO				1.3				
DFP	IV								
Antagonist	IP								
	IM				400				
	SC								
	PO								
Cathartic	IV								
	IP								
	IM								
	SC								
[a]total g	PO					[a]2-4 [2273]	[a]8-25 [2273]		

IN VITRO

mg %		Cardiac	Vascular	Gut	Uterine	Visceral	Skeletal	Trachea	

MEBUTAMATE

(Dormate, Butatensin, Carbuten)

mg/kg		Mouse	Rat	Guinea Pig	Rabbit	Cat	Dog	Monkey	
Lethal Dose	IV								
Y-LD$_{50}$	IP	Y460 457	Y410 457						
Z-MLD	IM								
	SC								
	PO	Y550 457	Y1160 467						
Cardiovascular	IV					30 467	20 457		
	IP				18 457				
	IM								
	SC								
	PO		120 457						
Anticonvulsant	IV								
	IP	90 457							
	IM								
	SC								
	PO								
	IV								
	IP								
	IM								
	SC								
	PO								

IN VITRO

mg %	Cardiac	Vascular	Gut	Uterine	Visceral	Skeletal	Trachea	

MECAMYLAMINE

(Inversine, Mekamine, Revertina)

mg/kg		Mouse	Rat	Guinea Pig	Rabbit	Cat	Dog	Monkey
Lethal Dose	IV	[a]Y21 58						
Y-LD$_{50}$	IP	[a]Y39 58	[a]Y54 58	[a]Y52 58				
Z-MLD	IM							
[a] as base	SC	[a]Y93 58	[a]Y145 58	[a]Y127 58				
	PO	[a]Y92 58	[a]Y171 58	[a]Y144 58			[a]50 58	
Ganglionic	IV	[a]2.5 58	2 386			0.23 113	[a]1 58	
block	IP	[a]2.5 58	2 1896					
[a] as base	IM							
	SC							
	PO	[a]2.5 58					[a]2 58	
Cardiovascular	IV				10 1133	0.15 867	1 458	
	IP						[a]0.01 1742	
[a]total mg	IM							
i. cerebral	SC							
	PO							
Neuromuscular	IV						10 214	
block	IP							
	IM							
	SC							
	PO							
Behavioral	IV							
	IP	2.5 878						
	IM	5 1440						
	SC							
	PO	5 935						
Decreased	IV					2.5 1015		
Renshaw	IP							
Cell Activity	IM							
	SC							
	PO							
	IV							
	IP							
	IM							
	SC							
	PO							
	IV							
	IP							
	IM							
	SC							
	PO							
	IV							
	IP							
	IM							
	SC							
	PO							

MECLOFENAMATE

(Arquel, Meclomen)

mg/kg		Mouse	Rat	Guinea Pig	Rabbit	Cat	Dog	Monkey	
Lethal Dose	IV								
Y-LD$_{50}$	IP								
Z-MLD	IM								
	SC								
	PO								
Gastrointestinal	IV						10 $_{1838}$		
	IP								
	IM								
	SC								
	PO								
Circulatory	IV						5 $_{1897}$		
	IP								
	IM								
	SC								
	PO								
Renal	IV						5 $_{1898}$		
	IP								
	IM								
	SC								
	PO		10 $_{1840}$						

IN VITRO

mg %	Cardiac	Vascular	Gut	Uterine	Visceral	Skeletal	Hepatocytes	
Rat							0.296 $_{1829}$	

MEPENZOLATE
(Cantil, Cantril, Trancolon)

mg/kg		Mouse	Rat	Guinea Pig	Rabbit	Cat	Dog	Monkey	
Lethal Dose	IV	Y9.8 460	Y21.8 460						
Y-LD$_{50}$	IP								
Z-MLD	IM								
	SC								
	PO	Y900 460	Y1100 460						
Anticholinergic	IV					0.02 460	0.02 460		
	IP		5 460		0.015 460				
	IM								
	SC								
	PO								
	IV								
	IP								
	IM								
	SC								
	PO								
	IV								
	IP								
	IM								
	SC								
	PO								

IN VITRO

mg %	Cardiac	Vascular	Gut	Uterine	Visceral	Skeletal	Trachea	
Anticholinergic			0.2 460					
Antihistamine			200 460					

MEPERIDINE

(Demerol, Mepadin, Pethidine)

mg/kg		Mouse	Rat	Guinea Pig	Rabbit	Cat	Dog	Monkey
Lethal Dose Y-LD$_{50}$ Z-MLD	IV	Y50 $_{579}$	Y34 $_{580}$		Y30 $_{579}$		100	
	IP	Y150	Y93 $_{580}$					
	IM							
	SC	Y195 $_{579}$	Y200 $_{579}$					
	PO	Y178 $_{579}$	Y170		Y500 $_{579}$			
Analgesia [a]ICV [b]Total μg IT	IV	20 $_{1043}$	10 $_{269}$		10 $_{191}$		2	
	IP	40	50 $_{580}$	51.8 $_{22}$				
	IM	[a]3.2 $_{1899}$	[b]74 $_{1752}$	2 $_{1235}$		5 $_{2272}$	10 $_{2272}$	
	SC	3.8 $_{1907}$	43.6 $_{581}$	20.4 $_{1044}$		11 $_{1232}$	25	
	PO	46.9 $_{1126}$	150 $_{580}$			11 $_{24}$	11 $_{24}$	
Thermoregulatory	IV							
	IP							
	IM							
	SC	5 $_{1613}$	1 $_{1496}$					
	PO							
Behavioral	IV							
	IP							
	IM							0.3 $_{1900}$
	SC	0.75 $_{1483}$						
	PO							
Antibradykinin	IV						0.8 $_{1311}$	
	IP							
	IM							
	SC							
	PO							
Inhibit urinary bladder [a]total mg ICV	IV		[a]0.044 $_{1743}$					
	IP							
	IM							
	SC							
	PO							
Spinal Reflex Depressant	IV					13 $_{510}$		
	IP							
	IM							
	SC		100 $_{269}$					
	PO							
Cardiovascular	IV						2 $_{860}$	
	IP							
	IM							
	SC							
	PO							
Increase 5HT levels in reserpinized animal	IV							
	IP	45 $_{1708}$						
	IM							
	SC							
	PO							

MEPERIDINE (continued)

mg/kg		Mouse	Rat	Guinea Pig	Rabbit	Cat	Dog	Monkey
Suppress	IV							
ACh	IP							
writhing	IM							
	SC	4.6 1296						
	PO							
	IV							
	IP							
	IM							
	SC							
	PO							
	IV							
	IP							
	IM							
	SC							
	PO							
	IV							
	IP							
	IM							
	SC							
	PO							

IN VITRO

mg %	Cardiac	Vascular	Gut	Uterine	Visceral	Skeletal	Trachea
Cat	2.47 1754						
Rabbit	20		20				

257

MEPHENESIN

(Myanesin, Tolosate, Tolseron)

mg/kg		Mouse	Rat	Guinea Pig	Rabbit	Cat	Dog	Monkey	
Lethal Dose	IV	Y186 909			Y125 845				
Y-LD$_{50}$	IP	Y471 461	283 461						
Z-MLD	IM								
	SC	600 1221							
	PO	Y990 461	Y625 975						
Skeletal	IV	30.9 909			10-12 2275	20 845	10-20 2275	100 1073	
muscle	IP	400 204	120						
relaxant	IM					12 2275			
(central)	SC	180 1221				12 2275	200		
	PO	550 462					40-100 2275		
Strychnine	IV								
antagonist	IP	100							
	IM		80						
	SC	200							
	PO	225 1016							
Polysynaptic	IV		7 1142			20 1080	25 271		
reflex	IP								
inhibition	IM								
	SC								
	PO								
Righting	IV						150	125 1073	
reflex	IP	130 461	103 461						
loss	IM								
	SC								
	PO	462 461	580 461						
Behavioral	IV								
	IP								
	IM								
	SC								
	PO	400 935	430 975						
	IV								
	IP								
	IM								
	SC								
	PO								
	IV								
	IP								
	IM								
	SC								
	PO								
	IV								
	IP								
	IM								
	SC								
	PO								

MEPHENTERMINE

(Wyamine, Mephine, Vialin)

mg/kg		Mouse	Rat	Guinea Pig	Rabbit	Cat	Dog	Monkey	
Lethal Dose	IV								
Y-LD$_{50}$	IP	Y110 [464]							
Z-MLD	IM								
	SC								
	PO								
Cardiovascular	IV					1 [465]	4 [466]		
	IP								
	IM								
	SC								
	PO								
Increased	IV						1 [467]		
Coronary	IP								
Blood Flow	IM								
	SC								
	PO								
	IV								
	IP								
	IM								
	SC								
	PO								

IN VITRO

mg %	Cardiac	Vascular	Gut	Uterine	Visceral	Skeletal	Trachea	
Adrenolytic	0.1 [468]		1 [465]					

MEPHENYTOIN

(Mesantoin, Phenantoin, Sedantoinal)

mg/kg		Mouse	Rat	Guinea Pig	Rabbit	Cat	Dog	Monkey
Lethal Dose	IV							
Y-LD$_{50}$	IP		270 $_{475}$	Y215 $_{352}$				
Z-MLD	IM							
	SC							
	PO	Y560 $_{352}$			Y430 $_{352}$	Y190 $_{352}$		
Ataxic	IV							
	IP							
	IM							
	SC							
	PO	103 $_{352}$			33 $_{352}$	6.3 $_{352}$		
Behavioral	IV							
	IP	64 $_{1155}$						
	IM							
	SC							
	PO							
	IV							
	IP							
	IM							
	SC							
	PO							

IN VITRO

mg %		Cardiac	Vascular	Gut	Uterine	Visceral	Skeletal	Trachea	

MEPROBAMATE

(Equanil, Miltown, Meprospan, SK-Bamate)

mg/kg		Mouse	Rat	Guinea Pig	Rabbit	Cat	Dog	Monkey
Lethal Dose	IV	450_{211}	Y350		$Y260_{845}$			
Y-LD$_{50}$	IP	$Y710_{461}$	410_{461}					
Z-MLD	IM							
	SC	550_{17}						
	PO	$Y980_{461}$	918_{461}					
Behavioral	IV					30_{254}		
	IP	100_{469}	135_{470}			20_{145}		
	IM	100_{175}						150_{1017}
	SC	50_{1008}	300_{231}					400_{211}
	PO	200_{924}	115_{211}		20_{417}	50_{211}	100_{417}	100_{211}
Sedative	IV	200_{211}				45_{462}		
	IP	200_{211}	300_{463}			400_{1018}		
	IM							
	SC	180_{211}						
	PO	100	150_{117}	100_{472}		65_{557}	30_{557}	325_{473}
Spinal Cord depressant	IV					40_{1080}		
	IP							
	IM							
	SC							
	PO	185_{1016}						
Cardiovascular	IV				25_{471}		20_{839}	
	IP							
	IM							
	SC							
	PO							
Hypnotic	IV	270_{211}						
	IP	260_{211}						
	IM							
	SC	300_{211}						
	PO	348_{211}	659_{471}	300_{1019}				
Anticonvulsant	IV							
	IP	155_{461}			100_{474}	20_{110}		
	IM							
	SC							
	PO	200_{474}	20_{982}	20_{982}				
Barbiturate sleep potentiation	IV							
	IP	80_{469}						
	IM							
	SC					100_{142}		
	PO		200_{200}	100_{142}				
Paralytic	IV	200_{211}			110_{1171}	20_{1171}		
	IP	200_{211}	300_{463}					
	IM							
	SC	180_{211}						
	PO	302_{119}	382_{119}					

MEPROBAMATE (continued)

mg/kg		Mouse	Rat	Guinea Pig	Rabbit	Cat	Dog	Monkey	
EEG	IV				110 845	30 823			
	IP		40 1069						
	IM								
	SC								
	PO					160 1165			
Affect food intake	IV								
	IP		50.1 1528						
	IM								
	SC								
	PO	46 1391	28.2 1528						
Block stress reaction	IV								
	IP		25 1902						
	IM								
	SC								
	PO								
	IV								
	IP								
	IM								
	SC								
	PO								
	IV								
	IP								
	IM								
	SC								
	PO								
	IV								
	IP								
	IM								
	SC								
	PO								
	IV								
	IP								
	IM								
	SC								
	PO								
	IV								
	IP								
	IM								
	SC								
	PO								
	IV								
	IP								
	IM								
	SC								
	PO								

MERCAPTAMINE
(MEA, Cysteamine, L-1573)

mg/kg		Mouse	Rat	Guinea Pig	Rabbit	Cat	Dog	Monkey
Lethal Dose Y-LD$_{50}$ Z-MLD	IV							
	IP							
	IM							
	SC							
	PO							
Duodenal ulcer induction	IV							
	IP							
	IM							
	SC		300 1637					
	PO		280 1638					
	IV							
	IP							
	IM							
	SC							
	PO							
	IV							
	IP							
	IM							
	SC							
	PO							
	IV							
	IP							
	IM							
	SC							
	PO							
	IV							
	IP							
	IM							
	SC							
	PO							
	IV							
	IP							
	IM							
	SC							
	PO							
	IV							
	IP							
	IM							
	SC							
	PO							
	IV							
	IP							
	IM							
	SC							
	PO							

MERCAPTOPURINE

(Purinethol, NCS-755)

mg/kg		Mouse	Rat	Guinea Pig	Rabbit	Cat	Dog	Monkey
Lethal Dose Y-LD$_{50}$	IV							
	IP	Y250 $_{1903}$						
	IM							
	SC							
	PO							
Treat L 1210 leukemic cells	IV							
	IP	100 $_{1756}$						
	IM							
	SC							
	PO							
Completely suppress immune response [a]12 d	IV							
	IP							
	IM							
	SC							
	PO	[a]33 $_{1446}$						
Increase Ig and decrease glomerular cell [a]daily	IV							
	IP	[a]7.5 $_{1627}$						
	IM							
	SC							
	PO							
Induce sterility and reduce litter size in offspring [a]daily	IV							
	IP							
	IM							
	SC	[a]1.5 $_{1904}$						
	PO							
	IV							
	IP							
	IM							
	SC							
	PO							
	IV							
	IP							
	IM							
	SC							
	PO							
	IV							
	IP							
	IM							
	SC							
	PO							
	IV							
	IP							
	IM							
	SC							
	PO							

MESCALINE

(Mezcaline, Peyote)

mg/kg		Mouse	Rat	Guinea Pig	Rabbit	Cat	Dog	Monkey
Lethal Dose	IV							
Y-LD$_{50}$	IP	Y500 [115]						
Z-MLD	IM							
a caged	SC							
individually	PO	a Y1180 [960]						
CNS	IV				1.1 [159]		20 [478]	
	IP							
	IM							
	SC	30 [119]				50 [476]		
	PO							
Cardiovascular	IV				25 [157]	7.5 [477]	5 [478]	
Respiratory	IP							
	IM							
	SC							
	PO							
Behavioral	IV					1 [110]		
	IP		5 [921]					
	IM	50 [251]					70 [479]	
	SC							
	PO							
Decreased	IV							
spontaneous	IP	50 [813]						
motor activity	IM							
	SC							
	PO	100 [960]						
EEG	IV					20 [842]		
	IP							
	IM							
	SC							
	PO							
	IV							
	IP							
	IM							
	SC							
	PO							
	IV							
	IP							
	IM							
	SC							
	PO							
	IV							
	IP							
	IM							
	SC							
	PO							

METARAMINOL

(Aramine, Pressonex, Metaradrine)

mg/kg		Mouse	Rat	Guinea Pig	Rabbit	Cat	Dog	Monkey	
Lethal Dose	IV	[a]Y51 58							
Y-LD$_{50}$	IP		[a]Y41						
Z-MLD	IM								
[a] as base	SC	[a]Y92 58	[a]Y117 58						
	PO	[a]Y99 58	[a]Y240						
Cardiovascular	IV					0.1 2272	[a]0.07 58		
[a]as base	IP								
	IM					0.1 2272	0.1 2272		
	SC		[a]3 862						
	PO								
Catecholamine	IV						0.25 58		
depletion	IP	0.1 58		0.2 58					
	IM								
(heart)	SC								
	PO								
	IV								
	IP								
	IM								
	SC								
	PO								

IN VITRO

mg %	Cardiac	Vascular	Gut	Uterine	Visceral	Skeletal	Trachea	

METERGOLINE

(MCE, Methergoline, Liserdol)

mg/kg		Mouse	Rat	Guinea Pig	Rabbit	Cat	Dog	Monkey	
Lethal Dose	IV								
Y-LD$_{50}$	IP								
Z-MLD	IM								
	SC								
	PO								
Block	IV								
Serotonin-	IP	1 _1636							
induced	IM								
twitching	SC								
	PO								
Behavioral	IV								
	IP		0.036_1905						
	IM							0.3 _1554	
	SC								
	PO								
Vascular	IV					0.01 _1555			
	IP								
	IM								
	SC								
	PO								
	IV								
	IP								
	IM								
	SC								
	PO								
	IV								
	IP								
	IM								
	SC								
	PO								
	IV								
	IP								
	IM								
	SC								
	PO								
	IV								
	IP								
	IM								
	SC								
	PO								

METHACHOLINE
(Provocholine, Mecholin, Mecholyl)

mg/kg		Mouse	Rat	Guinea Pig	Rabbit	Cat	Dog	Monkey	
Lethal Dose	IV	Y15 [14]	Y20 [14]						
Y-LD$_{50}$	IP								
Z-MLD	IM								
	SC	Y90 [14]	Y75 [14]						
	PO	Y1100 [14]	Y750 [14]						
Cholinergic	IV		0.003 [1425]		0.002 [14]		0.011 [2275]	7 [4]	
	IP					0.15 [4]		10 [4]	
	IM				5	0.15 [4]		10 [4]	
	SC				0.2 [14]	0.15 [4]		10 [4]	
	PO				50 [14]				
Cathartic	IV								
	IP								
	IM								
	SC						0.05 [14]		
	PO						25 [14]		
	IV								
	IP								
	IM								
	SC								
	PO								

IN VITRO

mg %	Cardiac	Vascular	Gut	Uterine	Visceral	Skeletal	Trachea	
Rat				0.02 [1157]				
Rabbit	0.008 [1157]							
Dog							0.059 [1906]	

METHADONE

(Dolophine, Methadose, Mephenon)

mg/kg		Mouse	Rat	Guinea Pig	Rabbit	Cat	Dog	Monkey	
Lethal Dose Y-LD$_{50}$ Z-MLD	IV	Y17 $_{480}$	Y10 $_{481}$				26		
	IP	Y38 $_{480}$	Y23 $_{480}$						
	IM								
	SC	Y33 $_{480}$	Y12 $_{480}$	Y54 $_{480}$			52	Y15 $_{480}$	
	PO	Y93.7 $_{480}$	Y95						
Analgesic [a]total mg IT [b]ED$_{50}$	IV		[a]0.041 $_{1752}$						
	IP	5	20						
	IM						1 $_{2275}$		
	SC	[b]0.28 $_{1489}$	13 $_{482}$	10			4		
	PO						1.1 $_{24}$		
Cardiovascular Respiratory [a]daily	IV				3 $_{43}$	0.84 $_{1626}$	0.75 $_{1907}$		
	IP		[a]5 $_{1661}$						
	IM								
	SC								
	PO								
Behavioral [a]self admin- istration	IV					10 $_{1022}$		[a]0.179*	
	IP	2.5 $_{251}$	10 $_{483}$					0.3 $_{1625}$	
	IM								
	SC	1 $_{1021}$	4.5 $_{927}$						
	PO		30 $_{1908}$						
Central sympathetic [a]Anesthetic	IV						[a]10 $_{2275}$		
	IP		1 $_{1480}$						
	IM								
	SC	1 $_{1086}$					[a]15 $_{2275}$		
	PO						[a]35 $_{2275}$		
Thermoregulatory	IV								
	IP		2.5 $_{1909}$						
	IM								
	SC	10 $_{1613}$	1 $_{1496}$						
	PO								
Antibradykinin	IV								
	IP								
	IM								
	SC								
	PO						1.9 $_{1311}$		
Growth hormone release	IV								
	IP								
	IM								
	SC		2.5 $_{1910}$						
	PO								
Neuroendocrine function	IV								
	IP								
	IM								
	SC		5 $_{1911}$						
	PO								

*1677

METHADONE (continued)

mg/kg		Mouse	Rat	Guinea Pig	Rabbit	Cat	Dog	Monkey	
Liver function effects	IV								
	IP								
	IM								
	SC	10 1912							
	PO								
	IV								
	IP								
	IM								
	SC								
	PO								
	IV								
	IP								
	IM								
	SC								
	PO								
	IV								
	IP								
	IM								
	SC								
	PO								

IN VITRO

mg %	Cardiac	Vascular	Gut	Uterine	Visceral	Skeletal	Trachea	
Cat	3.46 1754							

METHAMPHETAMINE

(Desoxyn, Methampex, Methedrine)

mg/kg		Mouse	Rat	Guinea Pig	Rabbit	Cat	Dog	Monkey	
Lethal Dose	IV	Y10 [111]							
Y-LD[50]	IP	Y15 [111]	25 [485]						
Z-MLD	IM								
[a]caged	SC	180				50			
individually	PO	[a]Y232 [960]	4 [335]						
Increased	IV	0.5 [149]	1 [149]						
motor activity	IP	2 [149]	2 [149]						
	IM	1 [175]							
	SC	5 [484]	0.3 [200]			2 [149]			
	PO	2 [149]	2 [149]			2 [149]			
Behavioral	IV							[a]0.004*	
[a]self	IP	20 [177]	0.5 [1095]			5 [487]		[b]0.5 [1915]	
administration	IM								
[b]IV daily,	SC		3.2 [486]						
long term	PO		10 [973]			2 [1007]	1 [149]		
Analgesic	IV						0.5 [248]		
	IP								
	IM								
	SC	3.2 [1913]							
	PO								
Analeptic	IV				2 [111]				
	IP								
	IM								
	SC								
	PO								
Diuretic	IV								
	IP								
	IM								
	SC						4 [885]		
	PO								
Alter	IV								
brain	IP		17.5 [1847]						
chemistry	IM								
	SC		15 [1916]						
	PO								
Block	IV								
ovulation	IP								
	IM								
	SC		15 [1917]						
	PO								
	IV								
	IP								
	IM								
	SC								
	PO								

*1914

METHARBITAL
(Gemonil)

mg/kg		Mouse	Rat	Guinea Pig	Rabbit	Cat	Dog	Monkey	
Lethal Dose	IV								
Y-LD$_{50}$	IP	Y500[111]							
Z-MLD	IM								
	SC								
	PO	Y500[111]							
Anticonvulsant	IV				20[111]				
	IP								
	IM								
	SC								
	PO	25[111]			50[111]		50[111]		
Ataxic	IV								
	IP	150[111]							
	IM								
	SC								
	PO	200[111]							
	IV								
	IP								
	IM								
	SC								
	PO								

IN VITRO

mg %		Cardiac	Vascular	Gut	Uterine	Visceral	Skeletal	Trachea	

METHAZOLAMIDE
(Neptazane)

mg/kg		Mouse	Rat	Guinea Pig	Rabbit	Cat	Dog	Monkey	
Lethal Dose	IV								
Y-LD$_{50}$	IP								
Z-MLD	IM								
	SC								
	PO								
Anticonvulsant	IV	[a]19.2 $_{1670}$							
	IP	[a]27.9 $_{1292}$							
	IM								
[a]ED$_{50}$	SC								
	PO								
	IV								
	IP								
	IM								
	SC								
	PO								
	IV								
	IP								
	IM								
	SC								
	PO								
	IV								
	IP								
	IM								
	SC								
	PO								
	IV								
	IP								
	IM								
	SC								
	PO								
	IV								
	IP								
	IM								
	SC								
	PO								
	IV								
	IP								
	IM								
	SC								
	PO								
	IV								
	IP								
	IM								
	SC								
	PO								

METHOTREXATE

(Folex, Mexate, MTX)

mg/kg		Mouse	Rat	Guinea Pig	Rabbit	Cat	Dog	Monkey
Lethal Dose	IV	a 200 1359						
Y-LD$_{50}$	IP	b Y4.5 1918						
Z-MLD	IM							
[a]IP, LD$_{10}$	SC							
[b]7 d	PO							
Completely	IV							
suppress	IP	100 1919						
immune	IM							
response	SC							
	PO							
Hemopoietic	IV							
and GI	IP	4 1920						
damage	IM							
	SC							
	PO							
Antileukemic	IV							
	IP	a 3 1359						
[a]alternate days	IM							
	SC							
	PO							
Block humeral	IV							
immune	IP	1 1758						
response	IM							
(not cellular)	SC							
	PO							
Tolerance	IV							
(hemopoietic	IP							
and GI)	IM							
[a]µg/hr,	SC	a 0.2 1921						
2 months	PO							
Antiarthritic	IV							
	IP							
	IM							
	SC		0.25 1835					
	PO							
Antineoplastic	IV					b 0.3-0.8*	b 0.3-0.8*	
	IP							
	IM							
[a]daily	SC							
[b]weekly	PO					a 0.06 2273	a 0.06 2273	
	IV							
	IP							
	IM							
	SC							
	PO							

*2273

METHOXAMINE
(Vasoxyl, Pressomin, Vasylox)

mg/kg		Mouse	Rat	Guinea Pig	Rabbit	Cat	Dog	Monkey	
Lethal Dose	IV	15 [149]							
Y-LD$_{50}$	IP	Y92 [488]							
Z-MLD	IM								
	SC								
	PO	135 [149]							
Cardiovascular	IV		0.1 [1923]			0.2 [489]	0.1 [490]		
	IP	35 [856]					a0.01 [1922]		
	IM						3 [149]		
aIA	SC						0.8 [149]		
	PO						35 [149]		
Barbiturate	IV								
sleep	IP								
potentiation	IM								
	SC	8 [98]							
	PO								
Urinary	IV								
bladder	IP	a3 [1424]							
contraction	IM								
	SC								
atotal mg	PO								

IN VITRO

mg %	Cardiac	Vascular	Gut	Uterine	Visceral	Skeletal	Trachea	
Guinea Pig	0.5 [149]			1.24 [149]				
Rabbit			1.24 [149]	1.24 [149]				
Rat			0.025 [1583]					

METHOXSALEN

(Oxsoralen, Ammoidin, Xanthotoxin)

mg/kg		Mouse	Rat	Guinea Pig	Rabbit	Cat	Dog	Monkey	
Lethal Dose	IV								
Y-LD$_{50}$	IP								
Z-MLD	IM								
	SC								
	PO								
Block	IV								
acetaminophen	IP								
hepatotoxicosis	IM								
	SC								
	PO	54.05 1281							
Increase	IV								
hexobarbital	IP		10.81 1924						
sleeptime	IM								
	SC								
	PO								
Induce	IV								
drug	IP		50 1925						
metabolism	IM								
	SC								
	PO								

IN VITRO

mg %		Cardiac	Vascular	Gut	Uterine	Visceral	Skeletal	Trachea	

METHSCOPOLAMINE

(Pamine, Mescopil, Proscomide)

mg/kg		Mouse	Rat	Guinea Pig	Rabbit	Cat	Dog	Monkey	
Lethal Dose	IV								
Y-LD$_{50}$	IP								
Z-MLD	IM								
	SC								
	PO								
Anticholinergic	IV		0.002 [491]						
(antisecretory)	IP								
	IM				0.025 [491]		0.01 [491]		
	SC	1 [1087]	0.2 [491]						
	PO		14 [491]				1.5 [491]		
Neuromuscular	IV						25 [491]		
block	IP								
	IM								
	SC								
	PO								
Ganglionic	IV					5 [491]			
block	IP								
	IM								
	SC								
	PO								
CNS	IV								
(stimulant)	IP								
	IM								
	SC		5 [491]						
	PO		50 [491]						
	IV								
	IP								
	IM								
	SC								
	PO								
	IV								
	IP								
	IM								
	SC								
	PO								
	IV								
	IP								
	IM								
	SC								
	PO								
	IV								
	IP								
	IM								
	SC								
	PO								

METHYLATROPINE

(Eumydrin, Metropine, Ekomine)

mg/kg		Mouse	Rat	Guinea Pig	Rabbit	Cat	Dog	Monkey	
Lethal Dose	IV	Y7 1926							
Y-LD$_{50}$	IP	Y250							
Z-MLD	IM								
	SC								
	PO								
Anticholinergic	IV	1.39 1926	0.5 1572	2		^{a}0.1-0.2*	^{a}1-6 2275		
	IP	0.05 1927				^{a}0.1-0.2*	^{a}1-6 2275		
	IM					^{a}0.1-0.2*	^{a}1-6 2275		
^{a}total mg	SC					^{a}0.1-0.2*	^{a}1-6 2275		
	PO					^{a}0.1-0.2*	^{a}1-6 2275		
Behavioral	IV								
	IP		86.2 1435						
	IM								
	SC								
	PO								
CNS	IV					10 114			
	IP								
	IM								
	SC								
	PO								

*2275

IN VITRO

mg %	Cardiac	Vascular	Gut	Uterine	Visceral	Skeletal	Pancreas	
Rat							^{a}1.6 1434	
Guinea Pig			^{a}3.1 1434					
Anticholinergic	10		10					
^{a}nanomolar								
solution								

METHYLDOPA

(MK 351, Aldomet, Dopamet)

mg/kg		Mouse	Rat	Guinea Pig	Rabbit	Cat	Dog	Monkey
Lethal Dose	IV	Y1900 [58]						
Y-LD$_{50}$	IP	Y406 [58]	Y647 [58]					
Z-MLD	IM							
	SC							
	PO	Y5300 [58]	Y7490 [58]		Y713 [58]			
Decarboxylase	IV		20 [493]	100 [494]		100 [493]		
Inhibition	IP							
	IM							
	SC	100 [492]						
	PO							
Decreased	IV							
serotonin	IP							
(brain)	IM							
	SC	400 [492]		400 [492]				
	PO							
Catecholamine	IV	50 [58]					100 [58]	
depletion	IP		400 [1141]					
(heart)	IM							
	SC							
	PO							
Barbiturate	IV							
sleep	IP							
potentiation	IM							
	SC	100 [492]						
	PO							
Cardiovascular	IV		[a]0.19 [1928]			100 [1929]	50 [1930]	
	IP		50 [1243]				[b]5 [1930]	
[a] i. cardiac	IM							
[b] total mg, ICV	SC		213.8 [916]					
	PO		200 [1138]					
Increase	IV							
serum	IP		25 [1931]					
prolactin	IM							
	SC							
	PO							
Decrease	IV						100 [1929]	
plasma	IP							
renin	IM							
activity	SC							
	PO							
Restore	IV							
anticonvulsant	IP	[a]15.4 [1292]						
activity of	IM							
methazolamide	SC							
[a] reserpinized	PO							

METHYLDOPA HYDRAZINE

(MK 486)

mg/kg		Mouse	Rat	Guinea Pig	Rabbit	Cat	Dog	Monkey	
Lethal Dose	IV								
Y-LD$_{50}$	IP								
Z-MLD	IM								
	SC								
	PO								
Potentiate	IV								
L-dopa	IP	25 $_{1932}$							
	IM								
	SC								
	PO								
Inhibit	IV								
peripheral	IP	100 $_{1393}$							
decarboxylase	IM								
	SC								
	PO								
	IV								
	IP								
	IM								
	SC								
	PO								
	IV								
	IP								
	IM								
	SC								
	PO								
	IV								
	IP								
	IM								
	SC								
	PO								
	IV								
	IP								
	IM								
	SC								
	PO								
	IV								
	IP								
	IM								
	SC								
	PO								
	IV								
	IP								
	IM								
	SC								
	PO								

3,4-METHYLENEDIOXYMETHAMPHETAMINE
(MDMA)

mg/kg		Mouse	Rat	Guinea Pig	Rabbit	Cat	Dog	Monkey
Lethal Dose	IV							
Y-LD$_{50}$	IP							
Z-MLD	IM							
	SC							
	PO							
Neurotoxic	IV							
	IP							
	IM							
	SC		10 [1934]	20 [1933]				
	PO							
Alter brain chemistry	IV							
	IP							
	IM							
	SC		3.5 [1935]					
	PO							
Increase serum corticoids	IV							
	IP		10 [1936]					
	IM							
	SC							
	PO							
Increase serum prolactin	IV							
	IP		1 [1936]					
	IM							
	SC							
	PO							
	IV							
	IP							
	IM							
	SC							
	PO							
	IV							
	IP							
	IM							
	SC							
	PO							
	IV							
	IP							
	IM							
	SC							
	PO							
	IV							
	IP							
	IM							
	SC							
	PO							

METHYLERGONOVINE

(Methergine, Basofortina, Partergin)

mg/kg		Mouse	Rat	Guinea Pig	Rabbit	Cat	Dog	Monkey	
Lethal Dose	IV	Y85 352	Y23 352		Y2.6 352				
Y-LD$_{50}$	IP								
Z-MLD	IM								
	SC								
	PO	Y187 352	Y93 352						
Oxytocic	IV				0.2 352	0.125 352			
	IP								
	IM								
	SC								
	PO								
	IV								
	IP								
	IM								
	SC								
	PO								
	IV								
	IP								
	IM								
	SC								
	PO								

IN VITRO

mg %	Cardiac	Vascular	Gut	Uterine	Visceral	Skeletal	Trachea	

METHYLPHENIDATE
(Ritalin, Centedrin, Phenidylate)

mg/kg		Mouse	Rat	Guinea Pig	Rabbit	Cat	Dog	Monkey
Lethal Dose	IV	41 1025	Y48 115					
Y-LD$_{50}$	IP	Y450 174						
Z-MLD	IM							
[a]caged	SC	[a]Y470 1142						
individually	PO	[a]Y680 960	Y367 115					
CNS	IV				5 495		2 93	
(stimulant)	IP	30 174						
	IM							
	SC	10 93	3.19 85					10 89
	PO	50 960					10 93	
Antagonize	IV					10 497	20 497	
amphetamine	IP							
hypertension	IM							
	SC							
	PO							
Phentolamine	IV						15 498	
antagonist	IP							
	IM							
	SC							
	PO							
Cardiovascular	IV		5 157		5 495	5 496	5 496	
	IP							
	IM							
	SC							
	PO							
Behavioral	IV							
	IP	10 1131	1.7 1501					
	IM							
	SC	10 940	10 1026			2 1024		
	PO	80 935				2 1007		
Affect on	IV							
growth and	IP							
endocrine	IM							
function	SC		35 1937					
	PO							
	IV							
	IP							
	IM							
	SC							
	PO							
	IV							
	IP							
	IM							
	SC							
	PO							

METHYLPREDNISOLONE

(Medrol, Mepred, Medrone)

mg/kg		Mouse	Rat	Guinea Pig	Rabbit	Cat	Dog	Monkey
Lethal Dose	IV							
Y-LD$_{50}$	IP							
Z-MLD	IM							
	SC							
	PO							
Inhibit	IV		30 1938					
weight gains	IP							
and involute	IM							
thymus	SC							
	PO							
Antichemotactic	IV				4.6 1823			
	IP							
	IM							
	SC							
	PO							
Anti-	IV							
inflammatory	IP							
	IM					[a]2-20 2275	[a]2-40 2275	
[a]total mg	SC							
	PO					2-4 2275	2-4 2275	
	IV							
	IP							
	IM							
	SC							
	PO							
	IV							
	IP							
	IM							
	SC							
	PO							
	IV							
	IP							
	IM							
	SC							
	PO							
	IV							
	IP							
	IM							
	SC							
	PO							
	IV							
	IP							
	IM							
	SC							
	PO							

METHYL(METHYPHENYL)TETRAHYDROPYRIDINE
(MPTP)

mg/kg		Mouse	Rat	Guinea Pig	Rabbit	Cat	Dog	Monkey
Lethal Dose	IV							
Y-LD$_{50}$	IP							
Z-MLD	IM							
	SC							
	PO							
Neurotoxic	IV							
(dopamine	IP	10 $_{1939}$	30 $_{1940}$					
depletion)	IM							
	SC	50 $_{1941}$						
	PO							
	IV							
	IP							
	IM							
	SC							
	PO							
	IV							
	IP							
	IM							
	SC							
	PO							

IN VITRO

mg %	Cardiac	Vascular	Gut	Uterine	Visceral	Skeletal	Trachea	

A-METHYLTYROSINE

(A-MMT)

mg/kg		Mouse	Rat	Guinea Pig	Rabbit	Cat	Dog	Monkey
Lethal Dose	IV							
Y-LD$_{50}$	IP							
Z-MLD	IM							
	SC							
	PO							
Antagonize	IV							
amphetamine	IP	32 1392						
anorexia	IM							
	SC							
	PO							
Potentiate	IV							
morphine	IP	150 1708						
analgesia	IM							
	SC							
	PO							
Deplete	IV							
central	IP	200 1597						
norepine-	IM							
phrine and	SC							
dopamine	PO							
Antagonize	IV							
amphetamines	IP	[a]250 1810						
activity	IM							
[a]2 divided	SC							
doses	PO							
Induced	IV							
hypokinesia	IP	[a]250 1942						
	IM							
[a]2 divided	SC							
doses	PO							
	IV							
	IP							
	IM							
	SC							
	PO							
	IV							
	IP							
	IM							
	SC							
	PO							
	IV							
	IP							
	IM							
	SC							
	PO							

METHYSERGIDE

(Sansert, Deseril, Desernil)

mg/kg		Mouse	Rat	Guinea Pig	Rabbit	Cat	Dog	Monkey	
Lethal Dose	IV								
Y-LD$_{50}$	IP								
Z-MLD	IM								
	SC								
	PO								
Inhibit	IV		0.5 1595						
action of	IP	10 1945							
amphetamines	IM								
	SC								
	PO								
Antagonize	IV	[a]0.001*							
morphine	IP								
	IM								
[a]total mg, ICV	SC	0.05 1944							
	PO								
Behavioral	IV								
	IP	4 1488	2 1871						
	IM							0.1 1946	
	SC								
	PO								
Antagonize	IV					0.025 1555	0.1 1542		
serotonin	IP								
	IM								
	SC								
	PO								
Hypothermia	IV								
	IP	5 1413							
	IM								
	SC								
	PO								
Decrease	IV								
audiogenic	IP	20 1488							
seizure	IM								
	SC								
	PO								
Block 5HTP-	IV								
and L DOPA	IP								
induced	IM								
hypoglycemia	SC	0.1 1456							
	PO								
	IV								
	IP								
	IM								
	SC								
	PO								

*1943

METIAMIDE
(SKF 92058)

mg/kg		Mouse	Rat	Guinea Pig	Rabbit	Cat	Dog	Monkey	
Lethal Dose	IV								
$Y-LD_{50}$	IP								
$Z-MLD$	IM								
	SC								
	PO								
Histamine-	IV								
H_2 antagonism	IP	5 1322							
	IM								
	SC								
	PO								
	IV								
	IP								
	IM								
	SC								
	PO								
	IV								
	IP								
	IM								
	SC								
	PO								

IN VITRO

mg %	Cardiac	Vascular	Gut	Uterine	Visceral	Skeletal	Trachea	
Guinea Pig	a_{10}^{-4} 1314							
^{a}molar solution								

METOCLOPRAMIDE

(Reglan, Cerucal, Metoclol)

mg/kg		Mouse	Rat	Guinea Pig	Rabbit	Cat	Dog	Monkey
Lethal Dose	IV							
Y-LD$_{50}$	IP							
Z-MLD	IM							
	SC							
	PO							
Effects	IV							
on GI	IP							
secretion	IM		10 $_{1423}$					
	SC							
	PO							
Cardiovascular	IV						2 $_{1748}$	
	IP							
	IM							
	SC							
	PO							
Antiemetic	IV					[a]1-2 $_{2273}$	[a]1-2 $_{2273}$	
	IP							
[a]infuse	IM							
over 24 h	SC							
	PO					0.5 $_{2272}$	0.5 $_{2272}$	
	IV							
	IP							
	IM							
	SC							
	PO							
	IV							
	IP							
	IM							
	SC							
	PO							
	IV							
	IP							
	IM							
	SC							
	PO							
	IV							
	IP							
	IM							
	SC							
	PO							
	IV							
	IP							
	IM							
	SC							
	PO							

METOPROLOL

(Lopressor, Beloc, Prelis)

mg/kg		Mouse	Rat	Guinea Pig	Rabbit	Cat	Dog	Monkey	
Lethal Dose	IV								
Y-LD$_{50}$	IP								
Z-MLD	IM								
	SC								
	PO								
Cardiovascular	IV						0.75 $_{1947}$		
	IP								
	IM								
	SC								
	PO		30 $_{1873}$						
Antagonize	IV								
aspirin	IP								
antihypertensive	IM								
effects	SC								
	PO		1 $_{1308}$						
	IV								
	IP								
	IM								
	SC								
	PO								

IN VITRO

mg %	Cardiac	Vascular	Gut	Uterine	Visceral	Skeletal	Trachea	

MIANSERIN

(Org GB 94, Athymil, Norval)

mg/kg		Mouse	Rat	Guinea Pig	Rabbit	Cat	Dog	Monkey	
Lethal Dose	IV								
Y-LD$_{50}$	IP								
Z-MLD	IM								
	SC								
	PO								
Attenuates	IV								
morphine	IP		[1] 1948						
withdrawal	IM								
signs	SC								
	PO								
Upregulation	IV								
of GABA	IP								
receptors	IM								
	SC		[a]10 1366						
[a]daily	PO								
Behavioral	IV								
	IP								
	IM							0.1 1946	
	SC								
	PO								
Antagonize	IV								
LSD induced	IP		0.1 1949						
depression	IM								
	SC								
	PO								
	IV								
	IP								
	IM								
	SC								
	PO								
	IV								
	IP								
	IM								
	SC								
	PO								
	IV								
	IP								
	IM								
	SC								
	PO								
	IV								
	IP								
	IM								
	SC								
	PO								

MILRINONE
(WIN 47,203-2)

mg/kg		Mouse	Rat	Guinea Pig	Rabbit	Cat	Dog	Monkey	
Lethal Dose	IV								
Y-LD$_{50}$	IP								
Z-MLD	IM								
	SC								
	PO								
Cardiovascular	IV						[a]0.1 1950		
	IP								
[a]follow with	IM								
0.0017	SC								
mg/kg/min	PO						[1] 2272		
	IV								
	IP								
	IM								
	SC								
	PO								
	IV								
	IP								
	IM								
	SC								
	PO								

IN VITRO

mg %	Cardiac	Vascular	Gut	Uterine	Visceral	Skeletal	Resp. Tiss.	
Dog	[5] 1395							
Guinea Pig							[a]3.6×10^{-5}*	
[a]molar solution								

*1358

MOCLOBEMIDE

(Ro 11-1163/000)

mg/kg		Mouse	Rat	Guinea Pig	Rabbit	Cat	Dog	Monkey	
Lethal Dose	IV								
Y-LD$_{50}$	IP								
Z-MLD	IM								
	SC								
	PO								
Antagonize	IV								
reserpine	IP	0.56 1833							
	IM								
	SC								
	PO	3 1833	1.9 1833						
Behavioral	IV								
	IP								
	IM								
	SC								
	PO	10 1833							
Antagonize	IV								
Oxotremorine	IP								
	IM								
	SC								
	PO	100 1833							
Potentiate	IV								
5 HTP-	IP	0.15 1833							
induced	IM								
tremor	SC								
	PO	0.4 1833	1.3 1833						
Potentiate	IV								
L-DOPA	IP								
running	IM								
	SC								
	PO	1.5 1833							
	IV								
	IP								
	IM								
	SC								
	PO								
	IV								
	IP								
	IM								
	SC								
	PO								
	IV								
	IP								
	IM								
	SC								
	PO								

MOLINDONE

(Moban, EN-1733A, Lidone)

mg/kg		Mouse	Rat	Guinea Pig	Rabbit	Cat	Dog	Monkey	
Lethal Dose	IV								
Y-LD$_{50}$	IP								
Z-MLD	IM								
	SC								
	PO								
CNS	IV								
	IP		10 1951						
	IM								
	SC								
	PO								
Behavioral	IV								
	IP		0.6 1782						
	IM								
	SC								
	PO								
Vasodepressant	IV		1 1782						
	IP								
	IM								
	SC								
	PO								
	IV								
	IP								
	IM								
	SC								
	PO								
	IV								
	IP								
	IM								
	SC								
	PO								
	IV								
	IP								
	IM								
	SC								
	PO								
	IV								
	IP								
	IM								
	SC								
	PO								
	IV								
	IP								
	IM								
	SC								
	PO								

MORPHINE

(Astramorph, Duramorph, MS Contin)

mg/kg		Mouse	Rat	Guinea Pig	Rabbit	Cat	Dog	Monkey
Lethal Dose	IV	Y275 [307]	Y237 [481]					
Y-LD$_{50}$	IP	Y500	920 [500]		Y500 [500]			
Z-MLD	IM			Z400 [502]				
	SC	Y531 [499]	Y572 [501]	Y391 [480]	Y600 [109]	Z60	210 [109]	
	PO	Y745 [911]	Y905 [481]	Z1000 [502]				
Analgesic	IV	[a]0.014 [1944]	20 [503]		2 [1031]		4	0.5 [248]
Preanesthetic	IP	2.3 [309]	[b]5.3 [1955]	12.1 [22]	5			
[a]IT	IM		[a]0.001 [1954]	2-5 [1221]	2-5 [1221]		2-5 [1221]	0.5 [248]
[b]Total µg ICV	SC	7 [267]	1.6 [267]	5 [923]	10 [978]		4	3 [1491]
	PO	52.5 [267]	15.4 [267]	25 [978]				
Behavioral	IV		[c]0.65 [1387]		1 [1952]	1 [1027]		[c]0.25*
[a]total mg ICV	IP	10 [1029]	10.25 [505]			2 [926]		[b]0.3 [1741]
[b]ICV	IM		[d]0.09 [1979]			[a]0.2 [1953]		3 [1974]
[c]Self admin.	SC	50 [504]	1.3 [506]	25 [978]		1 [507]	5 [479]	
[d]total mg IT	PO	25.4 [701]	40 [1030]					
Cardiovascular	IV		0.33 [507]		0.56 [1133]	1	4	
	IP							
	IM							
	SC		1.1 [908]		2 [508]		10 [1028]	
	PO							
Catatonic	IV							20 [506]
	IP	100 [1156]	18 [1863]					
	IM							
	SC	40	125				10 [1028]	
	PO		500 [269]					
EEG	IV		50 [989]		2 [337]	3 [509]	20 [509]	
and	IP		10 [1213]					
ECP	IM							
	SC					0.3 [1205]		
	PO							
Affect	IV	[b]0.001 [1967]	0.45 [1614]			[a]0.2 [1953]	0.1 [1966]	
GI motility	IP		0.04 [1965]					
[a]total mg ICV	IM							
[b]total mg IT	SC							
[c]IG	PO	[c]5.5 [1691]						
Tolerance	IV				4 [1960]			
and/or	IP		15 [1948]					
dependency	IM							
[a]total mg, SC	SC	100 [1959]	10 [1969]		10 [1961]			
implant	PO		[a]75 [1956]					
Renal	IV		4 [1957]					
Effects	IP		[a]0.004 [1958]					
	IM							
[a]ICV	SC	20 [1959]						
	PO							

*1972

mg/kg		Mouse	Rat	Guinea Pig	Rabbit	Cat	Dog	Monkey
Respiratory	IV		3.5 1963		2 1960	0.18 1626		
Effects	IP							
	IM							
[a]SC, stimu-	SC	1.75 1913	4 1640					
latory effects	PO		[a]160 1962					
Ocular	IV				12 1971	0.06 1884		
	IP							
	IM							
	SC		1 1964					
	PO							
Anticonvulsive	IV							
	IP							
	IM							
[a]total mg, i.	SC		64 1968					
substantia nigra	PO		[a]0.014 1716					
Thermoregulatory	IV		[a]0.0002*					
	IP		0.75 1853					
[a]total mg ICV	IM							
[b]SC daily,	SC	40 1970	1 1496					
long term	PO		[b]300 1973					
Affect	IV							
liver	IP							
function	IM							
	SC	20 1912	5 1975					
	PO							
Alter	IV							
brain	IP		30 1701					
dopamine	IM							
	SC		0.5 1480					
	PO							
Endocrine	IV						0.01 1724	
effects	IP		8 1745					
[a]total mg, SC	IM							
implant	SC	2.5 1980	10 1976					
[b]total mg IT	PO	[b]0.013 1980	[a]75 1977					
Affect urinary	IV		1 1978					
bladder	IP		[b]0.01 1978					
motility	IM		[b]0.023 1743					
[a]total mg, IT	SC		1 1978					
[b]total µg ICV	PO							
Affect	IV		10 1981					
GI	IP		[a]0.003 1981					
secretions	IM							
	SC							
[a]ICV	PO							

mg/kg		Mouse	Rat	Guinea Pig	Rabbit	Cat	Dog	Monkey	
Convulsant	IV								
	IP								
	IM								
	SC		160 1135		500	20			
	PO								
Polysynaptic reflex inhibition	IV					0.4 828	1 849		
	IP								
	IM								
	SC		4 1030						
	PO								
Antibradykinin	IV								
	IP								
	IM								
	SC		1.1 908						
	PO								
Metabolic	IV								
	IP		50 1209						
	IM								
	SC		5 1227						
	PO								

IN VITRO

mg %	Cardiac	Vascular	Gut	Uterine	Visceral	Skeletal	Trachea	
Rabbit	1		5					
Rat			0.0029 1717					
Cat	2.85 1754							

MUSCARINE

mg/kg		Mouse	Rat	Guinea Pig	Rabbit	Cat	Dog	Monkey	
Lethal Dose	IV	Y0.23 [16]							
Y-LD$_{50}$	IP								
Z-MLD	IM								
	SC				30 [511]	2.8 [109]			
	PO	750			268 [511]	28.6 [109]			
Spasmogenic	IV			0.002 [16]	0.01 [16]	0.005 [16]	0.0005 [16]		
	IP								
	IM								
	SC								
	PO								
Cardiovascular	IV			0.005 [16]	0.005 [16]	0.001 [16]	0.0005 [16]		
	IP								
	IM								
	SC								
	PO								
EEG (activation)	IV				1.2 [1100]	0.0001 [826]			
	IP								
	IM								
	SC								
	PO								

IN VITRO

mg %	Cardiac	Vascular	Gut	Uterine	Visceral	Skeletal	Trachea	
Guinea Pig	0.002 [16]		0.002 [16]	0.01 [16]	0.002 [16]			
Rabbit	0.003 [16]		0.003 [16]	0.05 [16]	0.008 [16]			
Dog			0.0008 [16]	0.01 [16]	0.0003 [16]			

MUSCIMOL

mg/kg		Mouse	Rat	Guinea Pig	Rabbit	Cat	Dog	Monkey
Lethal Dose	IV							
Y-LD$_{50}$	IP							
Z-MLD	IM							
	SC							
	PO							
Convulsive	IV		$^a0.05_{1982}$					
	IP							
	IM							
^{a}total μg,	SC							
i. cranial	PO							
Affect dopamine	IV		$^a0.05_{1468}$					
activity in	IP		0.5_{1468}					
adrenals	IM							
^{a}total μg	SC							
daily, ICV	PO							
Affect ethanol	IV		$^a0.3_{1335}$					
withdrawal	IP							
	IM							
^{a}total μg,	SC							
i. cisternal	PO							
Modulate	IV		$^a0.034_{1983}$					
cholinergic	IP							
activity	IM							
^{a}total μg,	SC							
i. septal	PO							
	IV							
	IP							
	IM							
	SC							
	PO							
	IV							
	IP							
	IM							
	SC							
	PO							
	IV							
	IP							
	IM							
	SC							
	PO							
	IV							
	IP							
	IM							
	SC							
	PO							

NADOLOL

(SQ 11725, Corgard, Solgol)

mg/kg		Mouse	Rat	Guinea Pig	Rabbit	Cat	Dog	Monkey
Lethal Dose	IV							
Y-LD$_{50}$	IP							
Z-MLD	IM							
	SC							
	PO							
Cardiovascular	IV						[1] 1545	
	IP							
	IM							
	SC							
	PO		30 1873					
Coronary blood flow regulation	IV						[4] 1832	
	IP							
	IM							
	SC							
	PO							
	IV							
	IP							
	IM							
	SC							
	PO							
	IV							
	IP							
	IM							
	SC							
	PO							
	IV							
	IP							
	IM							
	SC							
	PO							
	IV							
	IP							
	IM							
	SC							
	PO							
	IV							
	IP							
	IM							
	SC							
	PO							
	IV							
	IP							
	IM							
	SC							
	PO							

NALBUPHINE

(Nubain, EN-2234A)

mg/kg		Mouse	Rat	Guinea Pig	Rabbit	Cat	Dog	Monkey	
Lethal Dose	IV								
Y-LD$_{50}$	IP								
Z-MLD	IM								
	SC								
	PO								
Analgesic	IV								
	IP								
	IM								
[a]ED50	SC	[a]0.37 $_{1482}$	0.24 $_{1500}$	[a]1.73 $_{1482}$					
	PO								
Behavioral	IV							0.2 $_{1497}$	
	IP								
	IM								
	SC								
	PO								
Thermoregulatory	IV								
	IP								
	IM								
	SC	0.5 $_{1495}$	1 $_{1496}$						
	PO								
	IV								
	IP								
	IM								
	SC								
	PO								
	IV								
	IP								
	IM								
	SC								
	PO								
	IV								
	IP								
	IM								
	SC								
	PO								
	IV								
	IP								
	IM								
	SC								
	PO								
	IV								
	IP								
	IM								
	SC								
	PO								

NALORPHINE

(Nalline, Allorphine, Lethidrone)

mg/kg		Mouse	Rat	Guinea Pig	Rabbit	Cat	Dog	Monkey
Lethal Dose	IV	Y190[58]						
Y-LD$_{50}$	IP	Y590[17]						
Z-MLD	IM							
	SC	Y670[58]						
	PO							
Morphine	IV				5[513]	3[514]	1[2272]	
antagonist	IP	5[512]	5			0.02[1032]		
	IM						0.4[97]	
	SC	5[1033]	2[58]				1[2272]	
	PO							
Analgesic	IV					8[891]		
	IP	13.8[17]	1.55[513]					
	IM							
	SC	100[515]	28.3[1284]					
	PO							
EEG	IV				0.004[516]	8[891]		
	IP							
	IM							
	SC							
	PO							
Antidepressant	IV							
	IP							
	IM							
	SC			10[90]				
	PO							
Decreased	IV						1[849]	
polysynaptic	IP							
reflex	IM							
	SC							
	PO							
Behavioral	IV							
	IP							
	IM							0.16[1494]
	SC							
	PO							
Thermoregulatory	IV							
	IP							
	IM							
	SC	2.5[1495]						
	PO							
Diuretic	IV							
	IP							
	IM							
	SC		20[1499]					
	PO							

mg/kg		Mouse	Rat	Guinea Pig	Rabbit	Cat	Dog	Monkey	
Suppress	IV								
ACh	IP								
writhing	IM								
[a]ED$_{50}$	SC	[a]0.3 1296							
	PO								
	IV								
	IP								
	IM								
	SC								
	PO								
	IV								
	IP								
	IM								
	SC								
	PO								
	IV								
	IP								
	IM								
	SC								
	PO								

IN VITRO

mg %	Cardiac	Vascular	Gut	Uterine	Visceral	Skeletal	Ocular	

NALOXONE
(Narcan, Nalone, Narcon)

mg/kg		Mouse	Rat	Guinea Pig	Rabbit	Cat	Dog	Monkey
Lethal Dose Y-LD$_{50}$ Z-MLD	IV							
	IP							
	IM							
	SC							
	PO							
Protect against shock	IV	1 [1653]	10 [1986]				0.5 [1795]	
	IP							
	IM							
	SC							
	PO							
Antagonize opioid behavioral effects	IV		0.2 [1988]					10.64 [1497]
	IP		1 [1987]					
	IM							
	SC		0.1 [1493]					
	PO							
Behavioral	IV				0.1 [1952]			
	IP	0.25 [1457]						
	IM							
	SC							
	PO							
Precipitate morphine withdrawal syndrome	IV							
	IP		5 [1948]					
	IM							
	SC	3 [1969]	3 [1969]					
	PO		1 [1956]					
Antagonize opioid urinary bladder effects	IV		0.25 [1750]					
	IP							
	IM							
	SC		0.5 [1978]					
	PO							
Antagonize opioid renal effects [a]ICV	IV		[a]0.004 [1958]					
	IP							
	IM							
	SC		10 [1939]					
	PO							
Antagonize opioid endocrine effects	IV						0.01 [1724]	
	IP		5 [1745]					
	IM							
	SC		10 [1976]					
	PO							
Antagonize opioid GI effects [a]ICV	IV		[a]0.03 [1993]		2 [1984]			
	IP		1 [1656]					
	IM							
	SC	2 [1967]	3 [1993]					
	PO							

mg/kg		Mouse	Rat	Guinea Pig	Rabbit	Cat	Dog	Monkey
Antagonize opioid emetic effects [a]Total mg ICV	IV					5 1401		
	IP					5 1401		
	IM					[a]1 1401		
	SC							
	PO							
Antagonize opioid respiratory effects	IV				0.125 1960	0.04 2272	0.04 2272	
	IP							
	IM					0.04 2273	0.04 2273	
	SC	2.7 1881	0.04 1962		0.04 2273	0.04 2275		
	PO							
Antagonize opioid ocular effects	IV				0.5 1971	0.001 1884		
	IP							
	IM							
	SC							
	PO							
Antagonize morphine effect on EMG	IV							
	IP		10 1999					
	IM							
	SC							
	PO							
Antagonize endogenous non-opioid substances [a]Subst. P	IV							
	IP		[a]10 1998					
	IM							
	SC							
	PO							
Antagonize non-opioid drugs [a]i. cardiac	IV		2 1997					
	IP		25 1863					
	IM		[a]0.15 1928					
	SC	0.1 1293	1 1293					
	PO							
Antagonize morphine effects on liver function	IV							
	IP							
	IM							
	SC	1 1912						
	PO							
Respiratory stimulation	IV							
	IP							
	IM							
	SC		0.63 1962					
	PO							
Convulsive	IV							
	IP							
	IM							32 1994
	SC							
	PO							

mg/kg		Mouse	Rat	Guinea Pig	Rabbit	Cat	Dog	Monkey	
Antagonize	IV				0.0885[1481]	1[1990]			
opioid	IP								
action on	IM								
spinal	SC	2[1991]							
reflexes	PO								
Antagonize	IV	[a]0.3[1725]			1[1419]			1[1992]	
endogenous	IP								
opioids	IM								
[a]Total μg ICV	SC								
	PO								
	IV								
	IP								
	IM								
	SC								
	PO								
	IV								
	IP								
	IM								
	SC								
	PO								

IN VITRO

mg %	Cardiac	Vascular	Gut	Uterine	Visceral	Skeletal	Ocular	
Rat			0.0033[1717]					
Rabbit			0.0327[1984]			0.3274[1985]		
Guinea Pig			0.0003[1862]					

NALTREXONE

(Trexan, EN-1639A)

mg/kg		Mouse	Rat	Guinea Pig	Rabbit	Cat	Dog	Monkey	
Lethal Dose	IV								
Y-LD$_{50}$	IP								
Z-MLD	IM								
	SC								
	PO								
Antagonize	IV		1 [1605]					0.05 [1972]	
opioid	IP		0.1 [2000]						
behavioral	IM							0.056 [1477]	
effects	SC	5 [1995]	1 [1996]						
	PO								
Cardiovascular	IV		[a]0.15 [1928]				5 [2002]		
	IP								
	IM								
[a]IC	SC		1.5 [2001]						
	PO								
Antagonize	IV								
opioid	IP								
sedative	IM								
effects	SC								
	PO	10 [1608]	10 [1608]						
Antagonize	IV								
opioid	IP								
GI	IM								
effects	SC		1 [2003]						
	PO								
Enhance	IV						0.01 [1724]		
adrenal	IP								
catcholamine	IM								
release	SC								
	PO								
	IV								
	IP								
	IM								
	SC								
	PO								
	IV								
	IP								
	IM								
	SC								
	PO								
	IV								
	IP								
	IM								
	SC								
	PO								

NAPROXEN

(Equiproxen, Naprosyn, Anaprox)

mg/kg		Mouse	Rat	Guinea Pig	Rabbit	Cat	Dog	Monkey
Lethal Dose Y-LD$_{50}$ Z-MLD	IV							
	IP							
	IM							
	SC							
	PO							
Anti-inflammatory	IV							
	IP							
	IM							
	SC							
	PO		14.5 [1283]					
Effects on renal prostaglandin synthesis	IV						10 [1286]	
	IP							
	IM							
	SC							
	PO							
	IV							
	IP							
	IM							
	SC							
	PO							
	IV							
	IP							
	IM							
	SC							
	PO							
	IV							
	IP							
	IM							
	SC							
	PO							
	IV							
	IP							
	IM							
	SC							
	PO							
	IV							
	IP							
	IM							
	SC							
	PO							
	IV							
	IP							
	IM							
	SC							
	PO							

NEOSTIGMINE

(Prostigmin, Proserin, Synstigmin)

mg/kg		Mouse	Rat	Guinea Pig	Rabbit	Cat	Dog	Monkey	
Lethal Dose	IV	Y0.36 [517]	Y0.16 [518]		0.25 [519]		20 [521]		
Y-LD$_{50}$	IP	Y0.62 [907]							
Z-MLD	IM	Y0.4 [1878]			Y0.31 [517]				
	SC	Y0.8 [517]	Y0.37 [518]		Z12.5 [520]		Z13.5 [520]		
	PO	Y14.4 [517]							
Cholinergic	IV					0.1 [1034]	0.025		
	IP		0.1 [1430]						
[a]total mg	IM					1 [1034]	[a]0.25-2.5*		
	SC		0.1 [1432]			0.01-0.075*	0.025		
	PO						[a]0.25-2.5*		
Anticurare	IV		0.1 [1143]		0.25	0.025	0.17		
	IP								
	IM					0.075 [2275]			
	SC		0.3			0.075 [2275]			
	PO								
Anticonvulsant	IV								
	IP								
	IM								
	SC	1 [957]							
	PO								

*2275

IN VITRO

mg %	Cardiac	Vascular	Gut	Uterine	Visceral	Skeletal		
Rabbit		0.25	0.25					
Rat			0.00628 [1430]		0.01 [1157]			

NIALAMIDE

(Espril, Niamid, Nyazin)

mg/kg		Mouse	Rat	Guinea Pig	Rabbit	Cat	Dog	Monkey
Lethal Dose	IV							
Y-LD$_{50}$	IP	Y742 $_{115}$						
Z-MLD	IM							
	SC							
	PO	Y1000$_{115}$	Y1700 $_{115}$					
Monoamine-	IV				100$_{522}$			
oxidase	IP		^{a}0.25 $_{1169}$	^{a}10 $_{1169}$				
inhibition	IM							25 $_{1170}$
(brain)	SC		30 $_{173}$			10 $_{173}$		
^{a} 6 days	PO							
Behavioral	IV							
	IP	40 $_{1890}$		150 $_{1036}$				
	IM							
	SC		100 $_{1010}$			10$_{173}$		
	PO							
Anticonvulsant	IV							
	IP	100 $_{523}$	35 $_{1035}$					
	IM							
	SC							
	PO							
EEG	IV							
(synchroni-	IP							
zation)	IM							
	SC					10 $_{173}$		
	PO							
CNS	IV					50 $_{861}$		
stimulant	IP							
	IM							
	SC							
	PO							
	IV							
	IP							
	IM							
	SC							
	PO							
	IV							
	IP							
	IM							
	SC							
	PO							
	IV							
	IP							
	IM							
	SC							
	PO							

NICARDIPINE

(YC-93, RS-69216, Nicodel, Perdipine)

mg/kg		Mouse	Rat	Guinea Pig	Rabbit	Cat	Dog	Monkey	
Lethal Dose	IV								
Y-LD$_{50}$	IP								
Z-MLD	IM								
	SC								
	PO								
Hypotensive	IV						0.03 $_{1537}$		
	IP								
	IM								
	SC								
	PO								
Release	IV						0.05 $_{1775}$		
adrenal	IP								
catecholamines	IM								
	SC								
	PO								
	IV								
	IP								
	IM								
	SC								
	PO								

IN VITRO

mg %	Cardiac	Vascular	Gut	Uterine	Visceral	Skeletal	Ocular	

NICORANDIL

(SG-75, Sigmart)

mg/kg		Mouse	Rat	Guinea Pig	Rabbit	Cat	Dog	Monkey	
Lethal Dose	IV								
Y-LD$_{50}$	IP								
Z-MLD	IM								
	SC								
	PO								
Hemodynamic	IV						[a]0.016$_{2004}$		
	IP								
	IM								
	SC								
[a]mg/kg/min	PO								
	IV								
	IP								
	IM								
	SC								
	PO								
	IV								
	IP								
	IM								
	SC								
	PO								

IN VITRO

mg %	Cardiac	Vascular	Gut	Uterine	Visceral	Skeletal		
Dog	0.02112$_{2005}$							

NICOTINE

mg/kg		Mouse	Rat	Guinea Pig	Rabbit	Cat	Dog	Monkey	
Lethal Dose	IV	Y7.1 524	Z1	Z4.5 527	Y9.4 524		Y5 524		
Y-LD$_{50}$	IP	10							
Z-MLD	IM								
	SC	Z16 525	Y33.5 526	Z27.5 528	20 528				
	PO	Z24 525	Y55						
Behavioral	IV	0.3 529	0.23 530		0.02 533	0.02 533	[a]0.03 1606	0.01 2009	
	IP	5 369	5 531						
[a] self	IM				0.2 967	0.05 1151	0.01 1599	0.01 1599	
administration	SC	0.4 1101	0.5 532				0.2 534		
	PO	10 935							
Cardiovascular	IV		[b]0.02 2010	0.3	0.1 535	0.2 101	0.25		
[a] total mg	IP						[a,d]0.03**		
[b] mg/kg/min	IM						[a,c]0.005*		
[c] i. cerebral	SC						0.1		
[d] i. carotid	PO								
EEG	IV		1 1150	1.5 1150	0.01 825	0.01 825	0.01 825	0.01 825	
	IP								
	IM								
	SC					0.2 1203			
	PO								
Gastrointestinal	IV					0.05 1093			
	IP								
	IM								
	SC		0.15 1242						
	PO								
Increased	IV	[a]2 2008				0.3 1037			
spinal cord	IP	[b]3.13 2006							
inhibition	IM								
[a] mg/kg/min	SC								
[b] ED$_{50}$	PO								
Effect on	IV								
prenatal	IP								
Catecholamine	IM								
systems	SC		[a]6 1669						
[a] infusion 16 d	PO								
Increased	IV		0.01 1896						
ACTH	IP		0.1 2014						
secretion	IM		[a]1 1896						
[a] IP, prenatal	SC								
	PO								
Effects on	IV								
prolactin	IP		0.75 2015						
	IM								
	SC								
	PO								

*1742 **2007

mg/kg		Mouse	Rat	Guinea Pig	Rabbit	Cat	Dog	Monkey	
Tolerance	IV	[a]4 2011							
	IP	2 2012							
[a]mg/kg/hr	IM								
	SC								
	PO								
Analgesic	IV								
	IP								
	IM								
	SC	2 2013	0.7 2013						
	PO								
	IV								
	IP								
	IM								
	SC								
	PO								
	IV								
	IP								
	IM								
	SC								
	PO								

IN VITRO

mg %	Cardiac	Vascular	Gut	Uterine	Visceral	Skeletal	Trachea	
Rabbit	0.1		0.25					
Guinea Pig			0.2 1157					
Rat			0.5 1157					
Spasmogenic			0.5 1233					

314

NIFEDIPINE

(Adalat, Procardia, Nifedin)

mg/kg		Mouse	Rat	Guinea Pig	Rabbit	Cat	Dog	Monkey	
Lethal Dose	IV								
Y-LD$_{50}$	IP								
Z-MLD	IM								
	SC								
	PO								
Cardiovascular	IV		[a]0.1 $_{2018}$		b 0.0935*		0.003$_{2016}$	0.0005**	
[a]mg/kg/hr	IP		[c]1 $_{2019}$						
[b]mg perfused IA	IM								
[c]IA	SC								
	PO								
Gastrointestinal	IV						0.2 $_{2020}$		
	IP								
	IM								
	SC								
	PO								
	IV								
	IP								
	IM								
	SC								
	PO								

*1687   **2017

IN VITRO

mg %	Cardiac	Vascular	Gut	Uterine	Visceral	Skeletal	Renal	
Rat	1 $_{2021}$	0.00009$_{1634}$					0.0173*	
Guinea Pig	0.0346 $_{1320}$	0.00024$_{2023}$						
Rabbit		0.0001$_{1682}$						
Monkey			0.00035$_{2020}$					

*2022

NIKETHAMIDE

(Anacardone, Coramine, Tonocard)

mg/kg		Mouse	Rat	Guinea Pig	Rabbit	Cat	Dog	Monkey
Lethal Dose Y-LD$_{50}$ Z-MLD	IV		Y191 $_{93}$		250 $_5$		175 $_{537}$	
	IP	Y174 $_{284}$	Y300 $_{537}$	250 $_{537}$	Y225 $_{537}$			
	IM						175 $_{537}$	
	SC	295 $_{536}$	Y470 $_{538}$	300 $_{537}$	350 $_{537}$			
	PO				650 $_{537}$			
Analeptic	IV	19 $_{1137}$			10	8-31 $_{2273}$	8-31 $_{2273}$	
	IP							
	IM					8-31 $_{2273}$	8-31 $_{2273}$	
	SC					8-31 $_{2273}$	8-31 $_{2273}$	
	PO							
Behavioral CNS	IV				45 $_{157}$		33 $_{24}$	
	IP							
	IM	100 $_{175}$						
	SC			50 $_{978}$			33 $_{24}$	
	PO							
Convulsant	IV							
	IP	145 $_{284}$						
	IM							
	SC	201 $_{284}$						
	PO							
Anti-5HT	IV			10 $_{92}$				
	IP							
	IM							
	SC							
	PO							
	IV							
	IP							
	IM							
	SC							
	PO							
	IV							
	IP							
	IM							
	SC							
	PO							
	IV							
	IP							
	IM							
	SC							
	PO							
	IV							
	IP							
	IM							
	SC							
	PO							

NIMODIPINE

(Nimotop, Bay e 9736)

mg/kg		Mouse	Rat	Guinea Pig	Rabbit	Cat	Dog	Monkey	
Lethal Dose	IV								
Y-LD$_{50}$	IP								
Z-MLD	IM								
	SC								
	PO								
Cardiovascular	IV		0.006 $_{2024}$	[a]0.0001$_{2025}$	[a]0.0001$_{2027}$	[a]0.001 $_{2026}$			
	IP								
	IM								
[a]mg/kg/min	SC								
	PO								
Respiratory	IV						0.2 $_{2028}$		
	IP								
[a]% in aerosol	IM								
	SC								
	PO						[a]0.1 $_{2028}$		
	IV								
	IP								
	IM								
	SC								
	PO								

IN VITRO

mg %	Cardiac	Vascular	Gut	Uterine	Visceral	Skeletal	Renal	
Rat							[a]4.7x10^{-5}*	
Dog			[a]1.4x10^{-8}**					
[a]molar solution								

*1639   **2029

NISOLDIPINE
(Bay K 5552)

mg/kg		Mouse	Rat	Guinea Pig	Rabbit	Cat	Dog	Monkey	
Lethal Dose	IV								
Y-LD$_{50}$	IP								
Z-MLD	IM								
	SC								
	PO								
Cardiovascular	IV		[a]0.0016$_{2030}$			[b] 0.001$_{2031}$			
	IP								
[a]mg/kg/min	IM								
[b]IA	SC								
	PO								
	IV								
	IP								
	IM								
	SC								
	PO								
	IV								
	IP								
	IM								
	SC								
	PO								

IN VITRO

mg %	Cardiac	Vascular	Gut	Uterine	Visceral	Skeletal		
Dog	[a]1×10^{-6}*							
[a]molar								
solution								

*1350

NITROGLYCERIN
(Glyceryl Trinitrate, Nitroglycerol, Deponit, Nitronet)

mg/kg		Mouse	Rat	Guinea Pig	Rabbit	Cat	Dog	Monkey	
Lethal Dose Y-LD$_{50}$ Z-MLD	IV				Z45 [346]				
	IP								
	IM		Z275 [346]		Z450 [346]				
	SC					500 [346]	200 [346]		
	PO		Z100						
Cardiovascular (anesthetized) ^{a}IA	IV						0.02 [2033]		
	IP						^{a}0.0003 [2032]		
	IM								
	SC						0.01		
	PO		20 [539]						
Cardiovascular (conscious) ^{a}mg/kg/min ^{b}total mg	IV						0.025 [1218]		
	IP						^{a}0.008 [2004]		
	IM								
	SC								
	PO					^{b}0.1	^{b}0.1-1		
	IV								
	IP								
	IM								
	SC								
	PO								

IN VITRO

mg %	Cardiac	Vascular	Gut	Uterine	Visceral	Skeletal		
Guinea Pig	0.0227 [1320]							

NIZATIDINE

(LY 139037)

mg/kg		Mouse	Rat	Guinea Pig	Rabbit	Cat	Dog	Monkey	
Lethal Dose Y-LD$_{50}$ Z-MLD	IV								
	IP								
	IM								
	SC								
	PO								
GI antisecretory ^{a}mg/kg/hr	IV						^{a}0.0331$_{1550}$		
	IP								
	IM								
	SC		0.1254$_{1550}$						
	PO						0.5826 $_{1551}$		
	IV								
	IP								
	IM								
	SC								
	PO								
	IV								
	IP								
	IM								
	SC								
	PO								

IN VITRO

mg %	Cardiac	Vascular	Gut	Uterine	Visceral	Skeletal		

NOMIFENSINE
(HOE 984, Merital, Alival)

mg/kg		Mouse	Rat	Guinea Pig	Rabbit	Cat	Dog	Monkey	
Lethal Dose	IV								
Y-LD$_{50}$	IP								
Z-MLD	IM								
	SC								
	PO								
Behavioral	IV		13.7 [1365]						
	IP		10 [2034]						
	IM								
	SC								
	PO		31.7 [1365]						
Antagonize	IV								
reserpine	IP	0.17 [1833]							
	IM								
	SC								
	PO	0.3 [1833]	3.8 [1833]						
Effect on	IV								
GABA binding	IP								
	IM								
[a]daily	SC		[a]5 [1366]						
	PO								

IN VITRO

mg %	Cardiac	Vascular	Gut	Uterine	Visceral	Skeletal	CNS	
Rabbit							0.2383*	

*1390

NOREPINEPHRINE

(Levophed, Arterenol, Levarterenol, Noradrenaline)

mg/kg		Mouse	Rat	Guinea Pig	Rabbit	Cat	Dog	Monkey	
Lethal Dose	IV	Y>2 [896]							
Y-LD_{50}	IP								
Z-MLD	IM								
	SC		Y29 [1128]						
	PO		Y132 [1128]						
Cardiovascular	IV	0.003 [97]	0.005 [1352]	0.003 [97]	0.015 [1419]	[a]0.0002 [1367]	0.00025 [1420]	0.001 [1079]	
	IP						[c]0.01 [1422]		
[a]mg/kg/min	IM								
[b]mg/kg/hr	SC		[b]0.1 [1421]						
[c]mg/kg/min IA	PO								
Behavioral	IV						0.01 [99]		
	IP	4 [939]							
	IM								
	SC	2 [940]							
	PO								
Barbiturate	IV								
sleep	IP	2 [98]							
potentiation	IM								
	SC								
	PO								
Antagonize	IV								
reserpine	IP	1 [78]							
ptosis	IM								
	SC	0.5 [1418]							
	PO								
Diuretic	IV						0.007 [866]		
[a]total mg	IP		[a]0.1 [1424]						
	IM								
	SC		0.25 [151]		1 [863]				
	PO								
Bronchiolar	IV								
dilatation	IP								
	IM								
	SC			0.4 [1081]					
	PO								
Metabolic	IV								
	IP								
	IM								
	SC		1 [864]		1 [863]				
	PO								
Gastrointestinal	IV		0.0005 [1423]	0.01 [1419]					
	IP								
	IM								
	SC								
	PO								

322

NORNICOTINE

mg/kg		Mouse	Rat	Guinea Pig	Rabbit	Cat	Dog	Monkey	
Lethal Dose	IV								
Y-LD$_{50}$	IP								
Z-MLD	IM								
	SC								
	PO								
Behavioral	IV								
	IP								
	IM							0.0148_{2036}	0.03_{1599}	
	SC								
	PO								
Thermoregulatory	IV							0.4446_{2036}		
	IP								
	IM								
	SC								
	PO								
	IV								
	IP								
	IM								
	SC								
	PO								

IN VITRO

mg %		Cardiac	Vascular	Gut	Uterine	Visceral	Skeletal	CNS	

NORTRIPTYLINE

(Aventyl, Pamelor, Noritren)

mg/kg		Mouse	Rat	Guinea Pig	Rabbit	Cat	Dog	Monkey
Lethal Dose	IV							
Y-LD$_{50}$	IP							
Z-MLD	IM							
	SC							
	PO							
Antagonize	IV							
tetrabenazine	IP	[a]2.4 $_{1371}$						
ptosis	IM							
[a]ED$_{50}$	SC							
	PO							
Potentiate	IV							
peripheral	IP	2.5 $_{1418}$						
action of	IM							
norepinephrine	SC							
	PO							
Antagonize	IV							
reserpine	IP	[a]5.4 $_{1371}$						
ptosis	IM							
	SC							
[a]ED$_{50}$	PO							
	IV							
	IP							
	IM							
	SC							
	PO							
	IV							
	IP							
	IM							
	SC							
	PO							
	IV							
	IP							
	IM							
	SC							
	PO							
	IV							
	IP							
	IM							
	SC							
	PO							
	IV							
	IP							
	IM							
	SC							
	PO							

OCTOPAMINE

(ND 50, Norsympatol, Norsynephrine, Norfen)

mg/kg		Mouse	Rat	Guinea Pig	Rabbit	Cat	Dog	Monkey	
Lethal Dose	IV								
Y-LD$_{50}$	IP								
Z-MLD	IM								
	SC								
	PO								
Cardiovascular	IV					0.3 $_{912}$	0.3 $_{912}$		
	IP								
	IM								
	SC								
	PO								
	IV								
	IP								
	IM								
	SC								
	PO								
	IV								
	IP								
	IM								
	SC								
	PO								

IN VITRO

mg %		Cardiac	Vascular	Gut	Uterine	Visceral	Skeletal	CNS	

OUABAIN

(Astrobain, Gratibain, G-Strophanthin)

mg/kg		Mouse	Rat	Guinea Pig	Rabbit	Cat	Dog	Monkey	
Lethal Dose $Y-LD_{50}$ $Z-MLD$	IV		17.2 540		0.2 303	Y0.11	0.12 542		
	IP	Y20							
	IM			Y0.26 541					
	SC	10 303	Y97 166	0.2 303	0.25 303	0.17 303	0.13 303		
	PO				14 303	2.4 109	1.5 109		
Cardiovascular ^{a}mg/kg/min IV ^{b}IA ^{c}total mg ICV	IV		^{b}0.25 1671	0.02	0.05	0.089 913	0.25 2037		
	IP		2 1671			^{a}0.001 2038	^{c}0.585 1568		
	IM						0.025 97		
	SC								
	PO								
Arrhythmic ^{a}30 min intervals	IV				0.05 1090	^{a}0.025 1796	0.0665 1535		
	IP								
	IM								
	SC								
	PO								
Emetic	IV					0.06 890	0.05 1013		
	IP								
	IM								
	SC								
	PO								

IN VITRO

mg %	Cardiac	Vascular	Gut	Uterine	Visceral	Skeletal	Vas Deferens	
Rabbit	0.063		0.05					
Guinea Pig	0.0585 2023						0.5846*	
Dog	0.0117 1857	0.0117 2039						

*1820

OXAZEPAM

(Serax, Bonare, Enidrel, Serenid)

mg/kg		Mouse	Rat	Guinea Pig	Rabbit	Cat	Dog	Monkey
Lethal Dose	IV							
Y-LD$_{50}$	IP	Y>1500$_{1659}$						
Z-MLD	IM							
	SC							
	PO	Y7500$_{2040}$						
Anticonvulsant	IV	^{a}0.342$_{1659}$						
	IP							
	IM							
	SC							
^{a}ED$_{50}$	PO							
Behavioral	IV							
	IP	10$_{1324}$						
	IM							
	SC							
	PO							
Antagonize	IV							
LiCl taste	IP		^{a}5.9$_{1528}$					
aversion	IM							
^{a}ED$_{50}$	SC							
	PO		^{a}7.1$_{1528}$					
Antagonize	IV							
morphine-	IP	1$_{2041}$						
increased	IM							
motor activity	SC							
	PO							
Increase	IV							
LD$_{50}$ of	IP	1$_{2042}$						
morphine	IM							
	SC							
	PO							
	IV							
	IP							
	IM							
	SC							
	PO							
	IV							
	IP							
	IM							
	SC							
	PO							
	IV							
	IP							
	IM							
	SC							
	PO							

OXILORPHAN

(levo-BC-2605)

mg/kg		Mouse	Rat	Guinea Pig	Rabbit	Cat	Dog	Monkey
Lethal Dose	IV	Y32 2043						
Y-LD$_{50}$	IP							
Z-MLD	IM							
	SC	Y315 2043						
	PO							
Opioid	IV							
antagonist	IP							
	IM							
^{a}ED$_{50}$	SC	^{a}0.19 2043						
	PO	^{a}3.9 2043						
Analgesic	IV							
	IP							
	IM							
^{a}ED$_{50}$	SC	^{a}4.16 1482		^{a}4.26 1482				
	PO							
Anticonvulsant	IV							
	IP							
	IM							
	SC	27 2043						
	PO							
Sedative	IV							
	IP							
	IM							
^{a}rotorod	SC	^{a}28.3 1482						
	PO							
	IV							
	IP							
	IM							
	SC							
	PO							
	IV							
	IP							
	IM							
	SC							
	PO							
	IV							
	IP							
	IM							
	SC							
	PO							
	IV							
	IP							
	IM							
	SC							
	PO							

OXOTREMORINE

mg/kg		Mouse	Rat	Guinea Pig	Rabbit	Cat	Dog	Monkey
Lethal Dose	IV							
Y-LD$_{50}$	IP	Y5 $_{2045}$						
Z-MLD	IM							
	SC							
	PO							
Tremor	IV							
	IP	2 $_{2048}$	[a]1.6 $_{2046}$					
	IM							
[a]ED$_{50}$	SC	0.2 $_{1442}$	0.25 $_{2047}$					
	PO							
Salivation	IV							
	IP	0.56 $_{1439}$	[a]1.3 $_{2046}$					
	IM							
[a]ED$_{50}$	SC	0.2 $_{1442}$						
	PO							
Behavioral	IV							
	IP	0.56 $_{1439}$	0.3 $_{1434}$					
	IM							
	SC							
	PO							
Analgesia	IV							
	IP							
	IM							
	SC		0.04 $_{1453}$					
	PO							
Hypothermia	IV							
	IP	0.5 $_{1441}$						
	IM							
	SC	0.1 $_{1882}$						
	PO							
Sweating	IV							
	IP	0.15 $_{2049}$						
	IM							
	SC							
	PO							
Inhibit naloxone jumping in morphine dependence	IV							
	IP	0.2 $_{2050}$						
	IM							
	SC							
	PO							
Effects on adrenal	IV							
	IP							
	IM							
	SC		0.5 $_{1468}$					
	PO							

OXOTREMORINE (continued)

mg/kg		Mouse	Rat	Guinea Pig	Rabbit	Cat	Dog	Monkey
Increase plasma norepinephrine	IV							
	IP							
	IM							
	SC		0.25 2047					
	PO							
	IV							
	IP							
	IM							
	SC							
	PO							
	IV							
	IP							
	IM							
	SC							
	PO							
	IV							
	IP							
	IM							
	SC							
	PO							

IN VITRO

mg %	Cardiac	Vascular	Gut	Uterine	Visceral	Skeletal	
Guinea Pig			0.0007 2051				

332

OXYMETAZOLINE

(Afrin, Allerest, Dristan, Sinarest)

mg/kg		Mouse	Rat	Guinea Pig	Rabbit	Cat	Dog	Monkey
Lethal Dose Y-LD$_{50}$ Z-MLD	IV							
	IP							
	IM							
	SC							
	PO							
Sedative	IV							
	IP							
	IM	10 $_{1440}$						
	SC							
	PO							
α-agonist (blood pressure)	IV		0.00005 $_{1351}$					
	IP							
	IM							
	SC							
	PO							
	IV							
	IP							
	IM							
	SC							
	PO							
	IV							
	IP							
	IM							
	SC							
	PO							
	IV							
	IP							
	IM							
	SC							
	PO							
	IV							
	IP							
	IM							
	SC							
	PO							
	IV							
	IP							
	IM							
	SC							
	PO							
	IV							
	IP							
	IM							
	SC							
	PO							

OXYMORPHONE
(Numorphan)

mg/kg		Mouse	Rat	Guinea Pig	Rabbit	Cat	Dog	Monkey
Lethal Dose	IV							
Y-LD$_{50}$	IP							
Z-MLD	IM							
	SC							
	PO							
Induce	IV							
Straub	IP							
tail	IM							
reaction	SC	2 1991						
	PO							
Analgesia	IV					0.1-0.2**	0.1-0.2**	
	IP							
	IM					0.1-0.2**	0.03-0.05*	
	SC		0.009 1500			0.1-0.2**	0.1-0.2**	
	PO							
Behavioral	IV							
	IP							
	IM							
	SC	0.07 1483						
	PO							
Thermoregulatory	IV							
	IP							
	IM							
	SC	20 1613						
	PO							
	IV							
	IP							
	IM							
	SC							
	PO							
	IV							
	IP							
	IM							
	SC							
	PO							
	IV							
	IP							
	IM							
	SC							
	PO							
	IV							
	IP							
	IM							
	SC							
	PO							

*2272   **2273

PANCURONIUM BROMIDE

(Pavulon, Org NA 97, Mioblock)

mg/kg		Mouse	Rat	Guinea Pig	Rabbit	Cat	Dog	Monkey	
Lethal Dose	IV								
Y-LD$_{50}$	IP								
Z-MLD	IM								
	SC								
	PO								
Ganglionic	IV					0.1 _1538_			
	IP								
	IM								
	SC								
	PO								
Skeletal	IV					0.12 _2052_	0.1 _1732_		
muscle	IP								
relaxation	IM								
	SC								
	PO								
	IV								
	IP								
	IM								
	SC								
	PO								
	IV								
	IP								
	IM								
	SC								
	PO								
	IV								
	IP								
	IM								
	SC								
	PO								
	IV								
	IP								
	IM								
	SC								
	PO								
	IV								
	IP								
	IM								
	SC								
	PO								
	IV								
	IP								
	IM								
	SC								
	PO								

335

PAPAVERINE
(Cerespan, Pavabid, Pavacap)

mg/kg		Mouse	Rat	Guinea Pig	Rabbit	Cat	Dog	Monkey	
Lethal Dose	IV	Y33.1 $_{543}$							
Y-LD$_{50}$	IP	Y750	Y63 $_{546}$						
Z-MLD	IM								
	SC	Z500 $_{544}$	Y420 $_{1128}$		Z250 $_{109}$				
	PO	Y2500 $_{545}$	Y745 $_{543}$						
Cardiovascular	IV			10					
	IP			50 $_{1219}$					
	IM								
	SC								
	PO	100 $_{1318}$							
Relax biliary	IV								
and urinary	IP								
muscle	IM						[b]15-65 $_{2275}$		
[a]total mg SO4	SC						[a]30-130 $_{2275}$		
[b]total mg HCl	PO						[a]30-130 $_{2275}$		
Behavioral	IV								
	IP	60 $_{1131}$							
[a]catatonic	IM								
	SC					[a]30 $_{476}$			
	PO								

IN VITRO

mg %	Cardiac	Vascular	Gut	Uterine	Visceral	Skeletal		
Guinea Pig	3.394 $_{2053}$		0.001					
Rabbit	3.394 $_{2053}$		7.5					
Anti-5HT			0.3 $_{92}$					
Cat	0.679 $_{2054}$							

PARALDEHYDE

(Paral)

mg/kg		Mouse	Rat	Guinea Pig	Rabbit	Cat	Dog	Monkey	
Lethal Dose	IV				Y450 [7]	Y450 [7]	Y500 [7]		
Y-LD$_{50}$	IP	Z1500 [547]		Y1230 [549]					
Z-MLD	IM								
	SC	Z1650 [547]							
	PO	Y1650 [548]			5000 [109]		Y3500 [109]		
Anesthetic	IV				300 [7]	300 [7]	300 [7]		
	IP								
	IM								
	SC								
	PO				1000		2000		
Anticonvulsant	IV								
	IP	500 [1018]							
	IM								
	SC	266 [1075]							
	PO	1000 [550]							
Behavioral	IV								
(ataxic)	IP								
	IM								
	SC	462 [1075]							
	PO	800 [935]							
Lose	IV								
righting	IP	[a]546 [1323]							
reflex	IM								
	SC								
[a]ED$_{50}$	PO								
	IV								
	IP								
	IM								
	SC								
	PO								
	IV								
	IP								
	IM								
	SC								
	PO								
	IV								
	IP								
	IM								
	SC								
	PO								
	IV								
	IP								
	IM								
	SC								
	PO								

PARGYLINE

(Eutonyl, Eudatin, Supirdyl)

mg/kg		Mouse	Rat	Guinea Pig	Rabbit	Cat	Dog	Monkey	
Lethal Dose	IV								
Y-LD$_{50}$	IP	Y370 551	Y142 551			Y200 551		Y150 551	
Z-MLD	IM								
	SC								
	PO	Y680 551	Y300 551				Y175 551		
Monoamine-	IV		10 1215		10 552		50 2275		
oxidase	IP	10 69	20 1118						
inhibition	IM		25 867				50 2275		
	SC		12 868				50 2275		
	PO	75 69							
Increased	IV				25 552				
tissue	IP	100 551	50 553		100 830	100 553			
norepinephrine	IM								
	SC								
	PO								
Reverse	IV				50 69		25 1130		
reserpine	IP								
depression	IM								
(with DOPA)	SC								
	PO							50 551	
Behavioral	IV								
	IP		25 1846						
	IM								
	SC								
	PO						100 554		
CNS	IV					30 861			
	IP								
	IM								
	SC		20 1366						
	PO								
Increased	IV								
brain	IP	65 1725	65 1541						
histamine	IM								
	SC								
	PO								
Effect on	IV								
sympathetic	IP			100 2055					
neurotrans-	IM								
mission	SC								
	PO								
Potentiate	IV								
meperidine	IP		75 2056						
analgesia	IM								
	SC								
	PO								

PAROXETINE

mg/kg		Mouse	Rat	Guinea Pig	Rabbit	Cat	Dog	Monkey
Lethal Dose	IV							
Y-LD$_{50}$	IP							
Z-MLD	IM							
	SC							
	PO							
Potentiate	IV							
5HTP	IP							
hypermotility	IM							
	SC	0.6 $_{1760}$						
	PO							
Anticonvulsant	IV							
	IP							
	IM							
^{a}ED$_{50}$	SC							
	PO	^{a}1.2 $_{2057}$						
	IV							
	IP							
	IM							
	SC							
	PO							
	IV							
	IP							
	IM							
	SC							
	PO							
	IV							
	IP							
	IM							
	SC							
	PO							
	IV							
	IP							
	IM							
	SC							
	PO							
	IV							
	IP							
	IM							
	SC							
	PO							
	IV							
	IP							
	IM							
	SC							
	PO							

PENFLURIDOL
(Semap, McN-JR-16341)

mg/kg		Mouse	Rat	Guinea Pig	Rabbit	Cat	Dog	Monkey
Lethal Dose Y-LD$_{50}$ Z-MLD	IV							
	IP							
	IM							
	SC							
	PO							
Neuroleptic	IV	0.5 2059						
	IP							
	IM							
	SC							
	PO							
Block apomorphine hypothermia	IV							
	IP							
	IM							
	SC							
	PO	3.2 1415						
Increase brain homovanillic acid	IV							
	IP	5 1547						
	IM							
	SC							
	PO							
	IV							
	IP							
	IM							
	SC							
	PO							
	IV							
	IP							
	IM							
	SC							
	PO							
	IV							
	IP							
	IM							
	SC							
	PO							
	IV							
	IP							
	IM							
	SC							
	PO							
	IV							
	IP							
	IM							
	SC							
	PO							

PENTAGASTRIN

(Peptavlon, ICI 50123, AY-6608, Gastrodiagnost)

mg/kg		Mouse	Rat	Guinea Pig	Rabbit	Cat	Dog	Monkey
Lethal Dose Y-LD$_{50}$ Z-MLD	IV							
	IP							
	IM							
	SC							
	PO							
Gastrointestinal secretions ^{a}mg/kg/min ^{b}mg/kg/hr	IV		^{a}0.001 2060				^{b}0.0015*	
	IP							
	IM							
	SC		0.5 1435					
	PO							
Increase gastric blood flow	IV						0.001 1799	
	IP							
	IM							
	SC							
	PO							
	IV							
	IP							
	IM							
	SC							
	PO							
	IV							
	IP							
	IM							
	SC							
	PO							
	IV							
	IP							
	IM							
	SC							
	PO							
	IV							
	IP							
	IM							
	SC							
	PO							
	IV							
	IP							
	IM							
	SC							
	PO							

*1462

PENTAZOCINE

(Fortral, Talwin, Fortalin, Pentagin)

mg/kg		Mouse	Rat	Guinea Pig	Rabbit	Cat	Dog	Monkey	
Lethal Dose	IV								
Y-LD$_{50}$	IP								
Z-MLD	IM								
	SC								
	PO								
Behavioral	IV							[a]2.68 [1497]	
	IP								
[a]self	IM							3 [2061]	
administration	SC	6 [1483]							
	PO								
Analgesia	IV								
	IP								
	IM						2-4 [2273]		
[a]ED$_{50}$	SC	[a]1.35 [2063]	10 [2062]	[a]1.54 [1482]					
	PO								
Thermoregulatory	IV								
	IP								
	IM								
	SC	10 [1495]	5 [1496]						
	PO								
Sedative	IV								
	IP								
	IM								
[a]rotorod	SC	[a]42.8 [1482]							
	PO								
Substitutes	IV								
for morphine	IP								
in dependency	IM								
	SC	5 [1969]	5 [1969]						
	PO								
Antagonize	IV								
Straub tail	IP								
reaction	IM								
	SC	12 [2064]							
	PO								
Potentiate	IV								
morphine	IP								
analgesia	IM								
	SC	0.1 [2063]							
	PO								
Suppress	IV								
ACh	IP								
writhing	IM								
	SC	2.1 [1296]							
	PO								

PENTAZOCINE (continued)

mg/kg		Mouse	Rat	Guinea Pig	Rabbit	Cat	Dog	Monkey
Respiratory depression	IV							
	IP							
	IM							
	SC	0.6 1881						
	PO							
	IV							
	IP							
	IM							
	SC							
	PO							
	IV							
	IP							
	IM							
	SC							
	PO							
	IV							
	IP							
	IM							
	SC							
	PO							

IN VITRO

mg %	Cardiac	Vascular	Gut	Uterine	Visceral	Skeletal	
Cat	2.854 1754						

PENTOBARBITAL

(Dorsital, Nembutal, Palapent, Carbrital)

mg/kg		Mouse	Rat	Guinea Pig	Rabbit	Cat	Dog	Monkey
Lethal Dose Y-LD$_{50}$ Z-MLD	IV	Y80 [555]	Z50		Y45 [394]		62 [111]	
	IP	Y130 [555]	Y75	Y50 [556]	Z65 [129]	Z60 [449]	Z50	
	IM	Y124 [555]		Y70 [1235]				
	SC	Y107 [1075]	125 [66]					
	PO	Y280 [555]	Y118		Y275 [394]	Y100 [558]		
Anesthetic a see 1121 for sex differences	IV	35 [111]	25 [111]	30 [111]	30 [111]	25 [111]	30 [111]	25 [111]
	IP	60 [111]	a50 [111]	35 [111]	40 [111]	38 [111]	38 [111]	30 [111]
	IM		50 [902]	20 [1235]		15 [557]		
	SC						30 [111]	
	PO	80 [111]	50 [111]	50 [111]	45 [111]	50 [111]	50 [111]	45 [111]
Behavioral	IV				5 562	3.4 563		12 564
	IP	27.8 903	10 470					15 185
	IM							20 289
	SC		20 231				8 895	20 977
	PO	35 561	5 232			15 1108		20 929
EEG and ECP	IV				10 559	5	10 560	5 945
	IP		5 1069					
	IM							
	SC							
	PO						40 560	
Cardiovascular aTotal mg i. cranial	IV					6 565	10 560	
	IP					a0.5 [1471]		
	IM							
	SC							
	PO							
Neuronal membrane stabilization	IV					10 566		
	IP							
	IM							
	SC							
	PO							
Ataxic	IV	12.9 566			15 562			
	IP							
	IM							
	SC	30 1075	5 567					
	PO					15 1108		
Tremor	IV							
	IP					30 568		
	IM							
	SC							
	PO							
Increased serotonin (brain)	IV							
	IP		50 31					
	IM							
	SC							
	PO							

mg/kg		Mouse	Rat	Guinea Pig	Rabbit	Cat	Dog	Monkey	
CNS	IV		0.31 1664				25		
	IP	21 1452							
	IM								
	SC								
	PO	36 1391							
Anticonvulsant	IV								
	IP	26 1115							
	IM	20 1349							
	SC								
	PO								
Increased brain acetylcholine	IV								
	IP	55 1785	50 1209						
	IM								
	SC								
	PO								
Tolerance/ dependence [a]daily [b]IG	IV								
	IP		[a]100 2066						
	IM								
	SC								
	PO					[b]40 2067			
Analgesic	IV	11.8 1533							
	IP								
	IM								
	SC								
	PO								
Renal	IV		35 2068						
	IP								
	IM								
	SC								
	PO								
Thermoregulatory [a]BID	IV								
	IP		[a]30 2069						
	IM								
	SC								
	PO								

IN VITRO

mg %	Cardiac	Vascular	Gut	Uterine	Visceral	Skeletal	CNS	
Rat							0.770 2065	

PENTOLINIUM

(Ansolysen, Pentolonum, Pentolonium, Pentilium)

mg/kg		Mouse	Rat	Guinea Pig	Rabbit	Cat	Dog	Monkey	
Lethal Dose	IV	Y29 [214]							
Y-LD$_{50}$	IP	Y36 [214]							
Z-MLD	IM								
	SC								
	PO	Y512 [214]							
Ganglionic	IV					0.07 [113]	0.5		
block	IP		5 [381]						
	IM								
	SC								
	PO								
Epinephrine	IV					0.24 [154]			
sensitization	IP								
	IM								
	SC								
	PO								
Neuromuscular	IV						10 [214]		
block	IP								
	IM								
	SC								
	PO								
Cardiovascular	IV				10 [1133]				
	IP								
	IM								
	SC								
	PO								
	IV								
	IP								
	IM								
	SC								
	PO								
	IV								
	IP								
	IM								
	SC								
	PO								
	IV								
	IP								
	IM								
	SC								
	PO								
	IV								
	IP								
	IM								
	SC								
	PO								

PENTYLENETETRAZOL

(Cardiazol, Leptazol, Metrazol, Pentetrazole)

mg/kg		Mouse	Rat	Guinea Pig	Rabbit	Cat	Dog	Monkey
Lethal Dose Y-LD50 Z-MLD	IV	Y51 [962]	50 [569]		Z70 [572]	80 [570]	40	
	IP	Y92 [569]	Y70 [962]	90 [570]				
	IM							
	SC	Y101 [962]	Y100 [571]	85 [570]	87.5 [570]	75 [570]		
	PO	Y162 [962]	140 [962]					
Convulsant aED99	IV	48 [121]	20 [573]		20	11	20 [134]	
	IP	40.5 [284]	64 [121]	47.5 [961]			60 [962]	
	IM	40 [251]	100			50 [918]		64 [575]
	SC	a85 [2070]						
	PO	68 [284]	175 [574]					
Analeptic	IV				60	5-10 [2275]	5-10 [2275]	
	IP	10 [961]	57.5 [571]	40 [961]				
	IM					5-10 [2275]	5-10 [2275]	
	SC	19 [284]				5-10 [2275]	5-10 [2275]	
	PO					5-10 [2275]	5-10 [2275]	
Cardiovascular	IV			15 [157]			50 [410]	
	IP							
	IM							
	SC							
	PO							
Behavioral a daily, for tolerance	IV							
	IP		20 [1145]			20 [1068]		
	IM	50 [175]						
	SC							
	PO	50 [935]	a100 [1532]					
EEG	IV				100 [974]	10 [1039]		
	IP							
	IM							
	SC							
	PO							
	IV							
	IP							
	IM							
	SC							
	PO							
	IV							
	IP							
	IM							
	SC							
	PO							

PERGOLIDE

(Permax, LY 141B, LY 127809)

mg/kg		Mouse	Rat	Guinea Pig	Rabbit	Cat	Dog	Monkey	
Lethal Dose	IV								
Y-LD$_{50}$	IP								
Z-MLD	IM								
	SC								
	PO								
Affects	IV								
dopamine	IP		0.5 $_{1381}$						
release	IM								
	SC		0.005 $_{1402}$						
	PO								
Cardiovascular	IV						0.03 $_{2072}$		
	IP						[a]0.001$_{1565}$		
	IM								
[a]i. cisternal	SC		50 $_{2071}$						
	PO								
	IV								
	IP								
	IM								
	SC								
	PO								
	IV								
	IP								
	IM								
	SC								
	PO								
	IV								
	IP								
	IM								
	SC								
	PO								
	IV								
	IP								
	IM								
	SC								
	PO								
	IV								
	IP								
	IM								
	SC								
	PO								
	IV								
	IP								
	IM								
	SC								
	PO								

PERHEXILINE

(Pexid, Perhexilene)

mg/kg		Mouse	Rat	Guinea Pig	Rabbit	Cat	Dog	Monkey
Lethal Dose Y-LD$_{50}$ Z-MLD	IV							
	IP							
	IM							
	SC							
	PO							
Anti-ischemic (cardiac) [a]daily [b]mg/kg/min	IV						3 2073	
	IP						[b] 0.4 2275	
	IM							
	SC							
	PO						[a]200 2073	
	IV							
	IP							
	IM							
	SC							
	PO							
	IV							
	IP							
	IM							
	SC							
	PO							
	IV							
	IP							
	IM							
	SC							
	PO							
	IV							
	IP							
	IM							
	SC							
	PO							
	IV							
	IP							
	IM							
	SC							
	PO							
	IV							
	IP							
	IM							
	SC							
	PO							
	IV							
	IP							
	IM							
	SC							
	PO							

PERPHENAZINE
(Trilafon, Fentazin, PZC)

mg/kg			Mouse	Rat	Guinea Pig	Rabbit	Cat	Dog	Monkey	
Lethal Dose Y-LD$_{50}$ Z-MLD		IV	37 228	38 228			35 417	51 228		
		IP	Y70 1131	124 228						
		IM								
		SC								
		PO	120 228	318 228				100 228		
"Tranquilize"		IV				1.2 844	1 2275	0.5 2275	0.05 2275	
		IP	3.8 1119							
		IM					1 2275	0.5 228	0.2 576	
		SC	0.1 223	0.1 223			0.1 223	0.1 223	0.1 223	
		PO	1 223	1 223			1 223	1 223	1.5 223	
Behavioral		IV								
		IP	1 986	0.25 577			4 417			
		IM								
		SC	0.75 1040	0.4 578				0.4 1040	0.15 1041	
		PO	10 417	2 417			10 417	10 417		
Preanesthetic medication		IV					0.55 97	0.55 97		
		IP								
		IM					0.55 97	0.55 97		
		SC								
		PO		10 417			0.88 97	0.88 97		
Adrenolytic		IV					1 417	1 417		
		IP								
		IM								
		SC								
		PO								
Cardiovascular		IV				1 471	2 417	2 417		
		IP								
		IM								
		SC								
		PO								
EEG		IV				3 417				
		IP								
		IM								
		SC								
		PO								
Shock protection		IV						1 228		
		IP								
		IM		1.5 228						
		SC								
		PO								
Ataxic		IV						2 417		
		IP								
		IM								
		SC		10 1042						
		PO								

PERPHENAZINE (continued)

mg/kg		Mouse	Rat	Guinea Pig	Rabbit	Cat	Dog	Monkey
Decerebrate rigidity abolished	IV					0.4 844		
	IP							
	IM							
	SC							
	PO							
Catalepsy	IV							
	IP		5 2048					
	IM							
	SC							
	PO							
Effects on endocrine function & growth [a]daily	IV							
	IP							
	IM							
	SC							
	PO		[a]10 2074					
	IV							
	IP							
	IM							
	SC							
	PO							
	IV							
	IP							
	IM							
	SC							
	PO							
	IV							
	IP							
	IM							
	SC							
	PO							
	IV							
	IP							
	IM							
	SC							
	PO							
	IV							
	IP							
	IM							
	SC							
	PO							

PHENACEMIDE

(Phenurone, Epiclase, Phenylacetylurea)

mg/kg		Mouse	Rat	Guinea Pig	Rabbit	Cat	Dog	Monkey	
Lethal Dose	IV								
Y-LD_{50}	IP								
Z-MLD	IM								
	SC								
	PO	Y5000 [111]			3500 [111]	2000 [111]	3500 [111]		
Anticonvulsant	IV								
	IP	80 [933]							
	IM								
	SC								
	PO	300 [111]	21 [851]		300 [111]	25-50 [2275]	25-50 [2275]		
Behavioral	IV								
	IP								
	IM								
	SC								
	PO	205							
Ataxic	IV								
	IP								
	IM								
	SC								
	PO	400 [111]							
	IV								
	IP								
	IM								
	SC								
	PO								
	IV								
	IP								
	IM								
	SC								
	PO								
	IV								
	IP								
	IM								
	SC								
	PO								
	IV								
	IP								
	IM								
	SC								
	PO								
	IV								
	IP								
	IM								
	SC								
	PO								

PHENACETIN

(Acetophenetidin, Acetphenetidin)

mg/kg		Mouse	Rat	Guinea Pig	Rabbit	Cat	Dog	Monkey	
Lethal Dose	IV								
Y-LD$_{50}$	IP								
Z-MLD	IM								
	SC								
	PO	Y2015 2075							
Inhibit	IV								
acetic	IP								
acid	IM								
writhing	SC								
	PO	132 1291							
Behavioral	IV								
[a]IG self	IP								
administration	IM								
	SC								
	PO							[a]5 1611	
Protects from	IV								
acetaminophen	IP	300 2076							
hepatotoxicosis	IM								
	SC								
	PO								
Analgesic	IV								
Antipyretic	IP								
	IM								
	SC								
	PO	100 2275	200 2275			10-15 2275	10-30 2275		
	IV								
	IP								
	IM								
	SC								
	PO								
	IV								
	IP								
	IM								
	SC								
	PO								
	IV								
	IP								
	IM								
	SC								
	PO								
	IV								
	IP								
	IM								
	SC								
	PO								

PHENCYCLIDINE
(Sernylan, PCP, Sernyl, CI-395)

mg/kg		Mouse	Rat	Guinea Pig	Rabbit	Cat	Dog	Monkey
Lethal Dose	IV							
Y-LD$_{50}$	IP	79.24 [1861]						
Z-MLD	IM							
	SC							
	PO							
Anesthetic	IV					1.1 [1232]		1 [1073]
	IP							
	IM					[a]0.5-1 [2275]	[a]5-7 [2275]	1.5 [1073]
[a]immobilize	SC							
	PO							
Convulsant	IV							4 [1073]
	IP	50 [1073]						
	IM							
	SC							
	PO							
Behavioral	IV		[b]0.5 [1866]				[a]0.00625*	[a]0.03 [1654]
	IP	5.12 [1761]	1 [2078]					
[a]self adminis.	IM							0.03 [2079]
[b]mg/kg/hr	SC							
	PO		8 [2077]					0.32 [1655]
Tolerance/	IV			[a]45 [2080]				[b]0.05 [2081]
dependence	IP							
[a]mg/kg/day	IM							0.01 [2081]
infusion	SC							
[b]mg/kg/hr,10days	PO							1.5 [1389]
Ataxia	IV							
	IP	4.93 [1861]						
	IM							
	SC							
	PO							
Alter	IV							
brain	IP	2 [2082]	4 [2083]					
chemistry	IM							
	SC							
	PO							

*1864

IN VITRO

mg %	Cardiac	Vascular	Gut	Uterine	Visceral	Skeletal	
Guinea Pig	0.28 [2085]				0.028 [2084]		
Rat	0.28 [2085]						

PHENELZINE

(Nardil, Nardelzine, Phenodyn)

mg/kg		Mouse	Rat	Guinea Pig	Rabbit	Cat	Dog	Monkey
Lethal Dose	IV	Y157 115						
Y-LD$_{50}$	IP							
Z-MLD	IM							
	SC	Y150 1046						
	PO	Y156 115	210 455					
Analgesic	IV							
	IP							
[a]opioid	IM							
interactions	SC	[a]100 2087						
	PO	12 582						
Respiratory	IV							
	IP	10 455						
	IM							
	SC							
	PO	15 455						
Monoamine	IV	48 608						
oxidase	IP	32 608	10 1118					
inhibition	IM							
[a]daily	SC		10 1046					
	PO		10 1046				[a]4.5 2086	
Cardiovascular	IV					0.6 608	5 583	
	IP					15 608		
	IM							
	SC							
	PO							
Behavioral	IV							
	IP		5 848					
	IM							
	SC							
	PO							
	IV							
	IP							
	IM							
	SC							
	PO							
	IV							
	IP							
	IM							
	SC							
	PO							
	IV							
	IP							
	IM							
	SC							
	PO							

PHENIPRAZINE

(Catron, Catral, Catroniazid)

mg/kg		Mouse	Rat	Guinea Pig	Rabbit	Cat	Dog	Monkey	
Lethal Dose Y-LD_{50} Z-MLD	IV	Y60.6 460	Y44.5 460			35 584			
	IP	Y122	50						
	IM								
	SC	Y95 460	Y45.3 460			35 584			
	PO	Y73 460	Y34.1 460						
Monoamine-oxidase inhibition	IV	3 430			3 430	1.5	5 372		
	IP	10 2088	20 584				15		
	IM		10 867						
	SC	3 430			2 430	1.5 91			
	PO								
CNS Behavioral	IV				5 584	25 584	10 586		
	IP	50 585	30 585				25 584		
	IM								
	SC		20 460		2 430	25 584			
	PO								
Cardiovascular	IV		10 218	5	5	5	5 372		
	IP								
	IM								
	SC								
	PO								
Barbiturate sleep potentiation	IV								
	IP	10 585	10 585						
	IM								
	SC								
	PO								
Reverse reserpine effects	IV								
	IP	13.5 1292							
	IM								
	SC								
	PO								
	IV								
	IP								
	IM								
	SC								
	PO								
	IV								
	IP								
	IM								
	SC								
	PO								
	IV								
	IP								
	IM								
	SC								
	PO								

PHENOBARBITAL
(Luminal, Solfoton, Gardenal)

mg/kg		Mouse	Rat	Guinea Pig	Rabbit	Cat	Dog	Monkey
Lethal Dose $Y\text{-}LD_{50}$ $Z\text{-}MLD$	IV				$Y185_{122}$	100_{1232}		
	IP	$Y340_{122}$	$Y190_{122}$		$Z150_{588}$	150_{1232}		
	IM				$Z150_{128}$			
	SC	$Y230$	$Y200_{68}$					
	PO	$Y325_{391}$	$Y660_{587}$		$Z150_{588}$	$Y175_{558}$		
Anesthetic [a] total mg	IV	134_{65}	100_{589}		200_{590}	$^{a}60_{97}$	80_{591}	
	IP			100		180	150	100
	IM					$^{a}60_{97}$	30_{557}	
	SC	96					30_{557}	
	PO	107		30_{76}		$^{a}60_{97}$	150	125
Anticonvulsant [a] total mg	IV				25_{594}	20_{846}	25_{594}	
	IP	22.8_{1452}	25_{592}					15_{595}
	IM							15_{1096}
	SC	12.5_{2089}	30_{414}		50			
	PO	25	25_{593}	70_{1047}		$^{a}45_{24}$	$^{a}150_{24}$	
Behavioral	IV						1_{947}	
	IP	100_{933}	15_{470}			40_{1147}		27_{1230}
	IM	40_{175}	30_{230}					
	SC		39_{596}					
	PO	90_{505}	80_{934}	4_{1047}		40_{1165}	75_{597}	
Cardiovascular [a] total mg/d, propranolol interaction	IV				50_{598}		20_{599}	
	IP							
	IM							
	SC							
	PO						$^{a}180_{2094}$	
Ataxic	IV							
	IP							
	IM							
	SC	69_{1075}	88_{596}					
	PO	250_{484}				40_{1165}		
Induction [a] 7 days	IV							
	IP		80_{1363}					
	IM							
	SC		$^{a}70_{2090}$					
	PO							
Antagonize LiCl taste aversion [a] ED_{50}	IV							
	IP		$^{a}21.7_{1528}$					
	IM							
	SC							
	PO		$^{a}10.8_{1528}$					
CNS [a] daily [b] neurotoxic TD_{50}	IV		80_{1664}					
	IP	$^{b}64.9_{1452}$	40_{1448}					
	IM							
	SC							
	PO		$^{a}2.5_{2091}$					

mg/kg		Mouse	Rat	Guinea Pig	Rabbit	Cat	Dog	Monkey	
Teratogenic	IV								
	IP								
	IM								
	SC								
	PO		80 2092						
Block	IV								
stress	IP		10 1902						
reaction	IM								
(corticoid	SC								
release)	PO								
Enhance	IV								
acetaminophen	IP								
toxicosis	IM								
	SC								
	PO	150 2093							
Antidiuretic	IV						40 591		
	IP								
	IM								
	SC				120 591				
	PO								
Reflex	IV					10 564			
depressant	IP								
	IM								
	SC								
	PO								
EEG	IV				40 1223	40 843			
	IP					20 1009			
	IM								
	SC								
	PO				40 1012				
Tranquilize	IV								
	IP								
	IM								
[a]ED_{50}	SC								
	PO	[a]40.5 1372							

IN VITRO

mg %	Cardiac	Vascular	Gut	Uterine	Visceral	Skeletal	CNS	
Rat							48.77 2065	

PHENOXYBENZAMINE

(Dibenyline, Dibenzyline, Dibenzyran)

mg/kg		Mouse	Rat	Guinea Pig	Rabbit	Cat	Dog	Monkey
Lethal Dose Y-LD$_{50}$ Z-MLD	IV						Z10 [82]	
	IP							
	IM							
	SC							
	PO	Y1535 [82]	Y2500 [82]	Y500 [82]				
Adrenolytic (α-block)	IV	5 [1197]	0.031 [253]	15 [220]	3 [404]	10 [2095]		
	IP		1 [383]					
	IM	10 [1440]						
	SC							
	PO					0.25-0.5*	0.25-0.5*	
CNS	IV				1.5 [87]	0.6 [873]		
	IP	5 [350]	1 [1243]			10 [1100]		
	IM							
	SC		5 [350]					
	PO							
Catecholamine depletion	IV			10 [901]	20 [816]			
	IP		10 [600]					
	IM							
	SC							
	PO							
Cardiovascular [a]mg/min IC	IV		2 [2096]		1 [1133]	5 [1085]	1 [2097]	
	IP		20 [2099]	100 [1219]			[a]0.37 [2098]	
	IM							
	SC							
	PO		50 [387]					
EEG (synchronization)	IV				1.5 [298]			
	IP							
	IM							
	SC							
	PO							
Shock (therapy)	IV						0.1	
	IP							
	IM							
	SC							
	PO							
Catecholamine interactions	IV				5 [1182]			
	IP	20 [1932]						
	IM							
	SC							
	PO							
Behavioral	IV							
	IP	20 [1890]	2.5 [1871]					
	IM							
	SC							
	PO	185 [1372]						

*2273

mg/kg		Mouse	Rat	Guinea Pig	Rabbit	Cat	Dog	Monkey	
Opiate interactions	IV								
	IP		10 1910						
	IM								
	SC	2.5 1308							
	PO								
	IV								
	IP								
	IM								
	SC								
	PO								
	IV								
	IP								
	IM								
	SC								
	PO								
	IV								
	IP								
	IM								
	SC								
	PO								

IN VITRO

mg %	Cardiac	Vascular	Gut	Uterine	Visceral	Skeletal		
Adrenolytic		0.005		0.005	0.006			
Spasmolytic			0.1 1223					
Dog		0.3038 1729						
Anti-5HT			0.03 92					

PHENTOLAMINE
(C-7337, Regitine, Rogitine)

mg/kg		Mouse	Rat	Guinea Pig	Rabbit	Cat	Dog	Monkey
Lethal Dose Y-LD$_{50}$ Z-MLD	IV		Y75[603]					
	IP							
	IM							
	SC		Y275[603]					
	PO	Y1000[119]	Y1250[603]					
Adrenolytic (α-block)	IV		10[218]		3[305]	2[497]	1[408]	
	IP	4[939]		10[1219]				
	IM	5[1440]	5[1423]					
	SC				1[603]	1[603]	1[603]	
	PO						20[1082]	
CNS	IV				0.25[914]			
	IP	5[1544]						
	IM							
	SC							
	PO	150[119]						
Cardiovascular [a]Total mg ICV	IV		10[2101]		5[2275]	0.5[821]	0.5[2102]	
	IP		25[2275]				[a]0.1[1568]	
	IM							
	SC							
	PO							
Anticonvulsant	IV							
	IP							
	IM							
	SC	10[957]						
	PO							
Bronchiole dilatation	IV							
	IP							
	IM							
	SC			4.5[1081]				
	PO							
Increase norepinephrine from spleen	IV					3[901]		
	IP							
	IM							
	SC							
	PO							
Antagonize morphine [a]total mg ICV	IV	[a]0.001[1943]						
	IP		10[1384]					
	IM							
	SC	0.05[1944]						
	PO							
Behavioral	IV							
	IP		2.5[1871]					
	IM							
	SC							
	PO							

mg/kg		Mouse	Rat	Guinea Pig	Rabbit	Cat	Dog	Monkey	
Antagonize cocaine hepatotoxicosis	IV								
	IP	5 1603							
	IM								
	SC								
	PO								
	IV								
	IP								
	IM								
	SC								
	PO								
	IV								
	IP								
	IM								
	SC								
	PO								
	IV								
	IP								
	IM								
	SC								
	PO								

IN VITRO

mg %	Cardiac	Vascular	Gut	Uterine	Visceral	Skeletal	Trachea	
Adrenolytic		0.008 1157	0.01 604					
Anti-5HT			0.1 92					
Rabbit		0.0281 2100	0.04 1157					
Dog		0.0281 2039					0.2814*	

*1800

PHENYLBUTAZONE

(Azolid, Butazolidin, Reudox)

mg/kg		Mouse	Rat	Guinea Pig	Rabbit	Cat	Dog	Monkey
Lethal Dose	IV	Y123 605						
Y-LD$_{50}$	IP	Y336 17	Y215 605					
Z-MLD	IM							
	SC							
	PO	417.5 1526	Y650 923					
Analgesic	IV				100 50		22 2273	
	IP	150 50						
	IM							
	SC	5.6 908						
	PO	200 923		300 923			10-15 2273	
Anti-inflammatory	IV						22 2273	
	IP		100 928					
	IM							
	SC		200 50					
	PO		90 326	1800 55				
Antipyretic	IV						22 2273	
	IP							
	IM							
	SC					20 905		
	PO	200 935	12.5 905				10-15 2273	
Antibradykinin	IV							
	IP		32 908					
	IM							
	SC							
	PO						15 1311	
Renal	IV						2 2104	
	IP							
	IM							
	SC							
	PO		3 1312					
Antiarthritic	IV							
	IP							
	IM							
	SC							
	PO		100 2103					

IN VITRO

mg %	Cardiac	Vascular	Gut	Uterine	Visceral	Skeletal	Liver
Rat			3.08 1845			10.48 1829	

PHENYLEPHRINE

(Efrin, Adrianol, Meta-Sympatol, Neosynephrine)

mg/kg		Mouse	Rat	Guinea Pig	Rabbit	Cat	Dog	Monkey	
Lethal Dose	IV	Y21 840	6.8 607						
Y-LD$_{50}$	IP	Y1000					16 840		
Z-MLD	IM								
	SC	Y70 840	Y92 1128						
	PO	Y120 840	Y350 1128						
Cardiovascular	IV		[a]3 2105	5 1579	0.05 1419	0.01 840	0.03 408	0.001 2017	
	IP	2 840					[a]0.012 1438		
[a]mg/kg/hr	IM						[b]0.008 2102		
[b]total mg,	SC								
perfused leg	PO	50 840							
CNS	IV								
(stimulant)	IP								
	IM								
	SC						0.5		
	PO								
	IV								
	IP								
	IM								
	SC								
	PO								

IN VITRO

mg %	Cardiac	Vascular	Gut	Uterine	Visceral	Skeletal		
Rabbit	0.04		0.01					
Rat			0.002 1583					
Monkey		0.0159 1569						
Dog		0.001 2107						

PHENYLPROPANOLAMINE

(Monydrin, Mydriatine, Propadrine)

mg/kg		Mouse	Rat	Guinea Pig	Rabbit	Cat	Dog	Monkey	
Lethal Dose	IV								
Y-LD$_{50}$	IP								
Z-MLD	IM								
	SC								
	PO								
Affect	IV								
food	IP								
intake	IM								
	SC								
[a]IG	PO							[a]1 2108	
Behavioral	IV							0.3 2108	
	IP								
	IM								
[a]IG	SC								
	PO							[a]30 2108	
CNS	IV								
dopamine	IP								
depletion	IM								
	SC		200 2108						
	PO								
Vasoconstriction	IV								
Bronchodilation	IP								
	IM					2 2275	4 2275		
	SC					2 2275	4 2275		
	PO						8 2275		
	IV								
	IP								
	IM								
	SC								
	PO								
	IV								
	IP								
	IM								
	SC								
	PO								
	IV								
	IP								
	IM								
	SC								
	PO								
	IV								
	IP								
	IM								
	SC								
	PO								

PHENYTOIN

(Dilantin, Diphenylhydantoin, Dilabid)

mg/kg		Mouse	Rat	Guinea Pig	Rabbit	Cat	Dog	Monkey
Lethal Dose Y-LD_{50} Z-MLD	IV			Z160 610	Y125 70		Z90 610	
	IP	Y200 609	Y280 70					
	IM							
	SC							
	PO	Y490 226	Z>2200 610					
Anticonvulsant [a]Q24h [b]Q8h	IV					30 613	10 2272	
	IP	20 611	135 612		60			
	IM							15 1097
	SC	25 2089	7.4 2089		55			
	PO	50	2200 610		35 1012	[a]2-3 2272	[b]30 2272	
Toxic dose (emesis)	IV							
	IP	800	200		40 1068			
	IM							
	SC							
	PO	84 226						
Tremorine antagonist	IV							
	IP							
	IM	99 140						
	SC							
	PO	60 1131						
Behavioral [a]2 consecutive days	IV						40 1048	
	IP		50 1145					
	IM		50 230			[a]15 1229		
	SC							
	PO							
Cardiovascular	IV				30 818	2-20 1211	5 818	
	IP							
	IM							
	SC							
	PO						8-15 2273	
Hepatic enzyme inhibition	IV							
	IP		10 2109					
	IM							
	SC							
	PO							
Teratogenic	IV							
	IP							
	IM							
	SC	50 2110						
	PO		200 2092					
Decrease humoral immunity	IV							
	IP							
	IM							
	SC							
	PO	100 2111						

mg/kg		Mouse	Rat	Guinea Pig	Rabbit	Cat	Dog	Monkey	
Antispastic	IV					[a]40 2112			
	IP								
	IM								
[a]decerebrate	SC								
	PO								
Quinidine	IV						16.3 2113		
interaction	IP								
(pharmaco-	IM								
kinetics)	SC								
[a]total mg daily	PO						[a]700 2113		
EEG	IV				40 1223	20 1222			
	IP								
	IM								
	SC								
	PO								
Vagus	IV						20 818		
nerve	IP								
depression	IM								
	SC								
	PO								
Respiratory	IV				30 818		20 818		
depression	IP								
	IM								
	SC								
	PO								
Uterine	IV				40 819		20 819		
activity	IP								
depression	IM								
	SC								
	PO								

IN VITRO

mg %	Cardiac	Vascular	Gut	Uterine	Visceral	Skeletal		
Rabbit				0.1 819				

PHYSOSTIGMINE

(Antilirium, Isopto Eserine, Eserine)

mg/kg		Mouse	Rat	Guinea Pig	Rabbit	Cat	Dog	Monkey	
Lethal Dose	IV	0.5 519				0.4 614	0.25 614		
Y-LD50	IP	Y1 907							
Z-MLD	IM								
	SC	Y0.54 2114			3 519				
	PO	Y3 115							
Cholinergic	IV		0.02 2275			0.3 1444	0.5		
	IP	0.5 1785							
[a]total mg	IM		0.1-1 2275			[a]0.3-0.5*	[a]0.3-2*		
	SC				1 88	0.5 944	[a]0.3-2*		
	PO					[a]0.3-0.5*	[a]0.3-2*		
EEG	IV				0.3 60	0.1 1034			
(desynchroni-	IP								
zation	IM								
	SC								
	PO								
Behavioral	IV					0.3 1034	0.1	0.3 871	
	IP	0.5 852	0.8 1144			0.2 1100			
	IM								
	SC	0.3 856	1 1049			10 944			
	PO	1 935							
Increased	IV					1.5 379			
spinal cord	IP								
inhibition	IM								
	SC								
	PO								
Bulbocapnine	IV				0.1 288				
potentiation	IP	0.05 615							
	IM								
	SC								
	PO								
Tremor	IV								
	IP	5 369	0.75 1118						
	IM								
	SC								
	PO								
Hypothermic	IV								
	IP	0.5 1087							
	IM								
	SC								
	PO								
Cardiovascular	IV		0.05 2115		[b]0.275 1315				
	IP		[a]0.005 2116						
	IM								
[a]total mg ICV	SC								
[b]mg% in situ	PO								

*2275

PHYSOSTIGMINE (continued)

mg/kg		Mouse	Rat	Guinea Pig	Rabbit	Cat	Dog	Monkey	
Opioid interactions [a]mg/kg/min	IV		0.08 1753		[a]0.005 2117				
	IP								
	IM								
	SC	0.5 2050							
	PO								
	IV								
	IP								
	IM								
	SC								
	PO								
	IV								
	IP								
	IM								
	SC								
	PO								
	IV								
	IP								
	IM								
	SC								
	PO								

IN VITRO

mg %	Cardiac	Vascular	Gut	Uterine	Visceral	Skeletal		
Rabbit	0.025		0.5					
Rat						0.01 1157		
Guinea Pig	0.08 1157							

PICENADOL

(LY 150720)

mg/kg		Mouse	Rat	Guinea Pig	Rabbit	Cat	Dog	Monkey	
Lethal Dose	IV								
Y-LD$_{50}$	IP								
Z-MLD	IM								
	SC								
	PO								
Analgesic	IV								
	IP								
^{a}ED$_{50}$	IM							0.1 $_{2118}$	
	SC	^{a}0.38 $_{1482}$	^{a}0.98 $_{1482}$						
	PO								
Sedative	IV								
	IP								
^{a}rotorod test	IM								
	SC	^{a}26.1 $_{1482}$							
	PO								
	IV								
	IP								
	IM								
	SC								
	PO								
	IV								
	IP								
	IM								
	SC								
	PO								
	IV								
	IP								
	IM								
	SC								
	PO								
	IV								
	IP								
	IM								
	SC								
	PO								
	IV								
	IP								
	IM								
	SC								
	PO								
	IV								
	IP								
	IM								
	SC								
	PO								

PICOLINIC ACID

mg/kg		Mouse	Rat	Guinea Pig	Rabbit	Cat	Dog	Monkey
Lethal Dose	IV							
Y-LD$_{50}$	IP							
Z-MLD	IM							
	SC							
	PO							
Restore	IV							
dopamine	IP	[a]36.7 $_{1292}$						
following L-dopa	IM							
[a]reserpinized	SC							
	PO							
Antagonize	IV							
anticonvulsant	IP	39.5 $_{2119}$						
action of	IM							
methazolamide	SC							
	PO							
	IV							
	IP							
	IM							
	SC							
	PO							
	IV							
	IP							
	IM							
	SC							
	PO							
	IV							
	IP							
	IM							
	SC							
	PO							
	IV							
	IP							
	IM							
	SC							
	PO							
	IV							
	IP							
	IM							
	SC							
	PO							
	IV							
	IP							
	IM							
	SC							
	PO							

PICROTOXIN

mg/kg		Mouse	Rat	Guinea Pig	Rabbit	Cat	Dog	Monkey
Lethal Dose Y-LD$_{50}$ Z-MLD	IV	Z4	Y3 $_{166}$		Z1.25 $_{617}$			
	IP	Y7.2 $_{284}$	Y6.5 $_{166}$					
	IM							
	SC	Y7.04 $_{284}$	4.7 $_{616}$	3 $_{109}$	Z2.5 $_{617}$		2.2 $_{109}$	
	PO	Y14.8 $_{284}$						
Analeptic	IV			12.6 $_{1235}$	3		0.3	
	IP	10 $_{123}$				1.5 $_{618}$	0.3	
	IM						0.3	
	SC	1.6 $_{284}$					0.3	
	PO							
CNS (stimulant) [a]total mg	IV	2.9 $_{121}$	2.9 $_{121}$		0.89 $_{121}$	0.2 $_{854}$	[a]2 $_{24}$	
	IP		9 $_{130}$			0.5 $_{1068}$		
	IM							
	SC	5.9 $_{121}$	3 $_{617}$					
	PO							
Convulsant	IV	1.95 $_{1470}$				0.3 $_{134}$		
	IP	12 $_{2122}$						
	IM							
	SC	3.14 $_{284}$			3 $_{869}$			
	PO	8.43 $_{284}$						
Behavioral	IV							
	IP							
	IM	1 $_{175}$						
	SC		0.5 $_{1050}$					
	PO							
Cardiovascular [a]IA [b]total mg ICV	IV					0.5 $_{2120}$	2 $_{886}$	
	IP					[a]0.2 $_{2121}$		
	IM					[b]0.6 $_{2121}$		
	SC							
	PO							
Effects on urinary bladder	IV		2 ^{1467}					
	IP							
	IM							
	SC							
	PO							
Sympathetic nervous effects	IV					0.25 $_{1469}$		
	IP							
	IM							
	SC							
	PO							
Motor neuron effects	IV					0.9 $_{1451}$		
	IP							
	IM							
	SC							
	PO							

PILOCARPINE

(Adsorbocarpine, Almocarpine, Isopto Carpine)

mg/kg		Mouse	Rat	Guinea Pig	Rabbit	Cat	Dog	Monkey	
Lethal Dose	IV				175 $_{109}$				
Y-LD$_{50}$	IP	Y500							
Z-MLD	IM								
	SC								
	PO								
Cholinergic	IV						3		
	IP								
^{a}total mg	IM					^{a}2 $_{24}$	^{a}12 $_{24}$		
	SC	2 $_{2048}$	160 $_{619}$		5	^{a}2 $_{24}$	0.75		
	PO					^{a}0.5-2 $_{2275}$			
Anticonvulsant	IV								
	IP								
	IM								
	SC	160 $_{620}$	26 $_{620}$						
	PO								
Spinal Cord	IV					80 $_{900}$			
inhibition	IP								
blocked	IM								
	SC								
	PO								
Hypothermic	IV								
	IP	10 $_{1087}$	5 $_{1111}$						
	IM								
	SC								
	PO								
EEG	IV				0.64 $_{1099}$				
(arousal)	IP								
	IM								
	SC								
	PO								
Decrease	IV		0.5 $_{2275}$						
blood	IP								
pressure	IM								
	SC								
	PO								

IN VITRO

mg %	Cardiac	Vascular	Gut	Uterine	Visceral	Skeletal		
Rabbit	0.5		1	1				

PIMOZIDE

(Orap, Opiran, R 6238)

mg/kg		Mouse	Rat	Guinea Pig	Rabbit	Cat	Dog	Monkey
Lethal Dose	IV							
Y-LD$_{50}$	IP							
Z-MLD	IM							
	SC							
	PO							
Behavioral	IV				0.308 1790			
	IP	0.4 1416	0.3 1595					
	IM							
	SC							
	PO							
Decreased	IV							
motor	IP	0.2 1416						
activity	IM							
	SC							
	PO							
Dopamine	IV							
blockade	IP							
	IM							
	SC	1.25 2123	0.25 2124					
	PO							
Alter	IV							
brain	IP	5 1547						
chemistry	IM							
	SC							
	PO							
Antagonize	IV							
apomorphine	IP	0.2 1414						
	IM							
	SC							
	PO							
Thermoregulatory	IV							
	IP	[a]4 1413	1 1337					
	IM							
[a]apomorphine	SC							
interaction	PO							
Opioid	IV							
interactions	IP	0.25 1417						
	IM							
	SC							
	PO							
Antagonize	IV							
L-dopa-induced	IP							
hypoglycemia	IM							
	SC	0.5 1456						
	PO							

PIPEROXAN

(Benzdioxane, 933F, Benodaine)

mg/kg		Mouse	Rat	Guinea Pig	Rabbit	Cat	Dog	Monkey	
Lethal Dose	IV								
Y-LD$_{50}$	IP								
Z-MLD	IM								
	SC								
	PO								
Behavioral	IV								
	IP		40 1575						
	IM								
	SC								
	PO								
Antagonize	IV								
antiaggressive	IP								
property	IM								
of clonidine	SC	5 1560							
	PO								
α-Adrenergic	IV								
antagonism	IP								
	IM	5 1440							
	SC								
	PO								
	IV								
	IP								
	IM								
	SC								
	PO								
	IV								
	IP								
	IM								
	SC								
	PO								
	IV								
	IP								
	IM								
	SC								
	PO								
	IV								
	IP								
	IM								
	SC								
	PO								
	IV								
	IP								
	IM								
	SC								
	PO								

PIPRADROL

(Meratonic, Metadin, Stimolag Fortis)

mg/kg		Mouse	Rat	Guinea Pig	Rabbit	Cat	Dog	Monkey	
Lethal Dose	IV		Y30 [115]		Y15 [117]				
Y-LD$_{50}$	IP	Y94 [115]							
Z-MLD	IM								
[a]caged	SC	Y240 [115]	Y240 [117]						
individually	PO	[a]Y365 [960]	Y180 [115]						
CNS	IV		6 [117]						
stimulant and	IP	10 [323]							
increased	IM								
motor activity	SC	20 [204]	2.74 [85]						
	PO	50 [960]							
Analeptic	IV				12.5 [117]		2 [133]		
	IP		20 [621]						
	IM								
	SC								
	PO								
Cardiovascular	IV					8 [117]			
	IP								
	IM								
	SC								
	PO								
Behavioral	IV								
	IP		5 [622]						
	IM								
	SC						1 [1051]		
	PO								
	IV								
	IP								
	IM								
	SC								
	PO								
	IV								
	IP								
	IM								
	SC								
	PO								
	IV								
	IP								
	IM								
	SC								
	PO								
	IV								
	IP								
	IM								
	SC								
	PO								

PIRIBEDIL

(EU-4200, ET-495, Trivastal)

mg/kg		Mouse	Rat	Guinea Pig	Rabbit	Cat	Dog	Monkey
Lethal Dose	IV							
Y-LD$_{50}$	IP							
Z-MLD	IM							
	SC							
	PO							
Stimulant	IV							
	IP	20 [1697]						
	IM							
	SC							
	PO							
Induce	IV							
circling	IP	40 [1697]						
	IM							
	SC							
	PO							
Reverse	IV							
reserpine-	IP	50 [1932]						
induced	IM							
akinesia	SC							
	PO							
Decrease	IV							
audiogenic	IP	100 [1697]						
seizure	IM							
	SC							
	PO							
	IV							
	IP							
	IM							
	SC							
	PO							
	IV							
	IP							
	IM							
	SC							
	PO							
	IV							
	IP							
	IM							
	SC							
	PO							
	IV							
	IP							
	IM							
	SC							
	PO							

PIROXICAM
(Feldene, CP-16171)

mg/kg		Mouse	Rat	Guinea Pig	Rabbit	Cat	Dog	Monkey
Lethal Dose	IV							
Y-LD$_{50}$	IP							
Z-MLD	IM							
	SC							
	PO							
Anti-inflammatory	IV		4.1 $_{1310}$					
	IP							
	IM							
	SC							
	PO							
Decrease bladder contraction	IV		0.11 $_{1310}$					
	IP							
	IM							
	SC							
	PO							
	IV							
	IP							
	IM							
	SC							
	PO							

IN VITRO

mg %	Cardiac	Vascular	Gut	Uterine	Visceral	Skeletal	Hepatocytes
Rat							13.25 $_{1829}$

POTASSIUM CYANIDE

mg/kg		Mouse	Rat	Guinea Pig	Rabbit	Cat	Dog	Monkey	
Lethal Dose	IV	Z2.5 108	Z2.5 195				5		
Y-LD$_{50}$	IP	Z6 109							
Z-MLD	IM		8						
	SC	Y6.02 273	Z17 195						
	PO	Y16 623	Z12.5 195		Y5		1.6 624		
Vagal	IV					0.03 625			
bradycardia	IP								
potentiation	IM								
	SC								
	PO								
Increased O$_2$	IV								
consumption	IP								
	IM								
	SC		9.6 826						
	PO								
	IV								
	IP								
	IM								
	SC								
	PO								

IN VITRO

mg %	Cardiac	Vascular	Gut	Uterine	Visceral	Skeletal	Hepatocytes	
							13.25 1829	

PRACTOLOL
(AY-21011 ICI, 50172, Dalzic, Eraldin)

mg/kg		Mouse	Rat	Guinea Pig	Rabbit	Cat	Dog	Monkey
Lethal Dose	IV							
Y-LD$_{50}$	IP							
Z-MLD	IM							
	SC							
	PO							
ß-Adrenergic	IV							
blockade	IP	30 [1670]						
	IM							
	SC							
	PO							
Cardiovascular	IV				1 [1427]		1 [2125]	
	IP							
	IM							
	SC							
	PO							
Ocular	IV							
toxicosis	IP							
	IM							
[a]daily	SC							
	PO						[a]100 [2126]	
Local	IV	[a]64 [2127]		[a]8.8 [2127]				
anesthetic	IP							
	IM							
	SC							
[a]mg/ml	PO							
Increase	IV			5 [2127]				
severity of	IP							
anaphylactic	IM							
bronchospasm	SC							
	PO							
50% decrease	IV					0.16 [2127]	0.61 [2127]	
in isoprenaline	IP							
tachycardia	IM							
	SC							
	PO					2 [2127]	64 [2127]	
50% decrease	IV					1.6 [2127]	5.3 [2127]	
in isoprenaline	IP							
diastolic	IM							
hypotension	SC							
	PO					45 [2127]	14 [2127]	
	IV							
	IP							
	IM							
	SC							
	PO							

PRACTOLOL (continued)

mg/kg		Mouse	Rat	Guinea Pig	Rabbit	Cat	Dog	Monkey
	IV							
	IP							
	IM							
	SC							
	PO							
	IV							
	IP							
	IM							
	SC							
	PO							
	IV							
	IP							
	IM							
	SC							
	PO							
	IV							
	IP							
	IM							
	SC							
	PO							

IN VITRO

mg %	Cardiac	Vascular	Gut	Uterine	Visceral	Skeletal		
Rat				0.266 1583				
Rabbit	15 2127							

381

PRAZOSIN

(Minipress, Hypovase, Sinetens)

mg/kg		Mouse	Rat	Guinea Pig	Rabbit	Cat	Dog	Monkey
Lethal Dose	IV							
Y-LD$_{50}$	IP							
Z-MLD	IM							
	SC							
	PO							
Cardiovascular	IV		0.1 $_{2128}$			1 $_{1868}$	0.1 $_{2129}$	
[a]mg/min IC	IP		[c]0.02 $_{1997}$	2 $_{1579}$			[a]0.1 $_{2098}$	
[b]i. cisternal	IM						[c]0.001$_{2130}$	
[c]ICV	SC							
[d]total mg	PO		1 $_{2132}$				[d] 1-2 $_{2272}$	
Tolerance	IV							
	IP							
	IM							
[a]daily	SC							
	PO		[a]3 $_{2132}$					
Effects on	IV							
GI	IP							
secretions	IM		5 $_{1423}$					
	SC							
	PO							
Effects on	IV		0.01 $_{1425}$					
salivation	IP							
	IM							
	SC							
	PO							
Antagonize	IV		[a]0.1 $_{1812}$					
clonidine	IP			[b]13.7 $_{1581}$				
	IM							
[a]bladder	SC							
[b]CNS	PO							
Antagonize	IV							
phencyclidine	IP		0.1 $_{2078}$					
behavioral	IM							
effects	SC							
	PO							
Antagonize	IV							
amphetamine	IP		10 $_{1384}$					
mydriasis	IM							
	SC							
	PO							
	IV							
	IP							
	IM							
	SC							
	PO							

mg/kg		Mouse	Rat	Guinea Pig	Rabbit	Cat	Dog	Monkey
	IV							
	IP							
	IM							
	SC							
	PO							
	IV							
	IP							
	IM							
	SC							
	PO							
	IV							
	IP							
	IM							
	SC							
	PO							
	IV							
	IP							
	IM							
	SC							
	PO							

IN VITRO

mg %	Cardiac	Vascular	Gut	Uterine	Visceral	Skeletal		
Rat		3.82×10^{-7}*		0.00765**				
Dog	0.382 $_{2107}$	0.00382 $_{1819}$						
Guinea Pig	0.0382 $_{1320}$							
Rabbit		0.00382 $_{1819}$						

*2131   **1583

PREDNISOLONE

(Delta-Cortef, Sterane, Meticortelone)

mg/kg		Mouse	Rat	Guinea Pig	Rabbit	Cat	Dog	Monkey	
Lethal Dose Y-LD$_{50}$ Z-MLD	IV								
	IP								
	IM								
	SC								
	PO								
Protect against Paf gastric damage	IV								
	IP								
	IM								
	SC		20 [1652]						
	PO								
Increase pancreatic glucagon secretion [a]total mg/d	IV								
	IP								
	IM								
	SC								
	PO	[a]0.2 [2133]							
Potential candidiasis [a]daily	IV								
	IP								
	IM								
	SC	[a]1 [2134]							
	PO								
Anti- inflammatory [a]total mg	IV								
	IP								
	IM					1 [2272]	1 [2272]		
	SC					[a]5-20 [2275]	[a]5-50 [2275]		
	PO					1 [2272]	1 [2272]		
Immuno- suppressive	IV								
	IP								
	IM								
	SC								
	PO					3 [2273]	2 [2273]		
	IV								
	IP								
	IM								
	SC								
	PO								
	IV								
	IP								
	IM								
	SC								
	PO								
	IV								
	IP								
	IM								
	SC								
	PO								

PREDNISONE

(Deltasone, Meticorten, Orasone, Zenadrid)

mg/kg		Mouse	Rat	Guinea Pig	Rabbit	Cat	Dog	Monkey
Lethal Dose	IV							
Y-LD$_{50}$	IP							
Z-MLD	IM							
	SC							
	PO							
Synergistic	IV							
effect with	IP	[a]20 2135						
allo-antibodies	IM							
[a]Q3d	SC							
	PO							
Protect	IV							
against UV-	IP							
induced skin	IM							
tumor	SC	[a]20 1445						
[a]PC, daily	PO							
Anti-	IV							
inflammatory	IP							
	IM					0.3-1 2273	0.3-1 2273	
	SC							
	PO					0.5 2272	0.5 2272	
	IV							
	IP							
	IM							
	SC							
	PO							
	IV							
	IP							
	IM							
	SC							
	PO							
	IV							
	IP							
	IM							
	SC							
	PO							
	IV							
	IP							
	IM							
	SC							
	PO							
	IV							
	IP							
	IM							
	SC							
	PO							

PRENALTEROL
(H 133/22, CGP 7760B, Hyprenan, Varbian)

mg/kg		Mouse	Rat	Guinea Pig	Rabbit	Cat	Dog	Monkey	
Lethal Dose	IV								
Y-LD$_{50}$	IP								
Z-MLD	IM								
	SC								
	PO								
Behavioral	IV								
	IP		30 $_{1558}$						
	IM								
	SC								
	PO								
Cardiovascular	IV						[a]0.004 $_{2125}$		
	IP								
[a]mg/kg/min	IM								
	SC								
	PO								
	IV								
	IP								
	IM								
	SC								
	PO								
	IV								
	IP								
	IM								
	SC								
	PO								
	IV								
	IP								
	IM								
	SC								
	PO								
	IV								
	IP								
	IM								
	SC								
	PO								
	IV								
	IP								
	IM								
	SC								
	PO								
	IV								
	IP								
	IM								
	SC								
	PO								

PROADIFEN
(SKF525-A, RP5171, NSC-39690)

mg/kg		Mouse	Rat	Guinea Pig	Rabbit	Cat	Dog	Monkey
Lethal Dose	IV	Y60 115						
Y-LD$_{50}$	IP	Y117.5 115	Y163 115					
Z-MLD	IM							
	SC							
	PO	Y538 115	Y2140 115					
Barbiturate	IV							
sleep	IP	10 681						
potentiation	IM							
	SC	50 118						
	PO							
Protects	IV							
against	IP			40 1231				
CCl$_4$	IM							
toxicity	SC							
	PO							
Decrease	IV							
THC LD$_{50}$	IP	30 2194						
	IM							
	SC							
	PO							
	IV							
	IP							
	IM							
	SC							
	PO							
	IV							
	IP							
	IM							
	SC							
	PO							
	IV							
	IP							
	IM							
	SC							
	PO							
	IV							
	IP							
	IM							
	SC							
	PO							
	IV							
	IP							
	IM							
	SC							
	PO							

PROBARBITAL

(Ipral)

mg/kg		Mouse	Rat	Guinea Pig	Rabbit	Cat	Dog	Monkey
Lethal Dose	IV				140 27			
Y-LD$_{50}$	IP	250 66	110 66		110 66			
Z-MLD	IM							
	SC		310 66					
	PO				160 66	140 66		
Anesthetic	IV							
	IP	75 66			66 66			
	IM							
	SC			225 66				
	PO							
	IV							
	IP							
	IM							
	SC							
	PO							
	IV							
	IP							
	IM							
	SC							
	PO							

IN VITRO

mg %	Cardiac	Vascular	Gut	Uterine	Visceral	Skeletal		

PROBENECID

(Benemid, Probecid, Proben)

mg/kg		Mouse	Rat	Guinea Pig	Rabbit	Cat	Dog	Monkey	
Lethal Dose	IV	Y458 627			Y304 627		Y270 627		
Y-LD$_{50}$	IP	Y230 2136	Y394 627						
Z-MLD	IM								
	SC	Y1156 627	Y611 627						
	PO	Y1666 627	Y1604 627						
Uricosuric	IV						16 58		
	IP								
	IM								
	SC								
	PO		300 58				30 58		
Potentiate	IV								
hyperglycemia/	IP	240 1765							
antifrusemide	IM								
	SC								
	PO								
Block active	IV				b50 1841				
transport	IP	a200 2137							
[a]Brain	IM								
[b]Renal tubules	SC								
[c]mg/1000U Pen G	PO						c1-2 2275		

IN VITRO

mg %	Cardiac	Vascular	Gut	Uterine	Visceral	Skeletal		

PROCAINAMIDE

(Procan, Pronestyl, Novocamid)

mg/kg		Mouse	Rat	Guinea Pig	Rabbit	Cat	Dog	Monkey	
Lethal Dose	IV								
25-LD$_{50}$	IP								
Z-MLD	IM								
	SC								
	PO								
Antiarrhythmic	IV						6 $_{2272}$		
	IP						^{a}0.01-0.04*		
	IM						11-22 $_{2273}$		
^{a}mg/kg/min	SC								
	PO						10-12 $_{2273}$		
	IV								
	IP								
	IM								
	SC								
	PO								
	IV								
	IP								
	IM								
	SC								
	PO								

*2272

IN VITRO

mg %	Cardiac	Vascular	Gut	Uterine	Visceral	Skeletal		
Guinea Pig	7.5 $_{2138}$							
Dog	3 $_{1885}$							

PROCAINE

(Novocain, Allocaine, Neocaine)

mg/kg		Mouse	Rat	Guinea Pig	Rabbit	Cat	Dog	Monkey	
Lethal Dose	IV	Y45 [111]	Y50	Y51 [629]	Y57 [249]	Z45	Y62.4 [7]		
Y-LD$_{50}$	IP	Y230 [111]	Y250 [166]	Z60					
Z-MLD	IM	Y630 [628]	Y1600 [111]						
	SC	Y800 [259]	Y2100 [259]	Z430	Z460	Z450	Z250		
	PO	Y500 [111]							
Convulsant	IV				30				
	IP								
	IM			100 [630]					
	SC						100		
	PO								
Block	IV					10 [292]	20 [441]		
afferent	IP								
nerve	IM								
discharge	SC								
	PO								
Decreased	IV					10 [440]			
intestinal	IP								
motility and	IM								
pain	SC								
	PO								
Cardiovascular	IV				20 [631]	20 [631]	20 [631]		
	IP								
	IM								
	SC								
	PO								
Analgesic	IV								
	IP								
	IM								
	SC		50 [1453]						
	PO								
	IV								
	IP								
	IM								
	SC								
	PO								
	IV								
	IP								
	IM								
	SC								
	PO								
	IV								
	IP								
	IM								
	SC								
	PO								

PROCHLORPERAZINE

(Compazine, Chlormeprazine, Stemetil)

mg/kg		Mouse	Rat	Guinea Pig	Rabbit	Cat	Dog	Monkey	
Lethal Dose	IV	Y92 982	20 235		5 235			Z100 82	
Y-LD$_{50}$	IP	Y125 982							
Z-MLD	IM								
	SC	Y350 982							
	PO	Y750 982	Y1800 82				Z102 82		
Behavioral	IV								
	IP		8 227						
	IM							0.1 1053	
	SC	10 561	1.3 95						
	PO	7.4 505	2.5 934						
Cardiovascular	IV					0.1 82	0.5 82		
	IP								
	IM								
	SC								
	PO		0.05 82						
Decreased	IV								
activity	IP	10 986							
	IM								
	SC	1 578							
	PO								
Catatonic	IV				30 1052				
	IP	11.3 1052	16.5 227						
	IM								
	SC		30 1042						
	PO								
EEG	IV				2 824				
(synchroni-	IP								
zation)	IM				5				
	SC								
	PO								
Hypothermic	IV								
	IP								
	IM								
	SC	8.5 983							
	PO								
Tranquilize	IV								
	IP								
[a]ED$_{50}$	IM								
	SC								
	PO	[a]24.6 1372							
Antiemetic	IV								
	IP								
	IM					0.13 2272	0.13 2272		
	SC								
	PO						2-5 2275		

mg/kg		Mouse	Rat	Guinea Pig	Rabbit	Cat	Dog	Monkey
	IV							
	IP							
	IM							
	SC							
	PO							
	IV							
	IP							
	IM							
	SC							
	PO							
	IV							
	IP							
	IM							
	SC							
	PO							
	IV							
	IP							
	IM							
	SC							
	PO							

IN VITRO

mg %	Cardiac	Vascular	Gut	Uterine	Visceral	Skeletal		
Spasmolytic			0.1					
Anticholinergic			$^a0.8_{235}$					
Antihistaminic		$^a0.11_{235}$	$^a0.002_{235}$					
Anti-5HT			$^a0.0005_{235}$					
^{a}total mg								

PRODILIDINE
(Cogesic, A-1981-12, CI-427)

mg/kg		Mouse	Rat	Guinea Pig	Rabbit	Cat	Dog	Monkey	
Lethal Dose Y-LD$_{50}$ Z-MLD	IV	Y91 [267]	Y74 [267]						
	IP								
	IM								
	SC	Y194 [267]	Y188 [267]						
	PO	Y318 [267]	Y253 [267]						
Analgesic	IV	30 [267]	11.2 [267]						
	IP								
	IM		26.3 [267]						
	SC	72.3 [267]	17.8 [267]						
	PO	84 [267]	17.3 [267]						
Emetic	IV								
	IP								
	IM						2.5 [267]		
	SC					60 [267]	10 [267]		
	PO					60 [267]	10 [267]		
Cardiovascular	IV					10 [267]	10 [267]		
	IP								
	IM								
	SC								
	PO								
Convulsant	IV								
	IP								
	IM								
	SC					80 [267]		60 [267]	
	PO								
	IV								
	IP								
	IM								
	SC								
	PO								
	IV								
	IP								
	IM								
	SC								
	PO								
	IV								
	IP								
	IM								
	SC								
	PO								
	IV								
	IP								
	IM								
	SC								
	PO								

PROFADOL

(Centrac, CI-572, A-2205)

mg/kg		Mouse	Rat	Guinea Pig	Rabbit	Cat	Dog	Monkey	
Lethal Dose	IV								
Y-LD$_{50}$	IP								
Z-MLD	IM								
	SC								
	PO								
Analgesic	IV								
	IP								
	IM								
[a]ED$_{50}$	SC	[a]0.96 1482	[a]1.38 1482						
	PO								
Sedative	IV								
	IP								
	IM								
[a]rotorod	SC	[a]39.9 1482							
test	PO								
	IV								
	IP								
	IM								
	SC								
	PO								
	IV								
	IP								
	IM								
	SC								
	PO								
	IV								
	IP								
	IM								
	SC								
	PO								
	IV								
	IP								
	IM								
	SC								
	PO								
	IV								
	IP								
	IM								
	SC								
	PO								

PROGABIDE

(Gabren, SL 76002)

mg/kg		Mouse	Rat	Guinea Pig	Rabbit	Cat	Dog	Monkey
Lethal Dose $Y-LD_{50}$ $Z-MLD$	IV							
	IP							
	IM							
	SC							
	PO							
Adrenal effects	IV							
	IP		100 1468					
	IM							
	SC							
	PO							
Neurotoxic [a]TD_{50}, rotorod	IV							
	IP	[a]603 1452						
	IM							
	SC							
	PO							
Anticonvulsant [a]ED_{50}, electroshock	IV							
	IP	[a]334 1452						
	IM							
	SC							
	PO							
GABA receptor regulation [a]daily	IV							
	IP		[a]100 1366					
	IM							
	SC							
	PO							
	IV							
	IP							
	IM							
	SC							
	PO							
	IV							
	IP							
	IM							
	SC							
	PO							
	IV							
	IP							
	IM							
	SC							
	PO							
	IV							
	IP							
	IM							
	SC							
	PO							

PROGLUMIDE

(Nulsa, Milid, Gastridene, Promid)

mg/kg		Mouse	Rat	Guinea Pig	Rabbit	Cat	Dog	Monkey	
Lethal Dose $Y-LD_{50}$ $Z-MLD$	IV								
	IP								
	IM								
	SC								
	PO								
Antisecretory and antiulcer	IV								
	IP		150 1302						
	IM								
	SC								
	PO		150 1302						
	IV								
	IP								
	IM								
	SC								
	PO								
	IV								
	IP								
	IM								
	SC								
	PO								
	IV								
	IP								
	IM								
	SC								
	PO								
	IV								
	IP								
	IM								
	SC								
	PO								
	IV								
	IP								
	IM								
	SC								
	PO								
	IV								
	IP								
	IM								
	SC								
	PO								
	IV								
	IP								
	IM								
	SC								
	PO								

PROMAZINE

(Sparine, Protactyl, Verophene)

mg/kg		Mouse	Rat	Guinea Pig	Rabbit	Cat	Dog	Monkey	
Lethal Dose Y-LD$_{50}$ Z-MLD	IV	Y38 235	Y29 235		Y21 235				
	IP								
	IM						Y4.4 557		
	SC								
	PO	Y485 226	Y650 986						
Sedative and EEG (synchronization	IV				2 632	3.3 97	1.5		
	IP								
	IM					3.3 97	5.5 557		
	SC								
	PO	40 119				3.3 97	9 557		
Behavioral	IV								
	IP	5 633	2.4 227					7 1230	
	IM								
	SC	15 1054	3 986						
	PO	10 986	200 986						
Adrenolytic	IV		0.041 253						
	IP	10 634							
	IM								
	SC								
	PO								
Analgesic	IV								
	IP	10 238	120 238						
	IM								
	SC								
	PO	100 231							
Flexor reflex depression	IV								
	IP				1 258				
	IM								
	SC								
	PO								
Barbiturate sleep potentiation	IV						2 425		
	IP								
	IM								
	SC	5 118				4.4 1232			
	PO	14.4 227	50 986						
Catatonic	IV								
	IP		3.3 227						
	IM								
	SC		25 1042						
	PO								
Anticonvulsant	IV								
	IP	5 982	5 982	5 982					
	IM								
	SC								
	PO								

mg/kg		Mouse	Rat	Guinea Pig	Rabbit	Cat	Dog	Monkey
Reverse	IV				[1] 835			
amphetamine	IP							
EEG	IM							
arousal	SC							
	PO							
	IV							
	IP							
	IM							
	SC							
	PO							
	IV							
	IP							
	IM							
	SC							
	PO							
	IV							
	IP							
	IM							
	SC							
	PO							

IN VITRO

mg %	Cardiac	Vascular	Gut	Uterine	Visceral	Skeletal	
Anticholinergic			[a]0.175 235				
Antihistaminic		[a]0.04 235	[a]0.004 235				
Anti-5HT			[a]0.0006 235				
Anti-BaCl$_2$			[a]0.0002 235				
[a]total mg							

PROMETHAZINE
(Anergan 25, Phenergan, Remsed)

mg/kg		Mouse	Rat	Guinea Pig	Rabbit	Cat	Dog	Monkey
Lethal Dose Y-LD$_{50}$ Z-MLD	IV	Y75 $_{235}$	Y45 $_{235}$	Y42.5 $_{629}$	Y19 $_{235}$			
	IP							
	IM							
	SC	Y750	Y225					
	PO	Y125 $_{88}$						
Anticonvulsant	IV							
	IP	40						
	IM							
	SC	72 $_{252}$						
	PO							
Barbiturate sleep potentiation	IV							
	IP	12.5 $_{1055}$						
	IM							
	SC	20 $_{88}$	10 $_{88}$				5 $_{88}$	
	PO							
Sympathomimetic sensitization	IV					15 $_{635}$	[a]1 $_{1545}$	
	IP	40 $_{251}$						
	IM							
	SC							
[a]cardiac	PO							
Motion sickness antagonist [a]total mg	IV							
	IP		28.2 $_{1055}$					
	IM						[a]125 $_{97}$	
	SC							
	PO		312 $_{1056}$				2 $_{2272}$	
EEG (synchronize)	IV				2 $_{824}$	1 $_{1057}$		
	IP							
	IM							
	SC		1-5 $_{2275}$		1-5 $_{2275}$			
	PO							
Behavioral	IV							
	IP	8 $_{1155}$						
	IM						0.1 $_{1377}$	
	SC		1-5 $_{2275}$		1-5 $_{2275}$			
	PO							
Block histamine hyperglycemia	IV							
	IP	1 $_{1544}$						
	IM							
	SC							
	PO							
	IV							
	IP							
	IM							
	SC							
	PO							

mg/kg		Mouse	Rat	Guinea Pig	Rabbit	Cat	Dog	Monkey	
	IV								
	IP								
	IM								
	SC								
	PO								
	IV								
	IP								
	IM								
	SC								
	PO								
	IV								
	IP								
	IM								
	SC								
	PO								
	IV								
	IP								
	IM								
	SC								
	PO								

IN VITRO

mg %	Cardiac	Vascular	Gut	Uterine	Visceral	Skeletal		
Antihistaminic		0.006 [235]	0.01					
Anticholinergic			1 [88]					
Anti-5HT			[a]0.0007 [235]					
Adrenolytic				0.1 [88]				
Anti-BaCl$_2$			0.5 [88]					

[a]total mg

PRONETALOL

(Alderlin, Nethalide, Pronethalol)

mg/kg		Mouse	Rat	Guinea Pig	Rabbit	Cat	Dog	Monkey	
Lethal Dose	IV	Y50 636	Y50 636						
Y-LD$_{50}$	IP	Y124 887							
Z-MLD	IM								
	SC								
	PO	Y900 636	Y900 636			300 636			
Adrenolytic	IV		1.9 887			5 636	5 636		
(ß-block)	IP	30 1670							
	IM								
	SC		20 1083						
	PO			6.8 887			10 636		
Decrease	IV								
norepinephrine	IP		2 919						
uptake	IM								
(heart)	SC								
	PO								
CNS	IV								
	IP	[a]52 2139							
[a]anticonvulsant	IM								
ED$_{50}$	SC								
	PO					300 636	250 636		

IN VITRO

mg %	Cardiac	Vascular	Gut	Uterine	Visceral	Skeletal		
Adrenolytic	0.01		1 636					

PROPANTHELINE

(Pro-Banthine, Neo-Metantyl, Pantheline)

mg/kg		Mouse	Rat	Guinea Pig	Rabbit	Cat	Dog	Monkey	
Lethal Dose	IV								
Y-LD$_{50}$	IP								
Z-MLD	IM								
	SC		Y298 $_{1128}$						
	PO		Y370 $_{1128}$						
Anticholinergic	IV								
	IP		5 $_{144}$						
	IM						5 $_{638}$		
^{a}total mg	SC		0.05 $_{637}$						
	PO					^{a}7.5 $_{2273}$	^{a}7.5-30*		
Ganglionic	IV					0.7 $_{113}$			
block	IP								
	IM								
	SC								
	PO								
Chromodac-	IV								
ryorrhetic	IP								
	IM		0.29 $_{103}$						
	SC								
	PO								
Antispasmodic	IV								
(GI, urinary)	IP								
	IM								
^{a}total mg	SC								
	PO					^{a}7.5 $_{2272}$	0.5-1 $_{2272}$		
	IV								
	IP								
	IM								
	SC								
	PO								
	IV								
	IP								
	IM								
	SC								
	PO								
	IV								
	IP								
	IM								
	SC								
	PO								
	IV								
	IP								
	IM								
	SC								
	PO								

*2273

PROPOXYPHENE

(Darvon, Dolene, SK-65)

mg/kg		Mouse	Rat	Guinea Pig	Rabbit	Cat	Dog	Monkey
Lethal Dose	IV							
Y-LD$_{50}$	IP							
Z-MLD	IM							
	SC	Y204 $_{2140}$	Y131 $_{2140}$					
	PO		Y354 $_{2140}$					
Analgesic	IV							
	IP		25 $_{2272}$					
	IM					2.2 $_{2272}$		
^{a}ED$_{50}$	SC	^{a}1.42 $_{1482}$	^{a}4.1 $_{1482}$	^{a}22.5 $_{1482}$				
	PO	40 $_{2140}$	30 $_{2140}$				1-2 $_{2272}$	
Sedative	IV							
	IP							
^{a}rotorod	IM							
	SC	^{a}36.4 $_{1482}$						
	PO							
Decrease	IV							
urine	IP							
output	IM							
	SC		40 $_{1492}$					
	PO							
	IV							
	IP							
	IM							
	SC							
	PO							
	IV							
	IP							
	IM							
	SC							
	PO							
	IV							
	IP							
	IM							
	SC							
	PO							
	IV							
	IP							
	IM							
	SC							
	PO							
	IV							
	IP							
	IM							
	SC							
	PO							

PROPRANOLOL

(Inderal, Inderex, Indobloc)

mg/kg		Mouse	Rat	Guinea Pig	Rabbit	Cat	Dog	Monkey
Lethal Dose	IV	Y27 2044						
Y-LD$_{50}$	IP	Y114 2141						
Z-MLD	IM							
	SC							
	PO	Y380 2141						
Adrenolytic	IV	5 1197	3 1709	2.5 1091	1 1112	3 1113	2 1088	
(ß-block)	IP	10 1153	50 1468					
	IM	2.5 1440	10 1423					
	SC	10 1152			5 1120			
	PO							
Cardiovascular	IV			0.1 1127			1 2142	
[a] ICV	IP	28 2057	1 1243				[b]1 2148	
[b] IV	IM		[a]1 2143				[c]0.011 2149	
[c] mg/kg/min IV	SC		0.5 1139					
[d] total mg	PO		30 1873			[d]2.5-7.5*	5-40 2272	
Antiarrythmic	IV			[a]0.01 2127	0.5 1090	[a]0.026 2127	10 1089	
	IP							
[a] isoprenaline-	IM							
induced	SC							
	PO					[a]0.082 2127	0.5 1194	
CNS	IV						3 1154	
(behavioral)	IP							
	IM							
	SC							
	PO		10 877					
Metabolic	IV						4 1216	
	IP							
	IM							
	SC							
	PO							
Anticonvulsant	IV	[a]8 2145	0.6 2150					
[a] ED$_{50}$	IP	[a]12 2139						
[b] IV, hyperbaric	IM	[b]16 2146						
seizures	SC							
	PO							
Local	IV							
anesthetic	IP							
	IM							
[a] mg/ml	SC	[a]3.6 2127		[a]0.42 2127				
	PO							
Effects	IV							
on erythro-	IP							
poiesis	IM							
	SC		10 2147					
	PO							

*2272

mg/kg		Mouse	Rat	Guinea Pig	Rabbit	Cat	Dog	Monkey	
Partial	IV								
block of	IP								
oxotremorine	IM								
	SC		2.5_{2047}						
	PO								
Effects on	IV		0.2_{1812}						
micturition	IP								
reflex	IM								
	SC								
	PO								
Suppress	IV								
ACh	IP								
writhing	IM								
	SC	10.3_{1296}							
	PO								
Block drug	IV			$^b0.009_{2127}$					
effects on	IP	$^a1_{1237}$							
respiration	IM								
^{a}ethanol	SC								
^{b}isoprenaline	PO								
Pulmonary	IV								
effects	IP								
	IM								
^{a}mg/kg/min	SC	50_{2152}	$^a0.0002_{2151}$						
	PO								
	IV								
	IP								
	IM								
	SC								
	PO								

IN VITRO

mg %	Cardiac	Vascular	Gut	Uterine	Visceral	Trachea	CNS	
Langendorff	$^a0.003_{1157}$							
Rat	0.013_{1856}	0.026_{1874}	0.259_{1583}	0.001_{1157}		0.0078_{1410}		
Rabbit	0.002_{1157}	0.15_{2127}	3_{1157}					
Dog	0.0519_{1857}	0.13_{2144}				0.259_{1800}		
^{a}total mg								

PROPYLTHIOURACIL

(Propacil, Procasil, Prothyran)

mg/kg		Mouse	Rat	Guinea Pig	Rabbit	Cat	Dog	Monkey
Lethal Dose	IV							
Y-LD$_{50}$	IP							
Z-MLD	IM							
	SC							
	PO							
Induce	IV							
immune-	IP							
mediated	IM							
disease	SC							
[a]total mg/d	PO					[a]150 2153	11 2273	
Inhibit	IV							
thyroid	IP							
hormone	IM							
synthesis	SC			[a]20 2154				
[a]daily	PO							
	IV							
	IP							
	IM							
	SC							
	PO							
	IV							
	IP							
	IM							
	SC							
	PO							
	IV							
	IP							
	IM							
	SC							
	PO							
	IV							
	IP							
	IM							
	SC							
	PO							
	IV							
	IP							
	IM							
	SC							
	PO							
	IV							
	IP							
	IM							
	SC							
	PO							

PROTOVERATRINE

(Protalba, Provell, Puroverine, Veralba)

mg/kg		Mouse	Rat	Guinea Pig	Rabbit	Cat	Dog	Monkey	
Lethal Dose	IV	Y0.05 639			Y0.05 641				
Y-LD$_{50}$	IP	Y0.4 640							
Z-MLD	IM								
	SC		Y0.6 639		Y0.11 639	Y0.5 641			
	PO		Y5.0 639						
Cardiovascular	IV					0.002 279	0.001 642		
	IP								
	IM								
	SC		0.14 916						
	PO								
Respiratory	IV						0.007 643		
(depression)	IP								
	IM								
	SC								
	PO								
	IV								
	IP								
	IM								
	SC								
	PO								

IN VITRO

mg %	Cardiac	Vascular	Gut	Uterine	Visceral	Skeletal		

PROTRIPTYLINE

(Vivactil, Concordin, Maximed)

mg/kg		Mouse	Rat	Guinea Pig	Rabbit	Cat	Dog	Monkey
Lethal Dose	IV	Y37 1844						
Y-LD$_{50}$	IP							
Z-MLD	IM							
	SC	Y192 1844						
	PO	Y269 1844						
Antagonize	IV							
tetrabenazine	IP	[a]0.2 1371						
ptosis	IM							
	SC							
[a]ED$_{50}$	PO							
Antagonize	IV							
reserpine	IP	[a]0.4 1371						
ptosis	IM							
	SC							
[a]ED$_{50}$	PO							
	IV							
	IP							
	IM							
	SC							
	PO							
	IV							
	IP							
	IM							
	SC							
	PO							
	IV							
	IP							
	IM							
	SC							
	PO							
	IV							
	IP							
	IM							
	SC							
	PO							
	IV							
	IP							
	IM							
	SC							
	PO							
	IV							
	IP							
	IM							
	SC							
	PO							

409

PROXORPHAN
(BL-5572 M)

mg/kg		Mouse	Rat	Guinea Pig	Rabbit	Cat	Dog	Monkey
Lethal Dose	IV							
Y-LD$_{50}$	IP							
Z-MLD	IM							
	SC							
	PO							
Analgesic	IV							
	IP							
	IM							
^{a}ED$_{50}$	SC	^{a}0.19$_{1482}$	^{a}0.067$_{1482}$	^{a}0.029$_{1482}$				
	PO							
Sedative	IV							
(rotorod)	IP							
	IM							
	SC	83$_{1482}$						
	PO							
Increase	IV							
urination	IP							
	IM							
	SC		1.25$_{1989}$					
	PO							
	IV							
	IP							
	IM							
	SC							
	PO							
	IV							
	IP							
	IM							
	SC							
	PO							
	IV							
	IP							
	IM							
	SC							
	PO							
	IV							
	IP							
	IM							
	SC							
	PO							
	IV							
	IP							
	IM							
	SC							
	PO							

PSEUDOEPHEDRINE

(Dorcol, Novafed, Sudafed)

mg/kg		Mouse	Rat	Guinea Pig	Rabbit	Cat	Dog	Monkey	
Lethal Dose	IV				85 [149]		125 [149]		
Y-LD$_{50}$	IP								
Z-MLD	IM								
	SC		650 [149]			400 [149]			
	PO	115.5 [149]							
Cardiovascular	IV					1 [149]			
	IP								
	IM								
	SC								
	PO								
Diuretic	IV						0.6 [149]		
	IP								
	IM								
	SC								
	PO								
	IV								
	IP								
	IM								
	SC								
	PO								

IN VITRO

mg %	Cardiac	Vascular	Gut	Uterine	Visceral	Skeletal		
Contractile				0.3 [149]	0.2 [149]			

PSILOCIN

(Psilocyn, 4-Hydroxy Psilocybin)

mg/kg		Mouse	Rat	Guinea Pig	Rabbit	Cat	Dog	Monkey	
Lethal Dose	IV	Y74 115	Y75 115						
Y-LD$_{50}$	IP								
Z-MLD	IM								
	SC								
	PO								
Cardiovascular	IV						100 158		
	IP								
	IM								
	SC								
	PO								
EEG	IV				2 906				
	IP								
	IM								
	SC								
	PO								
	IV								
	IP								
	IM								
	SC								
	PO								

IN VITRO

mg %	Cardiac	Vascular	Gut	Uterine	Visceral	Skeletal		
Anti-5HT			[a]0.0005 644	[a]0.00003 644				
[a]total mg								

PSILOCYBINE

(Psilocybin, CY 39, Indocybin)

mg/kg		Mouse	Rat	Guinea Pig	Rabbit	Cat	Dog	Monkey	
Lethal Dose	IV	Y285 115	Y280 115						
Y-LD$_{50}$	IP								
Z-MLD	IM								
	SC								
	PO								
Behavioral	IV								
	IP		0.25 921						
	IM								
	SC								
	PO								
Cardiovascular	IV						0.2 158		
	IP		0.15 155						
	IM								
	SC								
	PO								
Pentobarbital	IV				0.32 159				
EEG	IP								
antagonist	IM								
	SC								
	PO								
Respiratory	IV						0.5 645		
(depression)	IP								
	IM								
	SC								
	PO								
Increased	IV					0.2			
flexor	IP								
reflex	IM								
	SC								
	PO								
Decreased	IV								
catecholamines	IP		25 1239						
(brain)	IM								
	SC								
	PO								

IN VITRO

mg %		Cardiac	Vascular	Gut	Uterine	Visceral	Skeletal		
Anti-5HT				[a]0.006 644	0.001 644				
[a]total mg									

PYRAZOLE

mg/kg		Mouse	Rat	Guinea Pig	Rabbit	Cat	Dog	Monkey
Lethal Dose	IV							
Y-LD$_{50}$	IP							
Z-MLD	IM							
	SC							
	PO							
Alcohol	IV							
dependency	IP	68.08 $_{1330}$						
	IM							
	SC							
	PO							
Partial	IV							
inhibition	IP	68 $_{2170}$						
of alcohol	IM							
metabolism	SC							
	PO							
Inhibit	IV							
DA	IP		[a]200 $_{2171}$					
hydroxylase	IM							
	SC							
[a]daily, 3 d	PO							
Decrease	IV							
brain	IP		100 $_{1342}$					
norepi	IM							
	SC							
	PO		100 $_{1342}$					
	IV							
	IP							
	IM							
	SC							
	PO							
	IV							
	IP							
	IM							
	SC							
	PO							
	IV							
	IP							
	IM							
	SC							
	PO							
	IV							
	IP							
	IM							
	SC							
	PO							

PYRILAMINE

(Anthisan, Mepyramine, Neo-Antergan)

mg/kg		Mouse	Rat	Guinea Pig	Rabbit	Cat	Dog	Monkey
Lethal Dose	IV	Y30 324		Y24.4 629				
Y-LD$_{50}$	IP	Y102 646						
Z-MLD	IM							
	SC	Y150 324	Y150 647	Y70 324				
	PO	Y235 58						
Antihistaminic	IV			0.1 1122			5 649	
	IP							
	IM						75 97	
[a]total mg	SC			1.3 58			75 97	
	PO			11.3 648			[a]125 97	
Sympatho-	IV					5 144		
mimetic	IP							
(sensitization)	IM							
	SC							
	PO							
Anticonvulsant	IV							
	IP			0.5 930				
	IM							
	SC							
	PO							
Reverse	IV							
oxotremorine	IP	33.9 1441						
hypothermia	IM							
	SC							
	PO							
Cardiac	IV						1 1545	
	IP							
	IM							
	SC							
	PO							

IN VITRO

mg %	Cardiac	Vascular	Gut	Uterine	Visceral	Skeletal		
Antihistaminic						0.003		
Guinea Pig						0.002 1157		

PYROCATECHOL

(Catechol, Pyrocatechin)

mg/kg		Mouse	Rat	Guinea Pig	Rabbit	Cat	Dog	Monkey	
Lethal Dose	IV						45 651		
Y-LD$_{50}$	IP		100 1058	150 205					
Z-MLD	IM								
	SC	150 195	225 650	225 650					
	PO		Y3890		1000 346				
Cardiovascular	IV						100 652		
	IP		12 328						
	IM								
	SC								
	PO								
CNS	IV					5 653			
(stimulation)	IP								
	IM								
	SC								
	PO								
EEG	IV				6 832				
	IP		50 1058						
	IM								
	SC								
	PO								

IN VITRO

mg %	Cardiac	Vascular	Gut	Uterine	Visceral	Skeletal		
Langendorff	[a]30 652							
Depressant	[b]6 652							
[a]total mg								
[b]mMol/L								

PYROGALLOL

(Pyrogallic Acid)

mg/kg		Mouse	Rat	Guinea Pig	Rabbit	Cat	Dog	Monkey	
Lethal Dose	IV						Z90 651		
Y-LD$_{50}$	IP								
Z-MLD	IM								
	SC		Z650 650	Z1000 650			Z350 654		
	PO				Z1100 109		Z35 346		
Cardiovascular	IV		45			4 655	25 282		
	IP								
	IM								
	SC								
	PO								
Catechol-O-	IV					4 655			
methyl	IP	[a]10 656	200 811						
transferase	IM								
inhibition	SC								
[a]total mg	PO								
Chloral	IV								
hydrate	IP	50 342							
potentiation	IM								
	SC								
	PO								
Effect on	IV								
DA brain	IP		200 1706						
concentrations	IM								
	SC								
	PO								
	IV								
	IP								
	IM								
	SC								
	PO								
	IV								
	IP								
	IM								
	SC								
	PO								
	IV								
	IP								
	IM								
	SC								
	PO								
	IV								
	IP								
	IM								
	SC								
	PO								

QUADAZOCINE
(WIN 44441-3)

mg/kg		Mouse	Rat	Guinea Pig	Rabbit	Cat	Dog	Monkey	
Lethal Dose Y-LD$_{50}$ Z-MLD	IV								
	IP								
	IM								
	SC								
	PO								
Increase spinal reflexes	IV				0.0885 [1481]				
	IP								
	IM								
	SC								
	PO								
Antagonize morphine analgesia	IV								
	IP								
	IM								
	SC							0.1 [1762]	
	PO								
Antagonize bremazocine and ethylketazocine analgesia	IV								
	IP								
	IM								
	SC							1 [1762]	
	PO								
	IV								
	IP								
	IM								
	SC								
	PO								
	IV								
	IP								
	IM								
	SC								
	PO								
	IV								
	IP								
	IM								
	SC								
	PO								
	IV								
	IP								
	IM								
	SC								
	PO								
	IV								
	IP								
	IM								
	SC								
	PO								

QUINACRINE

(Atabrine, Chinacrin, Erion)

mg/kg		Mouse	Rat	Guinea Pig	Rabbit	Cat	Dog	Monkey	
Lethal Dose	IV								
Y-LD$_{50}$	IP								
Z-MLD	IM								
	SC								
	PO								
Myocardial	IV						[a]0.03 1837		
protection	IP								
	IM								
[a]mg/min IA	SC		75 2172						
	PO								
Antiprotozoal	IV								
	IP								
[a]total mg	IM								
	SC								
	PO						10 2272	[a]50-100*		
	IV								
	IP								
	IM								
	SC								
	PO								

*2272

IN VITRO

mg %	Cardiac	Vascular	Gut	Uterine	Visceral	Skeletal	

QUINIDINE

(Cin-Quin, Quinidex, Quinora)

mg/kg		Mouse	Rat	Guinea Pig	Rabbit	Cat	Dog	Monkey	
Lethal Dose	IV	Y69 555	Y23.1 363			Y21.6 658			
Y-LD$_{50}$	IP	Y190 555	Z174 657						
Z-MLD	IM	Y200							
	SC	Z400 657							
	PO	Y593.9 555	Y1000 363						
Block atrial	IV			5		2 659	3		
flutter	IP	72 858							
	IM								
	SC								
	PO								
Cardiovascular	IV				8.75 1090	10 659	15 363		
	IP								
	IM						8-20 2273		
	SC								
	PO					15 1134	30 1134		
Nictitating	IV					10 363	15 363		
membrane	IP								
relaxation	IM								
	SC								
	PO								
Carotid sinus	IV								
reflex	IP								
depressant	IM								
	SC								
	PO						30 363		
Cardiac	IV						[a]0.5 2176		
	IP								
[a]mg/kg/min	IM								
	SC								
	PO						6-20 2272		
Digoxin	IV						[a]0.18 2177		
interactions	IP								
	IM								
[a]mg/kg/min	SC								
[b]total mg TID	PO						[b]300 2178		

IN VITRO

mg %	Cardiac	Vascular	Gut	Uterine	Visceral	Skeletal		
Guinea Pig	0.0324 2174			2				
Rabbit	0.5 2175		1					
Cat	0.0324 2174							
Dog	0.5 2173							

QUINPIROLE

(LY-171555)

mg/kg		Mouse	Rat	Guinea Pig	Rabbit	Cat	Dog	Monkey	
Lethal Dose	IV								
Y-LD$_{50}$	IP								
Z-MLD	IM								
	SC								
	PO								
Cardiovascular	IV		0.01 $_{2179}$				[a]0.002$_{1748}$	0.001$_{2180}$	
	IP								
[a]mg/kg/min	IM								
	SC								
	PO								
	IV								
	IP								
	IM								
	SC								
	PO								
	IV								
	IP								
	IM								
	SC								
	PO								
	IV								
	IP								
	IM								
	SC								
	PO								
	IV								
	IP								
	IM								
	SC								
	PO								
	IV								
	IP								
	IM								
	SC								
	PO								
	IV								
	IP								
	IM								
	SC								
	PO								
	IV								
	IP								
	IM								
	SC								
	PO								

QUIPAZINE

(MA-1291)

mg/kg		Mouse	Rat	Guinea Pig	Rabbit	Cat	Dog	Monkey	
Lethal Dose	IV								
Y-LD$_{50}$	IP								
Z-MLD	IM								
	SC								
	PO								
Behavioral	IV								
	IP		1.6 1553						
	IM							0.1 1554	
	SC								
	PO		2.5 2181						
Activation	IV		0.3 2182						
of serotonin	IP								
receptors	IM								
	SC								
	PO								
	IV								
	IP								
	IM								
	SC								
	PO								
	IV								
	IP								
	IM								
	SC								
	PO								
	IV								
	IP								
	IM								
	SC								
	PO								
	IV								
	IP								
	IM								
	SC								
	PO								
	IV								
	IP								
	IM								
	SC								
	PO								
	IV								
	IP								
	IM								
	SC								
	PO								

RACEMETHORPHAN

(Dextromethorphan, Levomethorphan, Methorphan)

mg/kg		Mouse	Rat	Guinea Pig	Rabbit	Cat	Dog	Monkey
Lethal Dose	IV							
Y-LD$_{50}$	IP							
Z-MLD	IM							
	SC							
	PO							
Gastrointestinal	IV							
	IP		10 $_{1656}$					
	IM							
	SC							
	PO		10 $_{1656}$					
Antitussive	IV					0.51 $_{1626}$		
	IP							
	IM							
	SC							
	PO							
	IV							
	IP							
	IM							
	SC							
	PO							

IN VITRO

mg %	Cardiac	Vascular	Gut	Uterine	Visceral	Skeletal		
Guinea Pig			0.217 $_{1610}$					

RACEMORPHAN
(DL-3-Hydroxy-N-Methylmorphinan)

mg/kg		Mouse	Rat	Guinea Pig	Rabbit	Cat	Dog	Monkey
Lethal Dose Y-LD$_{50}$ Z-MLD	IV	41 [409]			19 [409]			
	IP	120 [409]						
	IM							
	SC	153 [409]	125 [409]					
	PO							
Analgesic	IV							
	IP							
	IM							
	SC		1 [409]					
	PO		10 [409]					
Respiratory depressant	IV				2 [409]			
	IP							
	IM							
	SC							
	PO							
Increased intestinal motility	IV						2 [409]	
	IP							
	IM							
	SC							
	PO							
Cardiovascular	IV					4 [409]	4 [409]	
	IP							
	IM							
	SC							
	PO							
	IV							
	IP							
	IM							
	SC							
	PO							
	IV							
	IP							
	IM							
	SC							
	PO							
	IV							
	IP							
	IM							
	SC							
	PO							
	IV							
	IP							
	IM							
	SC							
	PO							

RANITIDINE

(Zantac, AH 19065, Ranidil)

mg/kg		Mouse	Rat	Guinea Pig	Rabbit	Cat	Dog	Monkey	
Lethal Dose Y-LD$_{50}$ Z-MLD	IV								
	IP								
	IM								
	SC								
	PO								
Gastrointestinal antisecretory	IV						0.21 $_{1548}$		
	IP		6.1 $_{1548}$						
	IM								
	SC								
	PO		6.84 $_{1637}$				0.5 $_{1549}$		
Gastrointestinal antilesion	IV								
	IP								
	IM								
	SC								
	PO		10 $_{1637}$				0.05 $_{1303}$		
	IV								
	IP								
	IM								
	SC								
	PO								
	IV								
	IP								
	IM								
	SC								
	PO								
	IV								
	IP								
	IM								
	SC								
	PO								
	IV								
	IP								
	IM								
	SC								
	PO								
	IV								
	IP								
	IM								
	SC								
	PO								
	IV								
	IP								
	IM								
	SC								
	PO								

RAUWOLFIA SERPENTINA

(Raudixin, Rauverid, Wolfina, Rauwolscine)

mg/kg		Mouse	Rat	Guinea Pig	Rabbit	Cat	Dog	Monkey
Lethal Dose	IV							
Y-LD$_{50}$	IP							
Z-MLD	IM							
	SC							
	PO							
Antipressor	IV		0.5 1709				0.1 1922	
	IP							
	IM							
	SC							
	PO							
CNS	IV							
(kindling	IP		1 1580					
development)	IM							
	SC							
	PO							
	IV							
	IP							
	IM							
	SC							
	PO							
	IV							
	IP							
	IM							
	SC							
	PO							
	IV							
	IP							
	IM							
	SC							
	PO							
	IV							
	IP							
	IM							
	SC							
	PO							
	IV							
	IP							
	IM							
	SC							
	PO							
	IV							
	IP							
	IM							
	SC							
	PO							

RESERPINE

(Sandril, Serpasil, Serpasol)

mg/kg		Mouse	Rat	Guinea Pig	Rabbit	Cat	Dog	Monkey
Lethal Dose Y-LD_{50} Z-MLD	IV		Y18 93					Y0.5 93
	IP	Y70 1131						
	IM							
	SC							
	PO	Y500 176						
Sedative	IV		5 899		3.5 661	1 634	0.05	
	IP	2.5 79					0.05	5 161
	IM	2 477					0.01 2275	
	SC	2.5 93	5 660				0.01 2275	
	PO	10 474	2 1221	4		10 634	0.65 93	
Serotonin and norepinephrine depletion	IV		0.4 662		5 667	3 91	5	
	IP	1 861	5 663	2.3 665		3 668	0.1 669	
	IM							1 1170
	SC		5 664	0.1 666		5	5	
	PO							
Behavioral	IV		0.2 670	1 1023				
	IP	6 137	5 106		0.5 1068			
	IM		1 260			5 487		0.75 671
	SC	2 561	1.2 596					
	PO	5 935	2 1059		2 1059	2 1059	2 1059	
CNS	IV				2 509	1 306		
	IP	0.5 882	0.5 1172			0.2 447		
	IM							
	SC							
	PO							
Barbituate sleep potentiation	IV		5 233				0.5 822	
	IP	5 469	5 411					
	IM							
	SC	1 1060						
	PO							
Gastrointestinal [a]total mg ICV	IV		2.5 2185					
	IP		[a]0.05 2186					
	IM		5 2183					
	SC		5 2186	2.5 1781				
	PO							
Thermoregulatory (hypothermia)	IV							
	IP	0.5 1670						
	IM							
	SC	2 1439						
	PO							
Effects on smooth muscle [a]daily	IV							
	IP		[a]1 2187			[a]0.3 2188		
	IM							
	SC							
	PO							

RESERPINE (continued)

mg/kg		Mouse	Rat	Guinea Pig	Rabbit	Cat	Dog	Monkey	
Opioid interactions	IV								
	IP	2 1708							
	IM								
	SC		1 1910						
	PO								
Antagonize amphetamine [a]behavioral	IV								
	IP	2 1810				5 1385			
	IM								
	SC								
	PO	[a]15.7 1372							
Dopamine interactions	IV	4 1888							
	IP	10 1705							
	IM								
	SC								
	PO								
Catatonic	IV								
	IP	5 1707	5 165						
	IM								
	SC								
	PO								
Cardiovascular	IV		1.5 985	0.1 2183	1 640	1 634	1 640	0.1 1646	
	IP		5 1609	10 1219	0.55 457		0.5 1819		
	IM						0.5 1819		
	SC		0.13 916						
	PO							1 640	
Metabolic	IV		1 884						
	IP								
	IM								
	SC								
	PO								
Anticonvulsant	IV								
	IP	4 1115	1.25 2184						
	IM								
	SC	1 957							
	PO								

IN VITRO

mg %	Cardiac	Vascular	Gut	Uterine	Visceral	Skeletal	
Rabbit Anti-5IIT			0.1				
			3 92				
Rat	0.061 1609						

428

RIOPROSTIL

(TR-4698, ORF-15927)

mg/kg		Mouse	Rat	Guinea Pig	Rabbit	Cat	Dog	Monkey	
Lethal Dose	IV								
Y-LD$_{50}$	IP								
Z-MLD	IM								
	SC								
	PO								
Gastrointestinal	IV		0.9 [1549]						
antisecretory	IP								
	IM		[a]3.7 [1549]						
[a]i. duodenal	SC		1.8 [1549]						
	PO		2.9 [1549]				0.016 [1549]	7 [1549]	
Gastrointestinal	IV								
antilesion	IP								
	IM								
	SC		0.012 [1549]						
	PO		0.0015 [1549]				0.0016 [1549]		
	IV								
	IP								
	IM								
	SC								
	PO								
	IV								
	IP								
	IM								
	SC								
	PO								
	IV								
	IP								
	IM								
	SC								
	PO								
	IV								
	IP								
	IM								
	SC								
	PO								
	IV								
	IP								
	IM								
	SC								
	PO								
	IV								
	IP								
	IM								
	SC								
	PO								

RITANSERIN

(R-55667)

mg/kg		Mouse	Rat	Guinea Pig	Rabbit	Cat	Dog	Monkey
Lethal Dose	IV							
Y-LD$_{50}$	IP							
Z-MLD	IM							
	SC							
	PO							
Decrease	IV		1 $_{1867}$					
blood pressure	IP							
and heart rate	IM							
	SC							
	PO							
Blocks 5HT-	IV		0.001 $_{1867}$					
induced blood	IP							
pressure	IM							
increase	SC							
	PO							
Behavioral	IV							
(PCP and	IP							
chloroamphet-	IM							
amine	SC		1 $_{1539}$					
interaction)	PO							
	IV							
	IP							
	IM							
	SC							
	PO							
	IV							
	IP							
	IM							
	SC							
	PO							
	IV							
	IP							
	IM							
	SC							
	PO							
	IV							
	IP							
	IM							
	SC							
	PO							
	IV							
	IP							
	IM							
	SC							
	PO							

SALICYLIC ACID

(Fomac, Ionil, Keralyt)

mg/kg		Mouse	Rat	Guinea Pig	Rabbit	Cat	Dog	Monkey	
Lethal Dose	IV								
Y-LD$_{50}$	IP								
Z-MLD	IM								
	SC								
	PO								
Inorganic	IV		75 2191						
sulfate	IP		^{a}0.26 2191						
excretion	IM								
^{a}mg/kg/min IV	SC								
	PO								
Antiseptic,	IV								
antifermentive	IP								
	IM								
	SC								
	PO							0.1-1 2275		
	IV								
	IP								
	IM								
	SC								
	PO								

IN VITRO

mg %	Cardiac	Vascular	Gut	Uterine	Visceral	Skeletal	Hepatic	
Rat							8.98 1829	

SARALASIN

(Sarenin, P-113, Sar, Ala-Angiotensin II)

mg/kg		Mouse	Rat	Guinea Pig	Rabbit	Cat	Dog	Monkey
Lethal Dose $Y-LD_{50}$ $Z-MLD$	IV							
	IP							
	IM							
	SC							
	PO							
Cardiovascular ^{a}mg/kg/min	IV		^{a}0.01 $_{1513}$					
	IP							
	IM							
	SC							
	PO							
Block AT II brain receptors ^{a}μg/hr ICV	IV		^{a}12 $_{2192}$					
	IP							
	IM							
	SC							
	PO							
Effect on renal blood flow ^{a}IA	IV						^{a}0.0005 $_{1519}$	
	IP							
	IM							
	SC							
	PO							
	IV							
	IP							
	IM							
	SC							
	PO							
	IV							
	IP							
	IM							
	SC							
	PO							
	IV							
	IP							
	IM							
	SC							
	PO							
	IV							
	IP							
	IM							
	SC							
	PO							
	IV							
	IP							
	IM							
	SC							
	PO							

SCOPOLAMINE

(Hyoscine, Skopolate, Skopyl, Transderm-V)

mg/kg		Mouse	Rat	Guinea Pig	Rabbit	Cat	Dog	Monkey
Lethal Dose	IV	Y153.5 [1926]						
Y-LD$_{50}$	IP							
Z-MLD	IM							
	SC	Y590 [672]						
	PO							
Anticholinergic	IV						0.06 [915]	
	IP	0.07 [915]	10 [1118]					
[a]total mg	IM						0.01-0.02*	
	SC	5 [673]				0.5	0.01-0.02*	
	PO		1.5 [144]				[a]0.3-1.5**	
Sedative	IV						1	
	IP							
	IM							
	SC	450 [672]	13 [674]				1	
	PO							
Increased	IV							
muscle	IP							
activity	IM							
	SC	20 [176]	5 [491]					
	PO		10 [491]					
EEG	IV				0.08 [675]	0.1 [184]		
(synchroni-	IP							
zation)	IM							1.5 [945]
	SC		1.05 [1173]				1.5 [945]	
	PO							
Behavioral	IV				0.05 [1161]		0.32 [915]	0.1 [1163]
	IP	1 [852]	1.8 [104]			0.6 [1068]		0.1 [185]
	IM		0.6 [1174]					
	SC	1 [856]	1 [1016]				1.5 [945]	
	PO						1.5 [945]	
Anticonvulsant	IV							
[a]anti-	IP	5 [251]						
oxotremorine	IM							
tremor	SC			[a]0.5				
	PO							
Increased	IV				0.1 [831]			
EEG	IP							
arousal	IM							
threshold	SC							
	PO							
CNS	IV							
anticholinergic	IP	5 [1458]						
	IM							
	SC							
	PO							

*2273 **2275

mg/kg		Mouse	Rat	Guinea Pig	Rabbit	Cat	Dog	Monkey
Mydriatic	IV							
	IP							
	IM							
	SC	[1] 1439						
	PO							
	IV							
	IP							
	IM							
	SC							
	PO							
	IV							
	IP							
	IM							
	SC							
	PO							
	IV							
	IP							
	IM							
	SC							
	PO							

IN VITRO

mg %	Cardiac	Vascular	Gut	Uterine	Visceral	Skeletal		
Anticholinergic					[a]2.5×10^{-10}			
Antihistaminic					[a]7×10^{-5}			
Anti-BaCl$_2$					[a]1×10^{-4}			
[a]molar solution								

SECOBARBITAL
(Seconal, Bipenal, Seotal)

mg/kg		Mouse	Rat	Guinea Pig	Rabbit	Cat	Dog	Monkey	
Lethal Dose	IV	Z80 63	Z35 63	Z35 63	Z45 63	Z50 63			
Y-LD$_{50}$	IP	Z140 63	Z110 63	Z40 63	Z50 63	Z75 63			
Z-MLD	IM								
	SC	Z160 63	Z140 63	Z60 63	Z90 63				
	PO		Z125 63			Y50 63	Z90 63		
Anesthetic	IV	30 63	17.5 63	20 63	22.5 72	25 63		17.5 63	
	IP	60 63	40 63	20 63	30 63	35 63			
	IM								
	SC	70 63	60 63	30 63	50 63				
	PO		65 63	15 76			40 63		
Sedative	IV								
	IP		40 63						
	IM								
	SC		60 63						
	PO		65 63			3 24	3 24		
Serotonin	IV								
increase	IP		40						
(brain)	IM								
	SC								
	PO								
Flexor	IV					5.4 34			
reflex	IP								
inhibition	IM								
	SC								
	PO								
	IV								
	IP								
	IM								
	SC								
	PO								
	IV								
	IP								
	IM								
	SC								
	PO								
	IV								
	IP								
	IM								
	SC								
	PO								
	IV								
	IP								
	IM								
	SC								
	PO								

SEMICARBAZIDE
(Aminourea, Carbamylhydrazine)

mg/kg		Mouse	Rat	Guinea Pig	Rabbit	Cat	Dog	Monkey	
Lethal Dose	IV	Y125.6 [550]							
Y-LD$_{50}$	IP	Y123.3 [550]							
Z-MLD	IM								
	SC	Y125.5 [550]							
	PO	Y176 [550]							
Convulsant	IV	111.7 [550]					10 [550]		
	IP	116.4 [550]	150 [550]	75 [550]	175 [550]	40 [550]		60 [550]	
	IM								
	SC	250 [1062]							
	PO								
	IV								
	IP								
	IM								
	SC								
	PO								
	IV								
	IP								
	IM								
	SC								
	PO								

IN VITRO

mg %	Cardiac	Vascular	Gut	Uterine	Visceral	Skeletal		

SEROTONIN

(Enteramine, Thrombocytin, Thrombotonin, 5HT)

mg/kg		Mouse	Rat	Guinea Pig	Rabbit	Cat	Dog	Monkey
Lethal Dose Y-LD$_{50}$ Z-MLD	IV	Y160 [814]	Y30 [814]					
	IP	Y868 [814]	Y117 [814]					
	IM	Y750 [119]						
	SC							
	PO							
Cardiovascular, respiratory [a] total mg IT [b] mg/kg/min IA	IV		0.003		0.02 [158]	0.014 [676]	0.05 [282]	[b]0.01 [2026]
	IP		[a]0.1 [2193]					
	IM							
	SC							
	PO							
Barbiturate sleep potentiation	IV		1.25 [677]					
	IP	8 [98]	10 [286]					
	IM							
	SC	50 [286]	50 [286]					
	PO							
EEG (desynchronization)	IV				0.065 [331]	0.05 [678]		
	IP							
	IM							
	SC							
	PO							
Anticonvulsant	IV							
	IP							
	IM							
	SC		50 [414]					
	PO							
Decreased cold exposure survival time	IV							
	IP							
	IM							
	SC		2 [679]					
	PO							
Gastrointestinal [a] mg/kg/min	IV						[a]0.03 [1870]	
	IP							
	IM							
	SC							
	PO							
Analgesic [a] total mg IT	IV		[a]0.1 [2193]					
	IP							
	IM							
	SC							
	PO							
Decrease endotoxin mortality	IV							
	IP	32.5 [1322]						
	IM							
	SC							
	PO							

mg/kg		Mouse	Rat	Guinea Pig	Rabbit	Cat	Dog	Monkey
Broncho-constriction	IV			0.006 $_{1295}$				
	IP							
	IM							
	SC							
	PO							
Increased vagal afferent activity	IV					0.05 $_{292}$	0.05 $_{631}$	
	IP							
	IM							
	SC							
	PO							
Behavioral	IV							
	IP	50 $_{954}$						
	IM							
	SC	40 $_{935}$	5 $_{1050}$					
	PO							
Decreased caloric intake	IV							
	IP							
	IM							
	SC		3 $_{680}$					
	PO							
Antagonize reserpine ptosis	IV							
	IP	12.5 $_{78}$						
	IM							
	SC							
	PO							
	IV							
	IP							
	IM							
	SC							
	PO							

IN VITRO

mg %	Cardiac	Vascular	Gut	Uterine	Visceral	Skeletal	Trachea	
Rat			0.008 $_{1157}$	0.012 $_{443}$				
Guinea Pig			0.02				0.08 $_{1157}$	
Rabbit	[a]0.02 $_{67}$	0.004 $_{1157}$						
Cat	[a]0.01 $_{292}$							
[a]total mg								

SERTRALINE
(CP-51974-1)

mg/kg		Mouse	Rat	Guinea Pig	Rabbit	Cat	Dog	Monkey
Lethal Dose	IV							
Y-LD$_{50}$	IP							
Z-MLD	IM							
	SC							
	PO							
Mydriasis	IV							
	IP							
	IM							
	SC	32 $_{1439}$						
	PO							
Oxotremorine Interaction	IV							
	IP							
	IM							
	SC	32 $_{1439}$						
	PO							
Reserpine interaction	IV							
	IP							
	IM							
	SC							
	PO	10 $_{1439}$						
5HT interaction (behavior)	IV							
	IP							
	IM							
	SC							
	PO	5.6 $_{1439}$						
	IV							
	IP							
	IM							
	SC							
	PO							
	IV							
	IP							
	IM							
	SC							
	PO							
	IV							
	IP							
	IM							
	SC							
	PO							
	IV							
	IP							
	IM							
	SC							
	PO							

SODIUM BROMIDE

(Sedoneural)

mg/kg		Mouse	Rat	Guinea Pig	Rabbit	Cat	Dog	Monkey
Lethal Dose	IV		Z1800 53					
Y-LD$_{50}$	IP							
Z-MLD	IM							
	SC	Y5020 1063						
	PO	Y7000 176	Y3500 682		Z580			
Sedative	IV						350	
	IP							
^{a}total mg	IM							
	SC						350	
	PO	3000 176			5000	^{a}30-325*	^{a}100-2000*	
Anticonvulsant	IV				50			
	IP							
	IM							
	SC	250 1063			150			
	PO	2000 550						
	IV							
	IP							
	IM							
	SC							
	PO							

*2275

IN VITRO

mg %	Cardiac	Vascular	Gut	Uterine	Visceral	Skeletal		

SODIUM FLUORIDE

(Fluorinse, Pediaflor, Zendium)

mg/kg		Mouse	Rat	Guinea Pig	Rabbit	Cat	Dog	Monkey	
Lethal Dose	IV				87.5 687		Z80 683		
Y-LD$_{50}$	IP	125 109	Z31 683						
Z-MLD	IM						Z40 683		
	SC	70 346	Z125 684	Z400 686		13.7 109	155 109		
	PO	80 346	Y200 685	Z250 686	Z200 684		Z75 683		
	IV								
	IP								
	IM								
	SC								
	PO								
	IV								
	IP								
	IM								
	SC								
	PO								
	IV								
	IP								
	IM								
	SC								
	PO								

IN VITRO

mg %		Cardiac	Vascular	Gut	Uterine	Visceral	Skeletal		

SODIUM NITRITE
(Erinitrit)

mg/kg		Mouse	Rat	Guinea Pig	Rabbit	Cat	Dog	Monkey	
Lethal Dose	IV				Z85 689		Z15		
Y-LD$_{50}$	IP								
Z-MLD	IM								
	SC		Z15 688		Z60 109	35 690	Z60 691		
	PO						Z330		
Cardiovascular	IV						10		
	IP		25 7						
[a]total mg	IM								
	SC		20 539				15		
	PO		40 7				[a]90		
Protect	IV	100 2275					[a]10-20 2275		
against CN	IP								
[a]use with	IM		10						
Na$_2$S$_2$O$_3$	SC								
IV, 500-1000	PO								
	IV								
	IP								
	IM								
	SC								
	PO								

IN VITRO

mg %	Cardiac	Vascular	Gut	Uterine	Visceral	Skeletal		
Rabbit		0.01	0.1					

SOTALOL

(Beta-Cardone, Sotacor, Sotalex)

mg/kg		Mouse	Rat	Guinea Pig	Rabbit	Cat	Dog	Monkey
Lethal Dose	IV							
Y-LD$_{50}$	IP	Y670 887	Y680 887				Y330 887	
Z-MLD	IM							
	SC							
	PO	Y2600 887	Y3450 887		Y1000 887			
Adrenolytic	IV		0.5 887					
(α-block)	IP							
	IM							
	SC		10 1083	10 1081				
	PO			0.4 887			18 1082	
Acute	IV						5 1858	
toxicosis	IP	40 887	93 887				54 887	
	IM							
	SC							
	PO	288 887	515 887					
Antiarrhythmic	IV						8 2195	
	IP							
	IM							
	SC							
	PO							

IN VITRO

mg %	Cardiac	Vascular	Gut	Uterine	Visceral	Skeletal		
Dog	10 1228							
Guinea Pig	0.0272 2196							
Rabbit	0.0272 2196							

SPARTEINE

(Lupinidine, Spartocin, Synastrin)

mg/kg		Mouse	Rat	Guinea Pig	Rabbit	Cat	Dog	Monkey	
Lethal Dose	IV				Z30 [109]				
Y-LD$_{50}$	IP								
Z-MLD	IM								
	SC	Z120 [692]			Z100 [109]				
	PO								
Cardiovascular	IV				5 [693]	5 [694]	5 [694]		
	IP								
	IM						10 [693]		
	SC						20 [693]		
	PO						60 [693]		
Ganglionic block	IV					1 [694]			
	IP								
	IM								
	SC								
	PO								
	IV								
	IP								
	IM								
	SC								
	PO								

IN VITRO

mg %	Cardiac	Vascular	Gut	Uterine	Visceral	Skeletal		

STREPTOZOCIN

(Zanosar, Streptozotocin, NSC-85998)

mg/kg		Mouse	Rat	Guinea Pig	Rabbit	Cat	Dog	Monkey	
Lethal Dose	IV								
Y-LD$_{50}$	IP								
Z-MLD	IM								
	SC								
	PO								
Induce	IV		55 2198				50 2275	50 2275	
diabetes	IP		60 2197						
	IM		22 1777						
	SC								
	PO								
Treat	IV						[a]14.5 2272		
hyperinsulinism	IP								
	IM								
	SC								
[a]daily	PO								
	IV								
	IP								
	IM								
	SC								
	PO								
	IV								
	IP								
	IM								
	SC								
	PO								
	IV								
	IP								
	IM								
	SC								
	PO								
	IV								
	IP								
	IM								
	SC								
	PO								
	IV								
	IP								
	IM								
	SC								
	PO								
	IV								
	IP								
	IM								
	SC								
	PO								

STRYCHNINE

mg/kg		Mouse	Rat	Guinea Pig	Rabbit	Cat	Dog	Monkey
Lethal Dose	IV	0.8 [176]	Z1.1 [695]		0.35 [109]	0.33 [109]	0.25 [109]	
Y-LD$_{50}$	IP	Y0.98 [284]	Y2.1 [696]					
Z-MLD	IM		Z4 [697]					
	SC	Y0.85 [284]	Y1.2 [697]	3.2 [109]	0.7 [109]	0.75 [109]	0.35 [109]	
	PO		Y16.2 [685]		15 [109]	0.75 [109]	1.1 [109]	
Convulsant	IV					0.5 [870]		
	IP	2.5 [924]	1.6 [1220]					
	IM		4					
	SC	1.33	8 [88]		0.4 [611]		0.07	
	PO	2 [935]						
Analeptic	IV				0.6			
	IP							
	IM							
[a]total mg	SC						[a]0.95 [97]	
	PO					[a]0.3 [97]	[a]0.95 [97]	
CNS	IV					0.1 [947]		
	IP					0.1 [1068]		
	IM							
	SC							
	PO							

IN VITRO

mg %	Cardiac	Vascular	Gut	Uterine	Visceral	Skeletal	
Rabbit		1	1				

SUBSTANCE K

(Neurokinin A)

mg/kg		Mouse	Rat	Guinea Pig	Rabbit	Cat	Dog	Monkey
Lethal Dose	IV							
Y-LD$_{50}$	IP							
Z-MLD	IM							
	SC							
	PO							
Activate	IV							
micturition	IP							
reflex	IM							
[a]total nMol	SC		[a]36 2199					
on bladder	PO							
Activate GI	IV		[a]0.83 1521					
motility	IP							
[a]nMol/kg	IM							
[b]total μmol	SC		[b]0.06 1521					
topical on gut	PO							
	IV							
	IP							
	IM							
	SC							
	PO							

IN VITRO

mg %	Cardiac	Vascular	Gut	Uterine	Visceral	Skeletal	Urinary Bladder
Rat							[a]2.9×10^{-8}*
[a]molar							
solution							

*2199

SUBSTANCE P

mg/kg		Mouse	Rat	Guinea Pig	Rabbit	Cat	Dog	Monkey
Lethal Dose $Y-LD_{50}$ $Z-MLD$	IV							
	IP							
	IM							
	SC							
	PO							
Salivation	IV		$0.003\ _{2200}$					
	IP							
	IM							
	SC							
	PO							
Cardiovascular [a]total μg IT	IV		[a]$4.45\ _{2101}$					
	IP							
	IM							
	SC							
	PO							
Effect on respiratory control system [a]ICV	IV		[a]0.003_{2201}					
	IP							
	IM							
	SC							
	PO							
Activate micturition reflex [a]total mg on bladder	IV							
	IP							
	IM							
	SC		[a]0.659_{2199}					
	PO							
Activate GI motility [a]total mg topical on gut	IV		0.0009_{1521}					
	IP							
	IM							
	SC		[a]0.485_{1521}					
	PO							
Decrease locomotor activity [a]total mg	IV							
	IP	[a]$5\ _{2205}$						
	IM							
	SC							
	PO							
Decrease 5HT & DA turnover [a]total mg	IV							
	IP	[a]$5\ _{2205}$						
	IM							
	SC							
	PO							
Suppress nalorphine-induced jumping [a]total mg	IV							
	IP							
	IM	[a]$10\ _{2206}$						
	SC							
	PO							

SUBSTANCE P (continued)

mg/kg		Mouse	Rat	Guinea Pig	Rabbit	Cat	Dog	Monkey	
	IV								
	IP								
	IM								
	SC								
	PO								
	IV								
	IP								
	IM								
	SC								
	PO								
	IV								
	IP								
	IM								
	SC								
	PO								
	IV								
	IP								
	IM								
	SC								
	PO								

IN VITRO

mg %	Cardiac	Vascular	Gut	Uterine	Visceral	Urinary Bladder	Trachea	
Rat						0.0061_{2199}		
Guinea Pig			0.0047_{2202}				$0.0013**$	
Dog			$1.3 \times 10^{-5}*$					

*2203   **2204

SUCCINYLCHOLINE

(Anectine, Quelicin, Suxamethonium, Sucostrin)

mg/kg		Mouse	Rat	Guinea Pig	Rabbit	Cat	Dog	Monkey	
Lethal Dose Y-LD$_{50}$ Z-MLD	IV	Y0.75 [111]			Y1 [281]		0.3 [281]		
	IP	Y4 [111]							
	IM								
	SC								
	PO	Y125 [111]							
Neuromuscular block	IV	0.45 [557]	0.45 [557]		0.25 [557]	0.08 [557]	0.1		
	IP					1			
	IM								
	SC								
	PO				0.1				
Ataxic and Respiratory depression	IV				0.075				
	IP								
	IM								
	SC						0.05		
	PO								
EEG	IV					0.1 [1175]			
	IP								
	IM								
	SC								
	PO								

IN VITRO

mg %	Cardiac	Vascular	Gut	Uterine	Visceral	Skeletal		
Rat						0.5 [1157]		

SUFENTANIL

(Sufenta, R-33800, Sufentanyl)

mg/kg		Mouse	Rat	Guinea Pig	Rabbit	Cat	Dog	Monkey	
Lethal Dose	IV								
Y-LD$_{50}$	IP								
Z-MLD	IM								
	SC								
	PO								
Inhibit	IV		[a]0.002$_{1743}$						
urinary	IP								
bladder	IM								
[a]total nmol	SC								
ICV	PO								
Cardiovascular	IV						0.02 $_{2207}$		
	IP								
	IM								
	SC								
	PO								
	IV								
	IP								
	IM								
	SC								
	PO								
	IV								
	IP								
	IM								
	SC								
	PO								
	IV								
	IP								
	IM								
	SC								
	PO								
	IV								
	IP								
	IM								
	SC								
	PO								
	IV								
	IP								
	IM								
	SC								
	PO								
	IV								
	IP								
	IM								
	SC								
	PO								

SULINDAC

(Clinoril)

mg/kg		Mouse	Rat	Guinea Pig	Rabbit	Cat	Dog	Monkey	
Lethal Dose	IV								
Y-LD$_{50}$	IP								
Z-MLD	IM								
	SC								
	PO								
Effect on	IV						[5] 1826		
renal PG	IP								
synthesis	IM								
	SC								
	PO								
Analgesic	IV								
	IP								
	IM								
[a]Freund's	SC		[a]2.56 1284						
adjuvant	PO								
	IV								
	IP								
	IM								
	SC								
	PO								
	IV								
	IP								
	IM								
	SC								
	PO								
	IV								
	IP								
	IM								
	SC								
	PO								
	IV								
	IP								
	IM								
	SC								
	PO								
	IV								
	IP								
	IM								
	SC								
	PO								
	IV								
	IP								
	IM								
	SC								
	PO								

SULPIRIDE

(Dogmatyl, Abilit, Coolspan)

mg/kg		Mouse	Rat	Guinea Pig	Rabbit	Cat	Dog	Monkey	
Lethal Dose	IV								
Y-LD$_{50}$	IP								
Z-MLD	IM								
	SC								
	PO								
Antagonize	IV								
apomorphine	IP	10 1414							
climbing	IM								
and hypothermia	SC								
	PO								
Cardiovascular	IV						1 1748		
	IP						0.25 1568		
	IM								
^{a}total mg ICV	SC								
	PO								
CNS Dopamine	IV								
receptor	IP		20 2209						
sensitivity	IM								
^{a}20 days,	SC		^{a}50 2208						
behavioral	PO								

IN VITRO

mg %	Cardiac	Vascular	Gut	Uterine	Visceral	Skeletal	CNS	
Rabbit		0.0102 2210					0.0003*	

*1411

SYNEPHRINE

(Analeptin, Oxedrine, Parasympatol)

mg/kg		Mouse	Rat	Guinea Pig	Rabbit	Cat	Dog	Monkey	
Lethal Dose	IV								
Y-LD$_{50}$	IP								
Z-MLD	IM								
	SC	750 $_{406}$							
	PO								
Cardiovascular	IV					[a]0.7 $_{266}$	0.25 $_{408}$		
	IP								
[a]total mg	IM								
	SC								
	PO								
Decrease	IV								
catecholamine	IP	40 $_{338}$							
binding	IM								
	SC								
	PO								
Oxytocic	IV		2.5 $_{407}$						
	IP								
	IM								
	SC								
	PO								
	IV								
	IP								
	IM								
	SC								
	PO								
	IV								
	IP								
	IM								
	SC								
	PO								
	IV								
	IP								
	IM								
	SC								
	PO								
	IV								
	IP								
	IM								
	SC								
	PO								
	IV								
	IP								
	IM								
	SC								
	PO								

SYROSINGOPINE

(Singoserp, Isotense, Siringina)

mg/kg		Mouse	Rat	Guinea Pig	Rabbit	Cat	Dog	Monkey	
Lethal Dose Y-LD$_{50}$ Z-MLD Z-MLD	IV		Y50 640				>3 640	>2 640	
	IP								
	IM								
	SC								
	PO								
Catecholamine depletion	IV				1 700	10 836	0.5 700		
	IP	5 698	40 699						
	IM								
	SC								
	PO								
Sedative	IV				4.5 700		5 640	2 640	
	IP		50 699						
	IM								
	SC	25 640							
	PO						>30 640		
Cardiovascular	IV						1 640		
	IP		0.95 699						
	IM								
	SC								
	PO						3 640		
	IV								
	IP								
	IM								
	SC								
	PO								
	IV								
	IP								
	IM								
	SC								
	PO								
	IV								
	IP								
	IM								
	SC								
	PO								
	IV								
	IP								
	IM								
	SC								
	PO								
	IV								
	IP								
	IM								
	SC								
	PO								

T-2 TOXIN

(Trichothecene mycotoxin)

mg/kg		Mouse	Rat	Guinea Pig	Rabbit	Cat	Dog	Monkey
Lethal Dose $Y-LD_{50}$ $Z-MLD$	IV		Y0.75 2211	Y1.3 2211				
	IP							
	IM							
	SC							
	PO							
Cardiovascular	IV		0.5 2211	0.5 2211				
	IP							
	IM							
	SC							
	PO							
	IV							
	IP							
	IM							
	SC							
	PO							
	IV							
	IP							
	IM							
	SC							
	PO							
	IV							
	IP							
	IM							
	SC							
	PO							
	IV							
	IP							
	IM							
	SC							
	PO							
	IV							
	IP							
	IM							
	SC							
	PO							
	IV							
	IP							
	IM							
	SC							
	PO							
	IV							
	IP							
	IM							
	SC							
	PO							

TERBUTALINE

(Brethaire, Brethine, Bricanyl)

mg/kg		Mouse	Rat	Guinea Pig	Rabbit	Cat	Dog	Monkey	
Lethal Dose Y-LD_{50} Z-MLD	IV								
	IP								
	IM								
	SC								
	PO								
Beta$_2$ stimulation after β_1 block [a]mg/kg/min	IV						[a]0.027_{1947}		
	IP								
	IM								
	SC								
	PO								
Pulmonary	IV								
	IP								
	IM								
	SC		0.01_{2151}						
	PO								
Decrease urinary bladder contraction [a] total mg	IV								
	IP		[a]3_{1424}						
	IM								
	SC								
	PO								
Broncho-dilation [a]total mg, Q8-12h	IV								
	IP								
	IM								
	SC								
	PO					[a]1.25_{2273}	[a]1.25-5_{2273}		
	IV								
	IP								
	IM								
	SC								
	PO								
	IV								
	IP								
	IM								
	SC								
	PO								
	IV								
	IP								
	IM								
	SC								
	PO								
	IV								
	IP								
	IM								
	SC								
	PO								

457

TERTATOL

(Servier 2395)

mg/kg		Mouse	Rat	Guinea Pig	Rabbit	Cat	Dog	Monkey	
Lethal Dose	IV								
Y-LD$_{50}$	IP								
Z-MLD	IM								
	SC								
	PO								
	IV								
	IP								
	IM								
	SC								
	PO								
	IV								
	IP								
	IM								
	SC								
	PO								
	IV								
	IP								
	IM								
	SC								
	PO								

IN VITRO

mg %	Cardiac	Vascular	Gut	Uterine	Visceral	Skeletal	Trachea	
Guinea Pig							$a_{3 \times 10^{-7}}$*	
Dog		$a_{1 \times 10^{-5}}$*						
a molar								
solution								

*2212

TETRABENAZINE

(Nitoman, RO-1-9569)

mg/kg		Mouse	Rat	Guinea Pig	Rabbit	Cat	Dog	Monkey	
Lethal Dose Y-LD$_{50}$ Z-MLD	IV	Y150 $_{115}$							
	IP								
	IM								
	SC	Y400 $_{115}$							
	PO								
Amine-depletion	IV				50 $_{601}$	80 $_{1202}$			
	IP	10 $_{861}$	2 $_{880}$						
	IM								
	SC								
	PO								
Barbiturate sleep potentiation	IV				50 $_{601}$				
	IP	40 $_{28}$							
	IM								
	SC								
	PO								
Behavioral [a]methamphetamine interaction	IV				40 $_{703}$				
	IP	200 $_{2213}$	0.5 $_{370}$						
	IM								
	SC		8 $_{702}$						
	PO	[a]82.6 $_{1372}$							
Sedative	IV								
	IP		20 $_{899}$						
	IM								
	SC							2 $_{702}$	
	PO								
Induce immobility and ptosis	IV								
	IP	40 $_{1371}$							
	IM								
	SC								
	PO								
	IV								
	IP								
	IM								
	SC								
	PO								
	IV								
	IP								
	IM								
	SC								
	PO								
	IV								
	IP								
	IM								
	SC								
	PO								

TETRACAINE

(Pontocaine, Amethocaine, Curtacain)

mg/kg		Mouse	Rat	Guinea Pig	Rabbit	Cat	Dog	Monkey	
Lethal Dose	IV	Y6.6 1349		Y15.6 629	8		Y4.3 704		
Y-LD$_{50}$	IP								
Z-MLD	IM			30 7					
	SC								
	PO								
Convulsant	IV	a2.95 1349	1.5 705						
	IP								
aED$_{50}$	IM								
	SC								
	PO								
Anticonvulsant	IV					0.8			
	IP								
	IM								
	SC	4.4 441							
	PO								
	IV								
	IP								
	IM								
	SC								
	PO								

IN VITRO

mg %		Cardiac	Vascular	Gut	Uterine	Visceral	Skeletal	Trachea	

TETRAETHYLAMMONIUM
(Etamon, TEA)

mg/kg		Mouse	Rat	Guinea Pig	Rabbit	Cat	Dog	Monkey	
Lethal Dose	IV	Y29 $_{214}$	Y63 $_{706}$		Y72 $_{706}$		Y55 $_{706}$		
Y-LD$_{50}$	IP	Y56 $_{214}$	Y115 $_{706}$						
Z-MLD	IM								
	SC	102 $_{707}$							
	PO	Y655 $_{214}$							
Ganglionic block	IV					10	10		
	IP								
	IM								
	SC								
	PO								
Cardiovascular	IV					3 $_{708}$	5 $_{708}$		
	IP								
	IM						2.5-7.5 $_{2275}$		
	SC								
	PO								
EKG	IV					25 $_{709}$	25 $_{709}$		
	IP								
	IM								
	SC								
	PO								
Catecholamine sensitization	IV				2.5 $_{395}$	2.5 $_{395}$			
	IP								
	IM								
	SC								
	PO								
Nictitating membrane potentiation	IV					2 $_{395}$			
	IP								
	IM								
	SC								
	PO								
Behavioral	IV								
	IP								
	IM								
	SC	80 $_{935}$							
	PO								
Anticonvulsant	IV								
	IP								
	IM								
	SC	30 $_{957}$							
	PO								
Decrease amphetamine hyperthermia	IV				15 $_{1182}$				
	IP								
	IM								
	SC								
	PO								

461

TETRAETHYLAMMONIUM (continued)

mg/kg		Mouse	Rat	Guinea Pig	Rabbit	Cat	Dog	Monkey	
	IV								
	IP								
	IM								
	SC								
	PO								
	IV								
	IP								
	IM								
	SC								
	PO								
	IV								
	IP								
	IM								
	SC								
	PO								
	IV								
	IP								
	IM								
	SC								
	PO								

IN VITRO

mg %	Cardiac	Vascular	Gut	Uterine	Visceral	Skeletal		
Contractile			0.75 388					
Adrenolytic			0.001 395					

Δ^1 -TETRAHYDROCANNABINOL

$(\Delta^1$ -THC)

mg/kg		Mouse	Rat	Guinea Pig	Rabbit	Cat	Dog	Monkey	
Lethal Dose	IV								
Y-LD$_{50}$	IP	^{a}Y270$_{2215}$							
Z-MLD	IM	^{b}Y519$_{2215}$							
^{a}isolated	SC								
^{b}IP, aggregat.	PO								
Barbiturate	IV								
sleep	IP	10$_{2214}$							
potentiation	IM								
	SC								
	PO								
Euphoria	IV							0.25$_{2275}$	
	IP								
	IM								
	SC								
	PO						0.5$_{2275}$		
	IV								
	IP								
	IM								
	SC								
	PO								
	IV								
	IP								
	IM								
	SC								
	PO								
	IV								
	IP								
	IM								
	SC								
	PO								
	IV								
	IP								
	IM								
	SC								
	PO								
	IV								
	IP								
	IM								
	SC								
	PO								
	IV								
	IP								
	IM								
	SC								
	PO								

463

Δ^9 -TETRAHYDROCANNABINOL
(Δ^9 -THC)

mg/kg		Mouse	Rat	Guinea Pig	Rabbit	Cat	Dog	Monkey	
Lethal Dose	IV								
Y-LD$_{50}$	IP	Y510$_{2194}$							
Z-MLD	IM	a200$_{1193}$							
a IP	SC								
	PO								
Cardiovascular	IV				0.05$_{2216}$	1$_{1185}$	6$_{1189}$	a0.5$_{2217}$	
a QID	IP					b3.25$_{2228}$			
b IV; CV &	IM								
respiratory	SC								
	PO								
Behavioral	IV		1$_{1187}$				0.062$_{2218}$	0.003$_{2220}$	
a locomotor	IP	25$_{1198}$	1$_{2219}$					b0.05$_{2226}$	
b mg/kg/hr IV,	IM							3$_{2218}$	
dependence	SC								
c daily	PO	5$_{2218}$	c50$_{1191}$	a3$_{2221}$			0.25$_{2218}$	c50$_{1191}$	
Hypothermic	IV								
	IP	10$_{1189}$							
	IM								
	SC		20$_{1227}$						
	PO								
Gastrointestinal	IV								
	IP								
	IM								
	SC	30$_{1238}$							
	PO								
Brain	IV	50$_{1541}$	50$_{1541}$						
chemistry	IP		10$_{2223}$						
effects	IM								
	SC	10$_{2222}$							
	PO								
Endocrine	IV		0.0625$_{2224}$						
effects	IP		10$_{2108}$						
(anti-LH)	IM								
	SC								
	PO								
Inhibit	IV								
naloxone-	IP	2.5$_{2225}$							
induced	IM								
withdrawal	SC								
	PO			3$_{2221}$					
Analgesic	IV								
	IP								
	IM								
	SC	20$_{2227}$							
	PO								

Δ^9 -TETRAHYDROCANNABINOL (continued)

mg/kg		Mouse	Rat	Guinea Pig	Rabbit	Cat	Dog	Monkey	
Anticonvulsant	IV								
	IP	40 2070							
	IM								
	SC								
	PO								
	IV								
	IP								
	IM								
	SC								
	PO								
	IV								
	IP								
	IM								
	SC								
	PO								
	IV								
	IP								
	IM								
	SC								
	PO								

IN VITRO

mg %	Cardiac	Vascular	Gut	Uterine	Visceral	Skeletal	CNS	
Rat							0.0031*	

*2229

TETRAMETHYLAMMONIUM
(TMA)

mg/kg		Mouse	Rat	Guinea Pig	Rabbit	Cat	Dog	Monkey	
Lethal Dose	IV				1.5 341				
Y-LD$_{50}$	IP								
Z-MLD	IM								
	SC	20 710			7 710				
	PO								
Ganglionic	IV					1	0.25		
stimulant	IP								
	IM								
	SC								
	PO								
Decrease	IV								
blood pressure	IP								
in experimental	IM								
hypertension	SC								
	PO		3 387						
	IV								
	IP								
	IM								
	SC								
	PO								

IN VITRO

mg %	Cardiac	Vascular	Gut	Uterine	Visceral	Skeletal		
Guinea Pig	8 1157		2 1157					

TETRODOTOXIN

(Maculotoxin, Spheroidine, Tarichatoxin, TTX)

mg/kg		Mouse	Rat	Guinea Pig	Rabbit	Cat	Dog	Monkey
Lethal Dose	IV							
Y-LD$_{50}$	IP							
Z-MLD	IM							
	SC							
	PO							
CNS	IV		$^a 50 \times 10^{-6}$*					
	IP							
	IM							
^{a}i. cranial	SC							
	PO							
Gastrointestinal	IV							
	IP							
^{a}Total μg,	IM							
topical	SC		$^a 20$ 1521					
	PO							
Urinary	IV							
bladder	IP							
motility	IM							
^{a}Total μg,	SC		$^a 20$ 2199					
topical	PO							

*1831

IN VITRO

mg %	Cardiac	Vascular	Gut	Uterine	Visceral	CNS	Renal	
Rat			0.002 1717		0.0096 1410	0.016 2230		
Guinea Pig	0.032 2164							
Dog	0.025 1353							

THALIDOMIDE

(Kevadon, Contergan, Distaval, K-17)

mg/kg		Mouse	Rat	Guinea Pig	Rabbit	Cat	Dog	Monkey
Lethal Dose	IV							
Y-LD$_{50}$	IP	>4000 [484]						
Z-MLD	IM							
	SC							
	PO	>5000 [484]						
CNS	IV							
(depression)	IP	500 [124]	550 [124]				65 [124]	
	IM					100 [557]	300 [557]	
	SC							
	PO	100 [484]		650 [484]				
Anticonvulsant	IV							
	IP	525 [124]						
	IM							
	SC							
	PO							
Decreased	IV							
motor activity	IP	1000 [711]	33 [2275]					
	IM							
[a]spontaneous	SC							
	PO	400 [484]	[a]8 [2231]	650 [484]		[a]8 [2231]		
Barbiturate	IV							
sleep	IP	1000 [711]						
potentiation	IM							
	SC							
	PO	1600 [484]						
Block	IV							
stress-induced	IP							
ulcer	IM							
	SC							
	PO	100 [712]						
Potentiate	IV							
chlorpromazine	IP							
and reserpine	IM							
catatonia	SC							
	PO	200 [484]						
Litter	IV							
malformation	IP							
or resorption	IM							
(fetal damage)	SC							
	PO	125-250*	150 [859]		100 [859]		100 [2275]	5-10 [2275]
	IV							
Increase REM	IP							
sleep	IM							
(not ataxic)	SC							
	PO		16 [2231]			2 [2231]		

*2275

THALIDOMIDE (continued)

mg/kg		Mouse	Rat	Guinea Pig	Rabbit	Cat	Dog	Monkey	
Respiratory depression and ataxia	IV								
	IP	30 $_{2231}$							
	IM								
	SC								
	PO								
	IV								
	IP								
	IM								
	SC								
	PO								
	IV								
	IP								
	IM								
	SC								
	PO								
	IV								
	IP								
	IM								
	SC								
	PO								

IN VITRO

mg %	Cardiac	Vascular	Gut	Uterine	Visceral	Skeletal		
Anticholinerg.			3 $_{484}$					
Antihistaminic			3 $_{484}$					

THEOPHYLLINE
(Duraphyl, Elixophyllin, Somophyllin, Theophyl)

mg/kg		Mouse	Rat	Guinea Pig	Rabbit	Cat	Dog	Monkey
Lethal Dose Y-LD$_{50}$ Z-MLD	IV		Z240		115 [109]			
	IP							
	IM							
	SC	Z200 [7]	Z325	185 [109]				
	PO				350 [109]	100 [109]		
Cardiovascular and diuretic ^{a}mg/min IA	IV				15	10	20 [898]	
	IP						^{a}1 [1837]	
	IM							
	SC							
	PO		30			3 [2272]	5-7 [2272]	
Increased motor activity ^{a}mg/min	IV		^{a}1.03 [2234]					
	IP							
	IM							
	SC		20 [180]					
	PO					50 [1007]		
Antagonize antinociception	IV		0.17 [1954]					
	IP							
	IM							
	SC							
	PO							
Behavioral	IV							
	IP	1.8 [2233]	45 [1501]					
	IM							
	SC				36 [1503]			
	PO				10 [2232]			
Increased prostaglandin excretion	IV							
	IP							
	IM							
	SC							
	PO		10 [1840]					
Respiratory effects	IV						20 [1907]	
	IP							
	IM							
	SC							
	PO					3 [2272]	5-7 [2272]	

IN VITRO

mg %	Cardiac	Vascular	Gut	Uterine	Visceral	Trachea	Fat	
Anti-5HT			8 [92]					
Guinea Pig	5.4 [2235]					2 [1157]		
Dog	0.9 [1321]							
Rat							5.95 [2236]	
Rabbit		0.18 [2237]						

THIOPENTAL

(Pentothal, Nesdonal, Thionembutal)

mg/kg		Mouse	Rat	Guinea Pig	Rabbit	Cat	Dog	Monkey	
Lethal Dose	IV	Y112 713	Y67.5 111	Y55 7	Y40 111		Y55 111		
Y-LD50	IP	Y200 111	Y120 111	Y57.5 714					
Z-MLD	IM								
	SC								
	PO	Y350 111			Y600 111		Y150 111		
Anesthetic	IV	25 111	20 111	20 111	20 111	28 24	25 716		
	IP		40 674	55 111		60 557			
	IM								
	SC								
	PO		70 715				100 111		
Behavioral	IV	17 933			5 562	5 889		0.5-4 1179	
	IP	15 1131							
	IM								
	SC				20 562				
	PO					50 953			
Depressed	IV					40 717			
spinal neuron	IP								
EPSP	IM								
	SC								
	PO								
EEG	IV				15 965	20 112	20 966	5 945	
	IP								
	IM								
	SC								
	PO								
Anticonvulsant	IV								
	IP								
	IM								
	SC	30 957							
	PO								
	IV								
	IP								
	IM								
	SC								
	PO								
	IV								
	IP								
	IM								
	SC								
	PO								
	IV								
	IP								
	IM								
	SC								
	PO								

THIOTHIXENE

(Navane, Tiotixene, Orbinamon)

mg/kg		Mouse	Rat	Guinea Pig	Rabbit	Cat	Dog	Monkey
Lethal Dose	IV							
Y-LD$_{50}$	IP							
Z-MLD	IM							
	SC							
	PO							
Tranquilize	IV							
	IP							
	IM							
	SC							
[a]ED$_{50}$	PO	[a]12.4 [1372]						
Decrease	IV							
methamphetamine	IP							
fighting	IM							
	SC							
	PO	1 [1372]						
Decrease	IV							
methamphetamine	IP							
hyperactivity	IM							
	SC							
	PO	5 [1372]						
	IV							
	IP							
	IM							
	SC							
	PO							
	IV							
	IP							
	IM							
	SC							
	PO							
	IV							
	IP							
	IM							
	SC							
	PO							
	IV							
	IP							
	IM							
	SC							
	PO							
	IV							
	IP							
	IM							
	SC							
	PO							

THYROTROPIN RELEASING HORMONE
(TRH)

mg/kg		Mouse	Rat	Guinea Pig	Rabbit	Cat	Dog	Monkey
Lethal Dose	IV							
Y-LD$_{50}$	IP	[a]30 2242						
Z-MLD	IM							
[a]Pentobarbital	SC							
interaction	PO							
Behavioral	IV	[a]0.26 2239						
	IP			20 2238				
[a]Induce forepaw	IM							
tremor	SC							
	PO							
Antagonize	IV	[a]2 2239	[b]1 1334					
depressants	IP							
[a]Barbiturate	IM							
[b]total μg i.	SC							
cisternal, ETOH	PO							
Cardiovascular	IV		[a]10 2240					
	IP							
[a]total μg IT	IM							
	SC							
	PO							
Increase	IV		10 2241					
brain	IP							
cGMP	IM							
	SC							
	PO							
Analeptic	IV							
	IP	3 2242						
	IM							
	SC							
	PO							
	IV							
	IP							
	IM							
	SC							
	PO							
	IV							
	IP							
	IM							
	SC							
	PO							
	IV							
	IP							
	IM							
	SC							
	PO							

TIFLUADOM

mg/kg		Mouse	Rat	Guinea Pig	Rabbit	Cat	Dog	Monkey	
Lethal Dose	IV								
Y-LD_{50}	IP								
Z-MLD	IM								
	SC								
	PO								
Analgesic	IV								
	IP								
[a]ED_{50}	IM								
	SC	[a]0.79 [1482]	0.12 [1500]	[a]0.02 [1482]				0.31 [1479]	
	PO								
Sedative	IV								
	IP								
[a]rotorod	IM								
	SC	[a]0.4 [1482]						0.1 [1479]	
	PO								
Behavioral	IV								
	IP								
	IM							0.056 [1477]	
	SC								
	PO								
Effects on	IV		[a]20 [1743]						
urinary bladder	IP								
	IM								
[a]nMol ICV	SC		5 [1478]					0.1 [1479]	
	PO								
Decrease	IV								
respiratory	IP								
rate	IM							0.3 [1880]	
	SC								
	PO								
Decrease	IV								
dopamine	IP								
release	IM								
in brain	SC		0.3 [1480]						
	PO								
Increase	IV								
corticoid	IP		0.2 [1745]						
release	IM								
(CNS effect)	SC								
	PO								
Increase	IV				0.1 [1481]				
spinal	IP								
reflexes	IM								
	SC								
	PO								

mg/kg		Mouse	Rat	Guinea Pig	Rabbit	Cat	Dog	Monkey	
	IV								
	IP								
	IM								
	SC								
	PO								
	IV								
	IP								
	IM								
	SC								
	PO								
	IV								
	IP								
	IM								
	SC								
	PO								
	IV								
	IP								
	IM								
	SC								
	PO								

IN VITRO

mg %	Cardiac	Vascular	Gut	Uterine	Visceral	Skeletal	CNS	
Rat							$^a 3 \times 10^{-6}$*	
^{a}molar								
solution								

*1464

TILORONE
(NSC-143969)

mg/kg		Mouse	Rat	Guinea Pig	Rabbit	Cat	Dog	Monkey
Lethal Dose	IV							
Y-LD$_{50}$	IP							
Z-MLD	IM							
	SC							
	PO							
Antiarthritic	IV							
	IP							
[a]daily	IM							
	SC							
	PO		[a]10 2103					
Antiedema	IV							
	IP							
	IM							
	SC							
	PO		100 2103					
	IV							
	IP							
	IM							
	SC							
	PO							
	IV							
	IP							
	IM							
	SC							
	PO							
	IV							
	IP							
	IM							
	SC							
	PO							
	IV							
	IP							
	IM							
	SC							
	PO							
	IV							
	IP							
	IM							
	SC							
	PO							
	IV							
	IP							
	IM							
	SC							
	PO							

TIMOLOL

(Blocadren, Timoptic, Timoptol)

mg/kg		Mouse	Rat	Guinea Pig	Rabbit	Cat	Dog	Monkey
Lethal Dose	IV							
Y-LD$_{50}$	IP							
Z-MLD	IM							
	SC							
	PO							
Antihypertensive	IV							
	IP							
	IM							
	SC							
	PO		30 1873					
	IV							
	IP							
	IM							
	SC							
	PO							
	IV							
	IP							
	IM							
	SC							
	PO							

IN VITRO

mg %	Cardiac	Vascular	Gut	Uterine	Visceral	Skeletal	Renal	
Rat		0.0032 1874					0.0284*	

*2230

TM-10

(Xylocholine)

mg/kg		Mouse	Rat	Guinea Pig	Rabbit	Cat	Dog	Monkey	
Lethal Dose	IV								
Y-LD$_{50}$	IP								
Z-MLD	IM								
	SC								
	PO	Y95$_{718}$							
Sympatholytic	IV					10 $_{719}$			
	IP								
	IM								
	SC								
	PO					17.5 $_{720}$			
Tyramine	IV					5			
potentiation	IP								
(B.P.)	IM								
	SC								
	PO								
Adrenal	IV								
medulla	IP								
catecholamine	IM								
depletion	SC		10 $_{721}$						
	PO								

IN VITRO

mg %	Cardiac	Vascular	Gut	Uterine	Visceral	Skeletal		
Adrenolytic $_{812}$			0.5					
Guinea Pig			5 $_{148}$					

ß-TM-10

(ß-Methyl Xylocholine)

mg/kg		Mouse	Rat	Guinea Pig	Rabbit	Cat	Dog	Monkey
Lethal Dose	IV	Y6.62 722						
Y-LD$_{50}$	IP							
Z-MLD	IM							
	SC							
	PO	1400 722						
Autonomic	IV	4.7 722				5 722	5 722	
	IP							
	IM							
	SC					3 722		
	PO					11.3 720		
Behavioral	IV							
	IP		30 722					
	IM							
	SC							
	PO							
	IV							
	IP							
	IM							
	SC							
	PO							

IN VITRO

mg %	Cardiac	Vascular	Gut	Uterine	Visceral	Skeletal	
Inhibition 812			10 722				

TOLAZOLINE

(Priscoline, Artonil, Vasodil)

mg/kg		Mouse	Rat	Guinea Pig	Rabbit	Cat	Dog	Monkey
Lethal Dose	IV		67_{640}					
Y-LD$_{50}$	IP	Y500						
Z-MLD	IM							
	SC							
	PO							
Adrenolytic	IV	5_{1197}		1		1	2.5	
	IP	20_{1118}	10_{219}	25_{1219}				
	IM	2.5_{1440}						
	SC							
	PO							
Cardiovascular	IV				2_{383}	1_{640}	1_{640}	
(reserpinized)	IP							
	IM							
	SC							
	PO							
CNS	IV		15_{350}					
[a]Increase	IP	$[a]30_{1670}$						
anticonvulsant	IM							
activity of	SC							
methazolamine	PO							

IN VITRO

mg %	Cardiac	Vascular	Gut	Uterine	Visceral	Skeletal		
Rabbit	0.5		1					
Rabbit Ear		2_{339}						
Guinea Pig			0.1_{1233}					

TOLMETIN

(Tolectin, McN-2559-21-98)

mg/kg		Mouse	Rat	Guinea Pig	Rabbit	Cat	Dog	Monkey
Lethal Dose Y-LD$_{50}$ Z-MLD	IV							
	IP							
	IM							
	SC							
	PO							
Anti-inflammatory	IV							
	IP							
	IM							
	SC							
	PO		56.7 1283					
Antidiuretic	IV							
	IP							
	IM							
	SC							
	PO		3 1312					
	IV							
	IP							
	IM							
	SC							
	PO							
	IV							
	IP							
	IM							
	SC							
	PO							
	IV							
	IP							
	IM							
	SC							
	PO							
	IV							
	IP							
	IM							
	SC							
	PO							
	IV							
	IP							
	IM							
	SC							
	PO							
	IV							
	IP							
	IM							
	SC							
	PO							

TRANYLCYPROMINE
(Parnate, Parnitene, Tylciprine)

mg/kg		Mouse	Rat	Guinea Pig	Rabbit	Cat	Dog	Monkey
Lethal Dose Y-LD$_{50}$ Z-MLD	IV	Y37 [115]						
	IP							
	IM							
	SC							
	PO	Y38 [115]						
Increased catecholamines (brain)	IV				5 [371]			
	IP	10 [433]	2 [1064]					
	IM		4 [1064]					
	SC		3 [868]					
	PO		5 [433]					
Reverse reserpine depression	IV							
	IP	2.5 [455]						
	IM							
	SC							
	PO	2.5 [455]						
EEG	IV				2 [331]		2 [1006]	
	IP							
	IM							
	SC							
	PO							
Cardiovascular	IV		5 [218]		2-5 [2275]			
	IP	2.5-10 [2275]	2.5-10 [2275]					
	IM							
	SC							
	PO	2.5-10 [2275]	2.5-10 [2275]	5 [2275]				
CNS stimulation and behavioral	IV					15 [861]	4 [160]	
	IP	5 [1064]						
	IM							
	SC							
	PO							
	IV							
	IP							
	IM							
	SC							
	PO							
	IV							
	IP							
	IM							
	SC							
	PO							

TRAZODONE

(Desyrel, Molipaxin, Pragmazone)

mg/kg		Mouse	Rat	Guinea Pig	Rabbit	Cat	Dog	Monkey
Lethal Dose	IV	Y96 1533						
Y-LD$_{50}$	IP							
Z-MLD	IM							
	SC							
	PO							
Analgesic	IV	a0.12 1533						
	IP							
aED$_{50}$	IM							
	SC							
	PO							
Ataxic	IV	a70.12 1533						
	IP							
aED$_{50}$	IM							
	SC							
	PO							
Anesthetic	IV	a57 1533						
	IP							
aED$_{50}$	IM							
	SC							
	PO							
GABA	IV							
receptor	IP							
regulation	IM							
	SC		a10 1366					
adaily	PO							
	IV							
	IP							
	IM							
	SC							
	PO							
	IV							
	IP							
	IM							
	SC							
	PO							
	IV							
	IP							
	IM							
	SC							
	PO							
	IV							
	IP							
	IM							
	SC							
	PO							

TREMORINE

mg/kg		Mouse	Rat	Guinea Pig	Rabbit	Cat	Dog	Monkey	
Lethal Dose	IV								
Y-LD$_{50}$	IP								
Z-MLD	IM								
	SC								
	PO								
Tremor and	IV	20 [723]	5-20 [724]	5-20 [724]		5-20 [724]	5-20 [724]	5-20 [724]	
decreased	IP	5-20 [724]	5-20 [724]	20 [724]		5-20 [724]	5 [723]	5-20 [724]	
brain amines	IM	5-20 [724]	5-20 [724]	5-20 [724]		5-20 [724]	5-20 [724]	5-20 [724]	
	SC	20 [76]	5-20 [724]	5-20 [724]		5-20 [724]	5-20 [724]	5-20 [724]	
	PO	20 [723]	5-20 [724]	5-20 [724]		5-20 [724]	5-20 [724]	5-20 [724]	
Increased	IV								
brain	IP								
histamine	IM								
	SC		100						
	PO								
Convulsant	IV								
	IP	5.8 [139]							
	IM								
	SC								
	PO								
Analgesic	IV								
	IP								
	IM	5							
	SC	6 [1066]							
	PO								
EEG	IV								
	IP					3 [725]			
	IM								
	SC								
	PO								
	IV								
	IP								
	IM								
	SC								
	PO								
	IV								
	IP								
	IM								
	SC								
	PO								
	IV								
	IP								
	IM								
	SC								
	PO								

TRIAMCINOLONE

(Aristocort, Kenacort, Tramacin, Triacet)

mg/kg		Mouse	Rat	Guinea Pig	Rabbit	Cat	Dog	Monkey	
Lethal Dose	IV								
Y-LD$_{50}$	IP								
Z-MLD	IM								
	SC								
	PO								
Effects on	IV								
spinal cord	IP								
function	IM					[a]8 2243			
[a]daily, 7 d	SC								
	PO								
Reduces plasma	IV								
ACTH and	IP								
cortisol	IM								
[a]total mg	SC						[a]15 2244		
topical	PO								
Anti-	IV								
inflammatory	IP								
[a]total mg	IM					[a]0.25-0.5*	0.25 2273		
	SC								
	PO					[a]0.25-0.5**	0.25 2272		
	IV								
	IP								
	IM								
	SC								
	PO								
	IV								
	IP								
	IM								
	SC								
	PO								
	IV								
	IP								
	IM								
	SC								
	PO								
	IV								
	IP								
	IM								
	SC								
	PO								
	IV								
	IP								
	IM								
	SC								
	PO								

*2273   **2272

485

TRIBROMOETHANOL

(Avertin, Bromethol, Narcolan)

mg/kg		Mouse	Rat	Guinea Pig	Rabbit	Cat	Dog	Monkey	
Lethal Dose	IV				135 66	300 557	300 557		
Y-LD$_{50}$	IP	600 66	550 726		400 66				
Z-MLD	IM								
	SC	500 66	730 727						
	PO		1000 728		2000 109	150 66			
Anesthetic	IV	120 66		100 66	80 66	100 557	125 557		
	IP	250 200	240 1685		225 66				
[a]Rectal	IM		400 547						
administration	SC				500 66	[a]300 2275			
	PO				600 66	100 66			
	IV								
	IP								
	IM								
	SC								
	PO								
	IV								
	IP								
	IM								
	SC								
	PO								

IN VITRO

mg %	Cardiac	Vascular	Gut	Uterine	Visceral	Skeletal		

TRIFLUOPERAZINE

(Stelazine, Eskazine, Terfluzine)

mg/kg		Mouse	Rat	Guinea Pig	Rabbit	Cat	Dog	Monkey	
Lethal Dose	IV	Y36 [82]					Y60 [82]		
Y-LD$_{50}$	IP								
Z-MLD	IM								
	SC								
	PO	Y442 [82]	Y740 [82]						
Behavioral	IV								
	IP		1 [577]						
	IM			0.3 [1053]				0.25 [1053]	
	SC		0.43 [95]						
	PO	1 [729]	12.8 [1056]						
Catatonic	IV								
	IP		165 [227]						
	IM								
	SC								
	PO	25 [730]	2.6 [730]				10 [1041]	20 [730]	
Decreased	IV								
spontaneous	IP								
motor activity	IM								
	SC								
	PO	10 [730]	2.5 [730]					10 [730]	
Barbiturate	IV								
sleep	IP	1 [227]							
Potentiation	IM								
	SC								
	PO								
EEG	IV				2 [824]				
	IP								
	IM								
	SC								
	PO								
Tranquilize	IV								
	IP								
[a]ED$_{50}$	IM								
	SC								
	PO	[a]8.3 [1372]							
Antagonize	IV						[a]0.1 [1398]		
angiotensin	IP								
(cardiac)	IM								
[a]IA	SC								
	PO								
CNS	IV								
	IP		1 [1982]						
	IM								
	SC								
	PO								

TRIFLUOPERAZINE (continued)

mg/kg		Mouse	Rat	Guinea Pig	Rabbit	Cat	Dog	Monkey	
Antiemetic	IV								
	IP								
	IM						0.03 2272		
	SC								
	PO								
	IV								
	IP								
	IM								
	SC								
	PO								
	IV								
	IP								
	IM								
	SC								
	PO								
	IV								
	IP								
	IM								
	SC								
	PO								

IN VITRO

mg %		Cardiac	Vascular	Gut	Uterine	Visceral	Skeletal	Renal	
Rat								0.0815*	

*1639

TRIMEBUTINE

mg/kg		Mouse	Rat	Guinea Pig	Rabbit	Cat	Dog	Monkey	
Lethal Dose	IV								
Y-LD$_{50}$	IP								
Z-MLD	IM								
	SC								
	PO								
Gastrointestinal	IV				2 [1984]	2 [1984]			
	IP								
	IM								
	SC								
	PO								
	IV								
	IP								
	IM								
	SC								
	PO								
	IV								
	IP								
	IM								
	SC								
	PO								

IN VITRO

mg %	Cardiac	Vascular	Gut	Uterine	Visceral	Skeletal		
Rabbit			[a]1×10^{-6}*					
[a]molar								
solution								

*1984

TRIMETHADIONE

(Tridione, Absentol, Trimedal)

mg/kg		Mouse	Rat	Guinea Pig	Rabbit	Cat	Dog	Monkey	
Lethal Dose	IV	Y2000 731			Y1500 731				
Y-LD$_{50}$	IP	Y1800 111			Y1500 731				
Z-MLD	IM								
	SC		Y2200 111						
	PO	Y2200 111							
Anticonvulsant	IV	275 881	200 111						
	IP	150 592	300 111		500				
	IM							50 1096	
	SC	225			500				
	PO	400	70 1038		942 1012	30 97	30 97		
Hypnotic	IV	1500			750 111				
	IP	1500							
	IM								
	SC		1500 63						
	PO	1500							
Behavioral	IV								
	IP								
	IM								
	SC								
	PO	800 935							
EEG	IV				200 1223	500 1222			
	IP								
	IM								
	SC								
	PO								
Teratogenic	IV								
	IP								
	IM								
	SC								
	PO		250 2092						
	IV								
	IP								
	IM								
	SC								
	PO								
	IV								
	IP								
	IM								
	SC								
	PO								
	IV								
	IP								
	IM								
	SC								
	PO								

TRIPELENNAMINE

(Pyribenzamine, Dehistin, Tonaril)

mg/kg		Mouse	Rat	Guinea Pig	Rabbit	Cat	Dog	Monkey	
Lethal Dose	IV	Y17 [732]	Y13 [732]		9		42.7		
Y-LD50	IP	Y70 [732]							
Z-MLD	IM								
	SC	Y75 [324]	Y225 [324]	Y30.2 [221]	33 [324]				
	PO	Y210 [324]	Y570 [324]	Y155 [221]					
Antihistaminic	IV			19 [221]		1 [2275]	1 [2275]		
	IP			10					
	IM			5		1 [2275]	1 [2275]		
	SC			5		1 [2275]	1 [2275]		
	PO			5.3 [648]		5.5 [97]	5.5 [97]		
Cardiovascular	IV		[a]2.5 [1974]			2 [496]	4 [263]		
potentiation	IP								
of aldehydes &	IM								
norepinephrine	SC								
[a]total mg	PO								
Behavioral	IV								
	IP		5.2 [848]						
	IM							0.1 [1377]	
	SC								
	PO								
Reverse	IV								
oxotremorine	IP	[a]30.9 [1441]							
hypothermia	IM								
[a]ED50	SC								
	PO								
Analgesic	IV								
	IP		20 [2062]						
	IM								
	SC								
	PO								
Substitute	IV								
for morphine	IP								
dependence	IM								
	SC	3 [1969]	3 [1969]						
	PO								

IN VITRO

mg %	Cardiac	Vascular	Gut	Uterine	Visceral	Skeletal	
Anti-5HT			0.1 [92]				
Antihistaminic			0.005 [93]				
Anticholinergic			6 [93]				

TUBOCURARINE

(Tubarine, Delacurarine, Tubadil)

mg/kg		Mouse	Rat	Guinea Pig	Rabbit	Cat	Dog	Monkey
Lethal Dose	IV	0.14 [733]		0.1 [736]	Y0.35 [735]		3	
Y-LD$_{50}$	IP	Y0.14 [734]	Y0.25 [735]					
Z-MLD	IM						10 [111]	
	SC	0.53 [733]	0.3	0.1 [109]	0.34 [109]	0.34 [109]	0.34 [109]	
	PO							
Neuromuscular	IV	0.075 [736]	0.075 [736]	0.035 [736]	0.12 [735]	0.07-0.1*	0.1-0.15*	0.75 [442]
Block	IP							
	IM				0.4 [736]	0.7 [557]	0.1-0.15*	
	SC				0.5 [361]		0.15	
	PO							
Cardiovascular	IV					0.1 [736]	0.1 [736]	
	IP							
	IM							
	SC							
	PO							
CNS	IV		0.05 [1000]			0.05 [1000]		
	IP							
	IM							
	SC							
	PO							

*2275

IN VITRO

mg %	Cardiac	Vascular	Gut	Uterine	Visceral	Skeletal		
Rat						0.05 [1157]		
Rabbit	0.1		0.1					

TYRAMINE

(Tyrosamine, Mydrial, Uteramin)

mg/kg		Mouse	Rat	Guinea Pig	Rabbit	Cat	Dog	Monkey	
Lethal Dose	IV				300 [109]				
Y-LD$_{50}$	IP								
Z-MLD	IM								
	SC	225 [109]				30 [109]			
	PO								
Cardiovascular	IV		0.1 [1352]		0.1	0.8 [2275]	0.25 [408]	1 [1646]	
	IP								
	IM								
	SC	30 [737]							
	PO								
Norepinephrine interactions	IV	5 [861]					10 [91]		
	IP	80 [338]	20 [879]						
	IM		20 [738]						
	SC								
	PO								
Neurotoxic	IV						1 [2086]		
	IP								
	IM								
	SC								
	PO								

IN VITRO

mg %	Cardiac	Vascular	Gut	Uterine	Visceral	Skeletal	Trachea	
Rat	0.002 [301]			0.17 [1157]				
Ear-Rabbit		[a]0.016 [339]						
Langendorff	[a]0.01 [739]							
Dog	1.37 [1321]						0.137 [1800]	
[a]total mg								

TYROSINE

mg/kg		Mouse	Rat	Guinea Pig	Rabbit	Cat	Dog	Monkey	
Lethal Dose	IV								
Y-LD$_{50}$	IP								
Z-MLD	IM								
	SC								
	PO								
Protect	IV								
against	IP		400 1638						
GI ulceration	IM								
	SC		256 1638						
	PO								
	IV								
	IP								
	IM								
	SC								
	PO								
	IV								
	IP								
	IM								
	SC								
	PO								

IN VITRO

mg %	Cardiac	Vascular	Gut	Uterine	Visceral	Skeletal	Trachea	

U-50,488H

mg/kg		Mouse	Rat	Guinea Pig	Rabbit	Cat	Dog	Monkey
Lethal Dose Y-LD$_{50}$ Z-MLD	IV							
	IP							
	IM							
	SC							
	PO							
Analgesic	IV							
	IP							
	IM							
	SC	2.5 1484	7 1484					
	PO							
Increase corticosteroids	IV							
	IP		2.3 1484					
	IM							
	SC							
	PO							
Renal effects	IV						5 2245	
	IP							
	IM							
	SC							
	PO							
	IV							
	IP							
	IM							
	SC							
	PO							
	IV							
	IP							
	IM							
	SC							
	PO							
	IV							
	IP							
	IM							
	SC							
	PO							
	IV							
	IP							
	IM							
	SC							
	PO							
	IV							
	IP							
	IM							
	SC							
	PO							

495

URAPIDIL

(Ebrantil, B-66256)

mg/kg		Mouse	Rat	Guinea Pig	Rabbit	Cat	Dog	Monkey	
Lethal Dose	IV								
Y-LD$_{50}$	IP								
Z-MLD	IM								
	SC								
	PO								
Vascular	IV		^{3} 2246						
(antipressor)	IP								
	IM								
	SC								
	PO								
Cardiac	IV						^{a}0.025$_{2130}$		
	IP								
^{a}i. cisternal	IM								
	SC								
	PO								
	IV								
	IP								
	IM								
	SC								
	PO								

IN VITRO

mg %		Cardiac	Vascular	Gut	Uterine	Visceral	Skeletal		
Rabbit			0.0116$_{2247}$						

URETHANE

(Ethyl Carbamate, NSC-746)

mg/kg		Mouse	Rat	Guinea Pig	Rabbit	Cat	Dog	Monkey
Lethal Dose Y-LD_{50} Z-MLD	IV				2000			
	IP	Z2150 194						
	IM							
	SC		1800					
	PO						2500	
Anesthetic [a] with chloralose, 35 IV	IV				1000	1000 2275	1000 413	
	IP		780 127	1500	1600 2275	1500 2275		
	IM		950 166			1800	1000	
	SC		950 166		1500	1000 740		
	PO					[a]750	1500 550	
Sedative [a] Total mg	IV							
	IP							
	IM							
	SC							
	PO	400 935				[a]1250 97	[a]1250 97	
Increase acetylcholine (brain)	IV							
	IP		1000 1209					
	IM							
	SC							
	PO							
Cardiovascular	IV							
	IP		1200 1572					
	IM							
	SC							
	PO							
	IV							
	IP							
	IM							
	SC							
	PO							
	IV							
	IP							
	IM							
	SC							
	PO							
	IV							
	IP							
	IM							
	SC							
	PO							
	IV							
	IP							
	IM							
	SC							
	PO							

VALPROIC ACID

(Depakene, Mylproin, DPA Sodium)

mg/kg		Mouse	Rat	Guinea Pig	Rabbit	Cat	Dog	Monkey	
Lethal Dose $Y-LD_{50}$ Z-MLD	IV								
	IP								
	IM								
	SC								
	PO								
Behavioral toxicosis [a]daily	IV								
	IP								
	IM								
	SC								
	PO								$^a7.5_{1738}$	
GABA receptor regulation [a]daily	IV								
	IP		$^a100_{1366}$						
	IM								
	SC								
	PO								
CNS	IV		640_{1664}						
	IP								
	IM								
	SC								
	PO								
Anticonvulsant	IV								
	IP	141_{1470}							
	IM								
	SC								
	PO						60_{2272}		
	IV								
	IP								
	IM								
	SC								
	PO								
	IV								
	IP								
	IM								
	SC								
	PO								
	IV								
	IP								
	IM								
	SC								
	PO								
	IV								
	IP								
	IM								
	SC								
	PO								

VANADATE

(Sodium Orthovanadate)

mg/kg		Mouse	Rat	Guinea Pig	Rabbit	Cat	Dog	Monkey
Lethal Dose	IV							
Y-LD$_{50}$	IP							
Z-MLD	IM							
	SC							
	PO							
Broncho-	IV			[1] 1295				
constriction	IP							
	IM							
	SC							
	PO							
Renal	IV		[a]0.036 2249					
(diuresis,	IP							
vasoconstriction	IM							
	SC							
[a]mg% perfusion	PO							
	IV							
	IP							
	IM							
	SC							
	PO							

IN VITRO

mg %	Cardiac	Vascular	Gut	Uterine	Visceral	Skeletal	Kidney	
Rat							17.89 2248	

VASOPRESSIN

(Antidiuretic Hormone, Pitressin, ADH)

mg/kg		Mouse	Rat	Guinea Pig	Rabbit	Cat	Dog	Monkey	
Lethal Dose	IV								
Y-LD$_{50}$	IP								
Z-MLD	IM								
	SC								
	PO								
Renal	IV		^{b}0.5 $_{1587}$			^{a}10 $_{2273}$	^{a}10 $_{2273}$	^{d}2 $_{2245}$	
^{a}total units	IP		^{c}0.027$_{1639}$						
^{b}μmol/kg	IM					^{a}10 $_{2273}$	^{a}10 $_{2273}$		
^{c}total nMol/Kid	SC								
^{d}pMol/kg/min	PO								
Cardiovascular	IV		$3 \times 10^{-5}$$_{1397}$						
	IP								
	IM								
	SC								
	PO								
Analgesic	IV	0.0085$_{2250}$							
	IP								
	IM								
	SC								
	PO								

IN VITRO

mg %	Cardiac	Vascular	Gut	Uterine	Visceral	Skeletal	Renal	
Rat							^{a}1$\times$10^{-10}*	
^{a}molar								
solution								

*1426

VERAPAMIL

(Iproveratril, Isoptin, Vasolan)

mg/kg		Mouse	Rat	Guinea Pig	Rabbit	Cat	Dog	Monkey
Lethal Dose	IV							
Y-LD_{50}	IP							
Z-MLD	IM							
	SC							
	PO							
Cardiovascular	IV		$^c1\ _{2021}$				0.01-0.3*	
^{a}mg/kg/min IV	IP		$20\ _{2254}$				$^a0.003\ _{2253}$	
^{b}mg/min IV(ECG)	IM						$^b1.5\ _{2255}$	
^{c}mg% perfused	SC							
heart	PO							
Antagonize	IV							
morphine	IP							
	IM							
	SC		$10\ _{1640}$					
	PO							
Antihyper-	IV							
sensitivity	IP			$8\ _{1680}$				
(pulmonary)	IM							
	SC							
	PO							

*2252

IN VITRO

mg %	Cardiac	Vascular	Gut	Uterine	Visceral	Skeletal	Pulmonary
Rat	$0.0045\ _{1609}$						
Guinea Pig	$0.0227\ _{2023}$					$0.61\ _{1801}$	
Rabbit	$0.0136\ _{1681}$	$0.0027\ _{1682}$				$0.4545\ _{1684}$	
Dog	$0.0454\ _{2251}$						

VERATRIDINE

(3-Veratroylveracevine, Veratrine)

mg/kg		Mouse	Rat	Guinea Pig	Rabbit	Cat	Dog	Monkey	
Lethal Dose	IV	Y0.42 $_{639}$							
Y-LD$_{50}$	IP	Y1.35 $_{640}$	Y3.5 $_{639}$						
Z-MLD	IM								
	SC								
	PO								
Cardiovascular	IV					[a]0.07 $_{741}$	0.005$_{742}$		
[a]Total mg	IP						[b]0.3 $_{2258}$		
[b]IV, in situ	IM								
	SC								
	PO								
Respiratory	IV								
(depression)	IP						0.6$_{643}$		
	IM								
	SC								
	PO								
	IV								
	IP								
	IM								
	SC								
	PO								

IN VITRO

mg %	Cardiac	Vascular	Gut	Uterine	Visceral	Skeletal	Renal	
Rat							[a]1×10^{-5}*	
[a]molar								
solution								

*2230

WARFARIN

(Coumadin, Panwarfin, Sofarin)

mg/kg		Mouse	Rat	Guinea Pig	Rabbit	Cat	Dog	Monkey	
Lethal Dose	IV	Y165 111	Y186 743		Y150 743		Y250 743		
Y-LD$_{50}$	IP								
Z-MLD	IM								
	SC								
	PO	Y374 743	Y323 743	Y182 743	Y800 743		Y250 743		
Antithrombotic	IV								
	IP								
	IM								
[a]Initial, then	SC								
0.05-1 daily	PO						[a]0.2 2272		
	IV								
	IP								
	IM								
	SC								
	PO								
	IV								
	IP								
	IM								
	SC								
	PO								

IN VITRO

mg %	Cardiac	Vascular	Gut	Uterine	Visceral	Skeletal		
Ionotropic(-)	25 744							

XYLAMINE

mg/kg		Mouse	Rat	Guinea Pig	Rabbit	Cat	Dog	Monkey
Lethal Dose	IV							
Y-LD$_{50}$	IP							
Z-MLD	IM							
	SC							
	PO							
CNS	IV							
(amine concen-	IP		12.5 ₂₂₅₆					
trations)	IM							
	SC							
	PO							
	IV							
	IP							
	IM							
	SC							
	PO							
	IV							
	IP							
	IM							
	SC							
	PO							

IN VITRO

mg %	Cardiac	Vascular	Gut	Uterine	Visceral	Skeletal	CNS	
Rat							[a]1×10^{-5}*	
[a]molar								
solution								

*2257

XYLAZINE

(Bay 1470, Rompun)

mg/kg		Mouse	Rat	Guinea Pig	Rabbit	Cat	Dog	Monkey
Lethal Dose	IV							
$Y-LD_{50}$	IP							
$Z-MLD$	IM							
	SC							
	PO							
Sedative	IV					$0.5-1_{2272}$	$0.5-1_{2272}$	
	IP							
	IM	$3-12_{1440}$				$1-2_{2272}$	$1-2_{2272}$	
	SC					$1.1-2.2_{2273}$	$1.1-2.2_{2273}$	
	PO							
Emetic	IV							
	IP							
$^{a}ED_{50}$	IM					1_{2274}		
	SC					$^{a}0.322_{2259}$		
	PO							
Behavioral	IV							
	IP		2.5_{1575}					
	IM							
	SC							
	PO							
Cardiovascular	IV						0.3_{2016}	
	IP							
	IM							
	SC							
	PO							
Analgesic	IV							
	IP							
	IM					1.1_{2274}	1.1_{2274}	
	SC					2.2_{2274}	2.2_{2274}	
	PO							
	IV							
	IP							
	IM							
	SC							
	PO							
	IV							
	IP							
	IM							
	SC							
	PO							
	IV							
	IP							
	IM							
	SC							
	PO							

YOHIMBINE

(Aphrodine, Corynine, Quebrachine)

mg/kg		Mouse	Rat	Guinea Pig	Rabbit	Cat	Dog	Monkey
Lethal Dose Y-LD$_{50}$ Z-MLD	IV	16 745			11 109			
	IP							
	IM							
	SC				50 109		20 346	
	PO	40 346						
Adrenolytic [a] mg/min IA	IV		5		2	0.5 1385	0.2 746	
	IP		1 2261				[a]0.01 2262	
	IM							
	SC							
	PO							
CNS	IV				8 1067			
	IP	5 350	1 1982	0.1 1581				
	IM							
	SC		5 350					
	PO							
Cardiovascular [a] ICV [b] mg/min IA [c] total mg IT [d] total mg	IV		1 2128				0.1 2102	
	IP		[c]0.01 1574				[a]0.1 2260	
	IM		[a]0.01 1997				[b]0.01 1728	
	SC		[a]0.001 1570					
	PO						[d]0.05-0.26*	
Antagonize [a] xylazine [b] clonidine	IV		[b]1 1577		[b]1 1577	[a]0.1 2276	[a]0.4 2278	
	IP		[a]10 1575					
	IM							
	SC	[b]1 2114				[a]0.103 2259		
	PO							
Gastrointestinal [a] salivary	IV		[a]0.3 1425					
	IP							
	IM		5 1423					
	SC							
	PO							
Opioid interactions [a] ICV	IV	[a]0.05 1944						
	IP		2.5 1910					
	IM							
	SC							
	PO							
Cocaine interactions	IV							
	IP	30 1603	5 1604					
	IM							
	SC							
	PO							
Antagonize [a] phencyclidine [b] ketamine	IV					[b]0.25 2277		
	IP		[a]0.3 2078					
	IM							
	SC							
	PO							

*2275

YOHIMBINE (continued)

mg/kg		Mouse	Rat	Guinea Pig	Rabbit	Cat	Dog	Monkey
Antagonize barbiturates	IV					0.4 [2274]	0.25 [2274]	
	IP							
	IM							
	SC							
	PO							
	IV							
	IP							
	IM							
	SC							
	PO							
	IV							
	IP							
	IM							
	SC							
	PO							
	IV							
	IP							
	IM							
	SC							
	PO							

IN VITRO

mg %	Cardiac	Vascular	Gut	Uterine	Visceral	Skeletal	CNS	
Anti-5HT			0.5 [92]					
Rat		0.00035 [2131]	0.0354 [1583]			0.0035*		
Dog	0.3544 [2107]							
Monkey		0.0083 [1569]						

*1410

ZIMELDINE

(Zimelidine, Normud, Zelmid)

mg/kg		Mouse	Rat	Guinea Pig	Rabbit	Cat	Dog	Monkey
Lethal Dose	IV							
Y-LD$_{50}$	IP							
Z-MLD	IM							
	SC							
	PO							
Anticonvulsant	IV							
^{a}ED$_{50}$	IP							
	IM							
	SC							
	PO	6 $_{1760}$						
GABA	IV							
receptor	IP							
regulation	IM							
	SC		10 $_{1366}$					
	PO							
Serotonin	IV							
interaction	IP							
	IM							
	SC							
	PO	11.2 $_{1439}$						
Reserpine	IV							
interaction	IP							
	IM							
	SC							
	PO	10 $_{1439}$						
	IV							
	IP							
	IM							
	SC							
	PO							
	IV							
	IP							
	IM							
	SC							
	PO							
	IV							
	IP							
	IM							
	SC							
	PO							
	IV							
	IP							
	IM							
	SC							
	PO							

ZOMEPIRAC

(Zomax, McN-2783-21-98)

mg/kg		Mouse	Rat	Guinea Pig	Rabbit	Cat	Dog	Monkey
Lethal Dose Y-LD$_{50}$ Z-MLD	IV							
	IP							
	IM							
	SC							
	PO							
Analgesic [a]PO, Freund's adjuvant [b]tooth pulp	IV							
	IP							
	IM							
	SC		[a]16.6 1284					
	PO		[b]2 1500					
Anti- inflammatory	IV							
	IP							
	IM							
	SC							
	PO		0.54 1283					
	IV							
	IP							
	IM							
	SC							
	PO							
	IV							
	IP							
	IM							
	SC							
	PO							
	IV							
	IP							
	IM							
	SC							
	PO							
	IV							
	IP							
	IM							
	SC							
	PO							
	IV							
	IP							
	IM							
	SC							
	PO							
	IV							
	IP							
	IM							
	SC							
	PO							

ZOPICLONE

(Imovance, RP-27267)

mg/kg		Mouse	Rat	Guinea Pig	Rabbit	Cat	Dog	Monkey	
Lethal Dose	IV								
Y-LD$_{50}$	IP								
Z-MLD	IM								
	SC								
	PO								
Behavioral	IV								
	IP		3 2263						
	IM							100 2264	
	SC								
	PO								
	IV								
	IP								
	IM								
	SC								
	PO								
	IV								
	IP								
	IM								
	SC								
	PO								
	IV								
	IP								
	IM								
	SC								
	PO								
	IV								
	IP								
	IM								
	SC								
	PO								
	IV								
	IP								
	IM								
	SC								
	PO								
	IV								
	IP								
	IM								
	SC								
	PO								
	IV								
	IP								
	IM								
	SC								
	PO								

ZOXAZOLAMINE

(Deflexol, Flexin, Zoxamin)

mg/kg		Mouse	Rat	Guinea Pig	Rabbit	Cat	Dog	Monkey
Lethal Dose	IV						Y117 1176	
Y-LD$_{50}$	IP	Y376 461	Y102 461					
Z-MLD	IM							
	SC							
	PO	Y825 461	Y376 461					
Loss of	IV						37 1176	
righting	IP	81 461	43 461					
reflex	IM							
	SC							
	PO	415 461	137 461					
Decrease	IV					30 191		
decerebrate	IP							
rigidity	IM							
	SC							
	PO	120 191						
Crossed-	IV					60		
extensor	IP							
reflex	IM							
depressant	SC							
	PO							
Antistrychnine	IV							
	IP	227 461						
	IM							
	SC							
	PO	120 1016						
Behavioral	IV					60 1016		
and	IP							
EEG	IM							
	SC							
	PO	200 935						
	IV							
	IP							
	IM							
	SC							
	PO							
	IV							
	IP							
	IM							
	SC							
	PO							
	IV							
	IP							
	IM							
	SC							
	PO							

HORMONE MAINTENANCE AND REPLACEMENT DOSAGE

Species	Effect of Hormone	Dose	Route	Reference

HYPOPHYSECTOMIZED

Species	Effect of Hormone	Dose	Route	Reference
MOUSE	Double Uterine Weight			
	Pregnant mare's serum gonadotrophin	1.8 IU	SC	754
RAT	Restore spermatogenesis			
	Testosterone propionate	3 mg/d/35 d	IP	755
	Stimulate ovarian growth			
	Diethylstilbestrol	1 mg/d/8 d	SC	756
	Estradiol	1 mg/d/8 d	SC	756
	Restore fatty acid synthesis			
	Thyroxine	0.1 mg/kg/d	IP	757
	ACTH	0.05 mg/d/14 d	IP	758
	Return O_2 consumption to normal			
	Thyroxine	0.01 mg/d	SC	759
	Corticosterone	1 mg/d/14 d	SC	760
	Cortisone Acetate	1 mg/d/14 d	SC	760
	Hydrocortisone Acetate	1 mg/d/14 d	SC	760
	Increase body weight to normal			
	Somatotropin	0.125 mg/12 h	SC	761
	(plus) Corticosterone	0.015 mg/12 h	SC	761
	(and) Thyroxine	0.003 mg/12 h	SC	761
DOG	Restore normal carbohydrate metabolism			
	Cortisone	1 mg/kg/d	IM	762
	Hydrocortisone	1 mg/kg/d	IM	762
	Produce hyperthyroid state			
	Thyroxin	0.4 mg/kg/d	IM	762

PANCREATECTOMIZED

Species	Effect of Hormone	Dose	Route	Reference
RAT	Maintain weight			
	Insulin	1 unit/12 h	SC	763
	Maintain glucosurea			
	Insulin	18 units/d	SC	764
	Maintain serum gamma globulin during stress			
	Insulin	0.033 unit/12 h	SC	765

Species	Effect of Hormone	Dose	Route	Reference

PANCREATECTOMIZED (con't.)

	Exacerbation of urinary glucose			
	Progesterone	50 mg/d	SC	766
	11-Desoxycorticosterone acetate	10 mg/d	SC	767
RABBIT	Maintain weight on carbohydrate diet			
	Insulin	12 units/d	SC	768
DOG	Decrease glucose content of blood			
	Testosterone propionate	40 mg	IM	769
BABOON	Control diabetes			
	Insulin	2.5 units/kg/d	IV	770

ADRENALECTOMIZED

Species	Effect of Hormone	Dose	Route	Reference
RAT	Maintenance dose			
	Hydrocortisone	0.1 mg/12 h	SC	771
	Cortexone acetate	0.1 mg/d	SC	772
	Diethylstilbestrol	0.1 mg/d	SC	773
	Return blood sugar to normal			
	Aldosterone	0.1 mg/d/9 d	SC	774
	Hydrocortisone acetate	15 mg/d/3 d	SC	775
	Return spontaneous activity to normal			
	Cortisone	5 mg/d/10 d	SC, PO	776
	Hydrocortisone	5 mg/d/10 d	SC	777
	Restore normal metabolism in adipose tissue			
	Dexamethasone	10 μg	IP	778
	Increase blood protein			
	Aldosterone	0.1 mg/d/12 d	SC	779
	Return plasma Na to normal			
	Aldosterone acetate	0.5 mg/kg	SC	780
	Block increase in antibody formation			
	Cortisone	80 mg/kg	SC	781
	Decrease heat loss on exposure to cold			
	Cortisone	1 mg/d	SC	782
	Adrenal cortical extract	0.25 mg/d	SC	782
	Prevent involution of pancreas acinar cells			
	Cortisone	0.5 mg/12 h	SC	783

Species	Effect of Hormone	Dose	Route	Reference

ADRENALECTOMIZED (con't.)

Species	Effect of Hormone	Dose	Route	Reference
GUINEA PIG	Maintenance dose			
	Deoxycorticosterone	1 mg/d	SC	784
	Anesthetic dose			
	Deoxycortisone glucoside	100 mg	SC	784
CAT	Retard salivary gland atrophy			
	Deoxycorticosterone	5 mg/kg/d	SC	782
DOG	Maintenance dose			
	Cortisone acetate	25 mg/d	PO	785
	(plus) Desoxycorticosterone acetate-1	2 mg/d	IM	785
	Desoxycorticosterone acetate	2.5 mg/d	IM	762
MONKEY	Maintenance dose			
	Hydrocortisone sodium succinate	50 mg/d x 1	IM	179
		20 mg/d x 3	IM	179
		10 mg/d (cont'd)	IM	1079

CASTRATED

Species	Effect of Hormone	Dose	Route	Reference
MOUSE	Maintenance dose			
	Testosterone phenylacetate	1 mg/10 d	SC	249
	Produce female-like mammary development			
	Estrone	92.5 μg	SC	786
RAT	Maintenance dose			
	Testosterone phenylacetate	50 mg/d	SC	787
	Increase weight of seminal vesicles			
	Testosterone	0.4 mg/d/7 d	SC	788
	Testosterone	1 mg/d/7 d	IP,PO	788
	Testosterone propionate	0.5 mg/d/20 d	SC	789
	Testosterone propionate	0.4 mg/d/7 d	IP	788
	Testosterone propionate	1 mg/d/7 d	PO	788
	Methyltestosterone	0.4 mg/d/7 d	SC,IP	
			PO	788

Species	Effect of Hormone	Dose	Route	Reference

CASTRATED (con't.)

	Inhibit calcium loss			
	Testosterone	2 mg/d	SC	790
	Return of spontaneous activity to normal			
	Testosterone propionate	20 mg/d/10 d	SC	776
	Prevent prostatic epithelial cell atrophy			
	Testosterone	100 μg/kg/d	SC	791

OVARIECTOMIZED

GUINEA PIG	Return seminal vesicle weight and metabolism to normal			
	Testosterone propionate	2 mg/d	SC	792
	Diminish the fall in hepatic glycogen			
	Testosterone	15 mg/2 d/30 d	SC	793
	Decrease nondirected hyperexcitability			
	Testosterone	250 μg/kg/d	SC	794
MICE	Induce mammary growth in immature			
	Estrone	0.006 μg/d/21 d	SC	795
RAT	Hormone replacement			
	Estradiol benzoate	0.015 mg/kg/d	SC	796
	Polyestradiol phosphate	20 mg/kg/d	SC	787
	Increase vaginal cornification and activity			
	Dienestral	1 μg/d/10 d	PO,SC	776
	Hexestral	1 μg/d/10 d	SC	776
	Hexestral	40 μg/d/10 d	PO	776
	Stilbestrol	1 μg/d/10 d	SC	776
	Stilbestrol	4 μg/d/10 d	PO	776
	Pregnancy maintenance			
	Acetonide	10 mg/d	SC,PO	797
	Acetophenone	20 mg/d	SC,PO	797
	Progesterone	20 mg/d	SC,PO	797
	Return spontaneous activity to normal			
	Estrone benzoate	1 mg/d/10 d	SC	776
	Lower ECS threshold			
	Estradiol	5 mg/kg/d/7 d	SC	798

Species	Effect of Hormone	Dose	Route	Reference

THYROIDECTOMIZED

Species	Effect of Hormone	Dose	Route	Reference
RAT	Maintenance dose			
	Thyroxine	0.005 mg/d	IP	799
	Return metabolic rate to normal			
	Thyroxine	0.015 mg/kg/d	IP	800
	Improve or normalize glucose tolerance			
	Triiodothyroxine	0.02 mg/d/4 d	SC	801
GUINEA PIG	Increase metabolism			
	Thyrotropic hormone	25 units/d/12 d	IM	802

THYROPARATHYROIDECTOMIZED

Species	Effect of Hormone	Dose	Route	Reference
RAT	Replacement therapy in lactating female			
	Thyroxin	30 μg/kg/d	SC	803
	(plus) Parathyroid hormone	300 USPU/kg/d	SC	803
	Produce arthritis			
	Deoxycorticosterone acetate	2 mg/d	SC	804
DOG	Return intestinal Ca absorption to normal			
	Parathyroid extract	500 IU	IV	805

PARATHYROIDECTOMIZED

Species	Effect of Hormone	Dose	Route	Reference
RAT	Increase excretion of urinary phosphate			
	Parathyroid hormone	20 USPU	SC	806
	Parathyroid hormone	1 IU/hour	SC	807
	Cortisone	10 mg/d	IP	808

PHYSIOLOGICAL SOLUTIONS
(grams/liter)

	NaCl	KCl	$CaCl_2$	$MgCl_2$	$NaHCO_3$	NaH_2PO_4	KH_2PO_4	$MgSO_4$	Glucose
Saline (Mammal)	9.00	--	--	--	--	--	--	--	--
Ringer (Mammal)	9.00	0.42	0.24	--	0.50	--	--	--	1.00
Ringer (by Cattell)	9.00	0.42	0.12	--	--	--	0.100	--	1.00
Ringer (by Dresel)	6.00	0.531	0.35	--	2.10	--	0.081	0.147	0.90
Ringer (by Evans)	--	0.42	0.12	0.200	--	--	--	--	1.00[a,b]
Ringer (by Genell)	8.00	0.42	0.24	0.005	1.00	--	--	--	0.50
Ringer (by Moran)	7.00	0.42	0.24	0.200	2.10	--	--	--	1.80
Ringer-Dale (by Stewart)	9.00	0.42	2.015	0.003	0.50	--	--	--	0.50
Ringer-Locke (same as Locke's)	9.00	0.42	0.24	--	0.15	--	--	--	1.75
Ringer-Locke (by Feldberg)	9.00	0.20	0.20	--	0.30	--	--	--	1.00
Ringer-Locke (by Gaddum)	9.00	0.42	0.06	--	0.50	--	--	--	0.50
Ringer-Locke (by Hukovic)	9.00	0.42	0.24	--	0.50	--	--	--	2.00
Locke's (by Burn)	9.00	0.42	0.24	0.005	0.50	--	--	--	0.50
Krebs-Henseleit	6.87	0.40	0.28	--	2.10	0.140	--	0.140	2.00
Krebs-Henseleit-Ringer	6.90	0.354	0.280	--	2.10	--	0.162	0.294	--
Krebs-Henseleit (by Furchgott)	6.90	0.354	0.282	--	2.10	--	0.162	0.294	1.80
Krebs (by Hukovic)	6.60	0.350	0.280	--	2.10	--	0.162	0.294	2.08
Beauvilain's	9.00	0.42	0.06	0.005	0.50	--	--	--	0.50
McEwan's	7.60	0.42	0.24	--	2.10	0.143	--	--	2.00[c]
Tyrode (Isolated Gut)	8.00	0.20	0.20	0.100	1.00	0.050	--	--	1.00
Feigen's (Isolated Heart)	9.00	0.42	0.62	--	0.60	--	--	--	1.00

[a]K_2SO_4 = 22.00 [b]$KHCO_3$ = 3.60 [c]Sucrose = 4.50

BIBLIOGRAPHY

1. Skog, E. A toxicological investigation of lower aliphatic aldehydes. I. Toxicity of formaldehyde, acetaldehyde, propionaldehyde and butyraldehyde; as well as of acrolein and crotonaldehyde. *Acta Pharmacol.* (Kbh.) 6: 299-318, 1950.

2. Stotz, E., *et al.* Behavioral and pharmacological studies of thiopropazate, a potent tranquilizing agent. *Arch. Int. Pharmacodyn.* 127: 85-103, 1960.

3. Supniewski, J.V. The toxic action of acetaldehyde on the organs of vertebrata. *J. Pharmacol. Exp. Ther.* 30: 429-437, 1927.

4. Sollmann, T.H. and P.J. Hanzlik. *Fundamentals of Experimental Pharmacology.* J.W. Stacey, Inc., San Francisco, 1940.

5. Eade, N.R. Mechanism of sympathomimetic action of aldehydes. *J. Pharmacol. Exp. Ther.* 127: 29-34, 1959.

6. Kreitmair, D.H. The pharmacological action of ephedrine. *Arch Exp. Path. Pharmakol.* 120: 189-228, 1927.

7. Anderson, H.H., *et al., Pharmacology and Experimental Therapeutics.* University of California Press, Berkeley and Los Angeles. 1947.

8. Smith, P.K. and W.E. Hambourger. The ratio of the toxicity of acetanilid to its antipyretic activity in rats. *J. Pharmacol. Exp. Ther.* 54: 159-160, 1935.

9. Smith, P.K. and W.E. Hambourger. The ratio of the toxicity of acetanilid and its antipyretic activity in rats. *J. Pharmacol. Exp. Ther.* 54: 346-351, 1935.

10. Lester, D. Formation of methemoglobin. *J. Pharmacol. Exp. Ther.* 77: 154-159, 1943.

11. Munch, J.D., *et al.* Acetanilid studies. I. Acute Toxicity. *J. Amer. Pharm. Ass.* 30: 91-98, 1941.

12. Karczmar, A.G. The effects of lethal doses of acetanilid in the dog. *Fed. Proc.* 6: 341-343, 1947.

13. Molitor, H. A comparative study of the effects of five choline compounds used in therapeutics: Acetylcholine chloride, acetyl beta-methylcholine chloride, carbaminoyl choline, ethyl ether beta-methyl-choline chloride, carbaminoyl beta-methylcholine chloride. *J. Pharmacol. Exp. Ther.* 58: 337-360, 1936.

14. Monnier, M. Electro-physiological actions of central nervous system stimulants. *Arch. Int. Pharmacodyn.* 124: 281-301, 1960.

15. Trendelenburg, U. and J.S. Gravenstein. Effect of reserpine pretreatment on stimulation of the accelerans nerve of the dog. *Science* 128: 901-902, 1958.

16. Fraser, P.J. Pharmacologic actions of pure muscarine chloride. *Brit. J. Pharmacol.* 12: 47-52, 1957.

Bibliography

17. Ben-Bassat, J., *et al.* Analgesimetry and ranking of analgesic drugs by the receptacle method. *Arch. Int. Pharmacodyn.* 122: 434-447, 1959.

18. Hart, E.R. The toxicity and analgetic potency of salicylamide and certain of its derivatives as compared with established analgetic-antipyretic drugs. *J. Pharmacol. Exp. Ther.* 89: 205-209, 1947.

19. Ichniowski, C.T. and W.C. Heuper. Pharmacological and toxicological studies on salicylamide. *J. Amer. Pharm. Ass.* 35: 225-230, 1946.

20. Eagle, E. and A.J. Carlson. Toxicity, antipyretic and analgesic studies on 39 compounds including aspirin, phenacetin and 27 derivatives of carbazole and tetrahydrocarbazole. *J. Pharmacol. Exp. Ther.* 99: 450-457, 1950.

21. Smith, C.S., *et al.* The analgesic properties of certain drugs and drug combinations. *J. Pharmacol. Exp. Ther.* 77: 184-193, 1943.

22. Winder, C.V. Quantitative evaluation of analgesic action in guinea pigs. Morphine, ethyl 1-methyl-4-phenylpiperidine-4-Carboxylate (demerol) and acetylsalicylic acid. *Arch. Int. Pharmacodyn.* 74: 219-226, 1947.

23. Eillinger, A. Aromatic hydrocarbons, phenols, aromatic acids, aromatic alcohols, aldehydes, ketones, quinines and nitro compounds. *Heffter's Hdb.* 1: 871-1048, 1923.

24. Jones, L.M. *Veterinary Pharmacology and Therapeutics.* The Iowa State College Press, Ames, Iowa, 1957.

25. Guerra, F. and G.H. Barbour. The mechanism of aspirin antipyresis in monkeys. *J. Pharmacol. Exp. Ther.* 79: 55-61, 1943.

26. Collier, H.O.J., *et al.* The bronchoconstrictor action of bradykinin in the guinea pig. *Brit. J. Pharmacol.* 15: 290-297, 1960.

27. Launey, L. Determination of toxicity and activity of several barbiturate derivatives. Principles of comparison. *J. Physiol. Path. gen.* 30: 364-378, 1932.

28. Pletscher, A., *et al.* Bensoquinolizine, a new compound with an action of 5-hydroxytryptamine and norepinephrine in the brain. *Arch. Exp. Path. Pharmakol.* 232: 499-509, 1958.

29. Barlow, O.W. Studies on the Pharmacology of ethyl alcohol. I. A comparative study of the pharmacologic effects of grain and synthetic ethyl alcohols. II. A correlation of the local irritant, anesthetic and toxic effects of three potable whiskeys with their alcoholic content. *J. Pharmacol. Exp. Ther.* 56: 117-146, 1936.

30. Alekseeva, I.A. The direct and conditioned reflex effects of inhibitory substances on the higher nervous activity of dogs with organic lesions of certain parts of the cerebral cortex. *Pavlov J. Higher Nerv. Activ.* 10: 737-744, 1960.

Bibliography

31. Bonnycastle, D.D., *et al.* The effect of a number of central depressant drugs upon brain 5-hydroxytryptamine levels in the rat. *J. Pharmacol. Exp. Ther.* 135: 17-20, 1962.

32. Miller, N.E. and H. Barry. Motivational effects of drugs: Some general problems in psychopharmacology. *Psychopharmacologia* 1: 169-199, 1960.

33. Lehman, A.J. Chemicals in food: A report to the Association of Food and Drug Officials on current developments. *Assoc. Food & Drug Officials U.S. Quart. Bull.* 15: 122-133, 1951.

34. Witkin, L.B., *et al.* A study of some central stimulants in mice. *Arch. Int. Pharmacodyn.* 124: 105-115, 1960.

35. Hanzlik, P.J., *et al.* Toxicity, fats and excretion of propylene glycol and some other glycols. *J. Pharmacol. Exp. Ther.* 67: 101-126, 1939.

36. Waisbren, B.A. Alloxan diabetes in mice. *Proc. Soc. Exp. Biol. (N.Y.)* 67: 154-156, 1948.

37. Gabe, M. Histological changes of the liver and heart following acute alloxan intoxication in the albino rat. *C.R. Soc. Biol. (Paris)* 142: 1335-1340, 1948.

38. Lazarow, A. Protective effect of glutathione against alloxan diabetes in the rat. *Proc. Soc. Exp. Biol. (N.Y.)* 61: 441-447, 1946.

39. Gomeri, G. and M.G. Goldner. Production of diabetes mellitus in rats with alloxan. *Proc. Soc. Exp. Biol. (N.Y.)* 54: 287-290, 1943.

40. Duff, G.L. and H. Starr. Experimental alloxan diabetes in hooded rats. *Proc. Soc. Exp. Biol. (N.Y.)* 57: 280-282, 1944.

41. Goldner, M.G. and G. Gomeri. Alloxan diabetes in the dog. *Endocrinology* 33: 297-308, 1943.

42. Gruber, C.M., *et al.* Studies on the pharmacology and toxicology of dl-α-1,3-dimethyl-4-phenyl-4-propionoxy piperidine (Nu-1196). *J. Pharmacol. Exp. Ther.* 99: 312-316, 1950.

43. Randall, L.O. and G. Lehman. Pharmacological properties of some neostigmine analogs. *J. Pharmacol. Exp. Ther.* 99: 16-32, 1950.

44. Maney, P.V., *et al.* Dihydroxypropyltheophylline: Its preparation and pharmacological clinical study. *J. Amer. Pharm. Ass., Sci. Ed.* 35: 266-272, 1946.

45. Thompson, C.R. and M.R. Warren. Acute and chronic toxicity studies on theophylline aminoisobutanol and theophylline ethylenediamine. *J. Lab. Clin. Med.* 31: 1337-1343, 1946.

Bibliography

46. Warecka, K. The influence of euphylline, chlorpromazine and reserpine on the pia mater blood vessels of cats and rabbits. *Acta Physiol. Pharmacol. Neerl.* 9: 452-460, 1960.

47. Christensen, J.M., *et al.* Ethylnorephrine: A unique bronchodilator. *Amer. Practit.* 9: 916-921, 1958.

48. Cameron, W.M., *et al.* Further evidences on the nature of the vasomotor actions of ethylnorsuprarenin. *J. Pharmacol. Exp. Ther.* 63: 340-351, 1938.

49. Koch, R. On the toxicity of pyramidon. *Med. Klin.* 45: 661-665, 1950.

50. Domenjoz, R. The pharmacology of phenylbutazone analogues. *Ann. N.Y. Acad. Sci.* 86: 263, 1960.

51. Rose, C.L. Detoxification of amidopyrine by sodium amytal. *Proc. Soc. Exp. Biol. (N.Y.)* 32: 1242-1243, 1935.

52. Hazelton, L.W., *et al.* Acute and chronic toxicity of butazolidin. *J. Pharmacol. Exp. Ther.* 109: 387-392, 1953.

53. Loeser, D. and A.L. Konwiser. A study of the toxicity of strontium and comparison with other cations employed in therapeutics. *J. Lab. Clin. Med.* 15: 35-41, 1929.

54. Horwitt, M.K., *et al.* Heat regulation and water exchange. *J. Pharmacol. Exp. Ther.* 48: 217-222, 1933.

55. Winder, C.V., *et al.* A study of pharmacological influences on ultraviolet erythema in guinea pigs. *Arch. Int. Pharmacodyn.* 116: 261, 1958.

56. Filehne, W. Pyramidon. *Z. Klin. Med.* 32: 569-577. 1897.

57. Biberfeld, J. Pharmacological studies on some pyrazolon derivatives. *Zschr. Exp. Path.* 5: 28-42, 1908.

58. Merck Institute. Personal communication.

59. Herr, F., *et al.* Tranquilizers and antidepressants: A pharmacological comparison. *Arch. Int Pharmacodyn.* 134: 328-342, 1961.

60. Steiner, W.G. and H.E. Himwich. Central cholinolytic action of chlorpromazine. *Science* 136: 873-875, 1962.

61. Feldman, S.A. Effect of decamethonium upon conditioned reflexes in rats. *Anaesthesia* 15: 55-60, 1960.

62. Amberg, S. and H.F. Helmholz. The fatal dose of various substances on intravenous injection in the guinea pig. *J. Pharmacol. Exp. Ther.* 6: 595, 1915.

63. Swanson, E.E. and W.E. Fry. A comparative study of two short acting barbituric acid derivatives. *J. Amer. Pharm. Ass.* 26: 1248-1249, 1937.

64. Holck, H.G. and M.A. Kanan. Intravenous lethal doses of amytal in the dog and rabbit and a table of animal dosages compiled from the literature. *J. Lab. Clin. Med.* 19: 1191-1205, 1934.

65. Butler, T.C. The delay in onset of intravenously injected anesthetics. *J. Pharmacol. Exp. Ther.* 74: 118-128, 1942.

66. Heubner, W. and J. Schuller. Narcotics of the aliphatic series. *Heffter's Hdb. E.* 2: 1-282, 1936.

67. Hirschfelder, A.D. and R.N. Bieter. Local anesthetics. *Physiol. Rev.* 12: 190-282, 1932.

68. Vogt, M. Comparative studies in circulatory damage and narcotic effect of various barbituric acid derivatives. *Arch Exp. Path. Pharmakol.* 152: 341-360, 1930.

69. Swett, L.R., *et al.* Structure-activity relations in the pargyline series. *Ann. N.Y. Acad. Sci.* 107: 891-898, 1963.

70. Gruber, C.M., *et al.* III. The toxic actions of sodium diphenyl hydantoinate (Dilantin) when injected intraperitoneally and intravenously in experimental animals. *J. Pharmacol. Exp. Ther.* 68: 433-436. 1940.

71. Maloney, A.H. Picrotoxin as an antidote in acute poisoning by the barbiturates. *J. Pharmacol. Exp. Ther.* 42: 267-268, 1931.

72. Gruber, C.M. and G.F. Keyser. A study on the development of tolerance and cross tolerance to barbiturates in experimental animals. *J. Pharmacol. Exp. Ther.* 86: 186-196, 1946.

73. Halpern, B.N. Toxicity and cardiovascular action of ß-phenylisopropylamine (benzedrine). *J. Physiol. Path. Gen.* 37: 597-614, 1939.

74. Heubner, W. and M. Stuhlman. A notice on benzedrine and pervitin. *Arch. Exp. Path. Pharmakol.* 202: 594-596, 1943.

75. Gunther, B. Toxicity of benzedrine sulfate in the white mouse and in the frog (Calyptocephalus gayi). *J. Pharmacol. Exp. Ther.* 76: 375-377, 1942.

76. Frommel, E., *et al.* Pharmacological study of dextrorotatory and levorotatory pheneturide. *Arch. Int. Pharmacodyn.* 122: 15-31, 1959.

77. Chen, A.L. Preliminary observations with theophylline mono-ethanolamine. *J. Pharmacol. Exp. Ther.* 45: 1-5, 1932.

78. Garattini, S., *et al.* Antagonists of reserpine induced eyelid ptosis. *Med. Exp. (Basel)* 3: 252-259, 1960.

Bibliography

79. Wilson, S.P. and R. Tislow. Differential antagonism of reserpine eyelid closure by imipramine and amphetamine. *Proc. Soc. Exp. Biol. (N.Y.)* 109: 847-848, 1962.

80. Swinyard, E.A., *et al.* Studies on the mechanism of amphetamine toxicity in aggregated mice. *J. Pharmacol. Exp. Ther.* 132: 97-102, 1961.

81. Ehrich, W.E. and K.B. Krumbhaar. The effects of large doses of benzedrine sulphate on the albino rat: Functional and tissue changes. *Ann. Intern. Med.* 10: 1874-1888, 1957.

82. Smith, Kline and French Laboratories. Personal Communication.

83. Ehrich, W.E., *et al.* Experimental studies upon the toxicity of benzedrine sulphate in various animals. *Amer J. Med. Sci.* 198: 784-803, 1939.

84. Searle, L.V. and C.W. Brown. Effect of subcutaneous injections of benzedrine sulfate on the activity of white rats. *J. Exptl. Psychol.* 22: 480-490, 1938.

85. Garberg, L. and F. Sandberg. A method for quantitative estimation of the stimulant effect of analeptics on the spontaneous motility of rats. *Acta Pharmacol. (Kbh).* 16: 367-373, 1960.

86. Esser, A. Clinical, anatomical and spectrographic investigations of the central nervous system in acute metal poisoning with particular consideration of their importance for forensic medicine and industrial pathology. *Dtsch. Z. Ges. Gerichtl. Med.* 25: 239-317, 1935.

87. Munoz, C. and L. Goldstein. Influence of adrenergic blocking drugs upon the EEG analeptic effect of dl-amphetamine in conscious unrestrained rabbits. *J. Pharmacol. Exp. Ther.* 132: 354-359, 1961.

88. Courvoisier, S. Pharmacodynamic properties of the chlorhydrate of chloro-3 (dimethyl-amino-3' propyl)-10 phenothiazine (4.560 R.P.) *Arch. Int. Pharmacodyn.* 92: 305-361, 1953.

89. Cole, J. and P. Glees. Some effects of methyl-phenidate (Ritalin) and amphetamine on normal and neucotomized monkeys. *J. Ment. Sci.* 103: 406-417, 1957.

90. Uyeda, A. and J.M. Fuster. The effects of amphetamine on tachistoscopic performance in the monkey. *Psychopharmacologia* 3: 463-467, 1962.

91. Hertting, G., *et al.* Effect of drugs on the uptake and metabolism of H^3-Norepinephrine. *J. Pharmacol. Exp. Ther.* 134: 146-153, 1961.

92. Jaques, R. 5-Hydroxytryptamine antagonists, with special reference to the importance of sympathomimetic amines and isopropyl-noradrenaline. *Helv. Physiol. Pharmacol. Acta.* 14: 269-278, 1956.

93. Ciba Pharmaceutical Company. Personal communication.

Bibliography

94.   Orahovats, P.D., *et al.* Pharmacology of ethyl-1-(4-aminophenethyl)-4-phenylisonipecotate, anileridine, a new potent synthetic analgesic. *J. Pharmacol. Exp. Ther.* 119: 26-34, 1957.

95.   Janssen, P.A.J., *et al.* Apomorphine-antagonism in rats. *Arzneimittel-Forsch.* 10: 1003-1005, 1960.

96.   Klee, P. and L. Laux. Further investigations on vomiting and the action of emetics. *Deut. Arch. Klin. Med.* 149: 189-208, 1925.

97.   Seiden, R. *Veterinary Drugs in Current Use.* Springer, New York, 1960.

98.   Dandiya, P.C. and E.A. Sellers. Mechanism of the hypnosis prolongation action of 5-hydroxytryptamine and some sympathomimetic amines. *Arch. Int. Pharmacodyn.* 130: 32-41, 1961.

99.   Cook, L., *et al.* Epinephrine, norepinephrine and acetylcholine as conditioned stimuli for avoidance behavior. *Science* 131: 990-991, 1960.

100.   Chang, V. and M.J. Rand. Transmission failure in sympathetic nerves produced by hemicholinium. *Brit. J. Pharmacol.* 15: 588-600, 1960.

101.   Cahen, R.L. and K. Tvede. Homatropine methyl-bromide: A pharmacological reevaluation. *J. Pharmacol. Exp. Ther.* 105: 166-177, 1952.

102.   Randall, L.O. and G. Lehmann. Pharmacological studies on analgesic piperidine derivatives. *J. Pharmacol. Exp. Ther.* 93: 314-328, 1948.

103.   Schwartz, A. A comparison of two in vivo methods used for assaying anti-ulcer potency. *Arch. Int. Pharmacodyn.* 127: 203-210, 1960.

104.   Willberg, M.A. Natural resistance of several animals toward atropine. *Biochem. Z.* 66: 389-407, 1914.

105.   Frommel, E. and C. Fleury. On the paradoxical mechanism of the potentiation of the soporific effect of barbiturates by belladonna. *Med. Exp. (Basel)* 3: 257-263, 1960.

106.   Domer, F.R. and F.M. Schueler. Investigations of the amnesic properties of scopolamine and related compounds. *Arch. Int. Pharmacodyn.* 127: 449-458, 1960.

107.   Ficklewirth, G. and A. Heffter. Resistance of the rabbit to atropine. *Biochem. Z.* 40: 36-47, 1912.

108.   White, R.P. and L.D. Boyajy. Neuropharmacological comparison of atropine, scopolamine, benactyzine, diphenhydramine and hydroxyzine. *Arch. Int. Pharmacodyn.* 127: 260-273, 1960.

109.   Flury, F. and F. Zernik. Classification of toxic and lethal doses for the commonly used poisons and research animals. *Abderhalden, Handbuch der biologischen Arbeitsmethoden. Abt. IV, Teil* 7B: 1289-1422, 1928.

Bibliography

110. Rice, W.B. and J.D. McColl. Antagonism of psychotomimetic agents in the conscious cat. *Arch. Int. Pharmacodyn.* 127: 249-259, 1960.

111. Abbott Laboratories. Personal Communication.

112. Loeb, C., *et al.* Electrophysiological analysis of the action of atropine on the central nervous system. *Rev. Arch. Ital. Biol.* 98: 293-307, 1960.

113. Bainbridge, J.G. and D.M. Brown. Ganglion-blocking properties of atropine-like drugs. *Brit. J. Pharmacol.* 15: 147-151, 1960.

114. Paul-David, J., *et al.* Quantification of effects of depressant drugs on EEG activation response. *J. Pharmacol. Exp. Ther.* 129: 69-74, 1960.

115. Usdin, E. and R.L.S. Amasi. Psychotropic and related compounds. *Psychopharmacology Service Center Bulletin* 2: 17-93, 1963.

116. Brown, B.B. The pharmacologic activity of α-(4-piperidyl)-benzhydrol hydrochloride (azacyclonol hydrochloride): An ataractic agent. *J. Pharmacol. Exp. Ther.* 118: 153-161, 1956.

117. Root, W.S. and F.G. Hofman. *Physiological Pharmacology.* Vol. 1: The Nervous System. Part A. Central Nervous System Drugs. Academic Press, New York and London, 1963.

118. Rumke, C.L. and J. Bout. The influence of previously introduced drugs on hexobarbital narcosis. *Arch. Exp. Path. Pharmakol.* 240: 218-223, 1960.

119. Tripod, J., *et al.* Experimental differentiation of a series of central nervous system inhibitors. *Arch. Int. Pharmacodyn.* 112: 319-341, 1957.

120. Dhawan, B.N. and G.P. Gupta. Hypothermic and antipyretic activity of 4-piperidyl diphenyl carbinol hydrochloride (azacyclonol). *Arch. Int. Pharmacodyn.* 137: 54-60, 1962.

121. Hahn, F. and A. Oberdorf. Comparative investigations on the antagonism of bemegride, pentylenetetrazol and picrotoxin. *Arch. Int. Pharmacodyn.* 135: 9-30, 1962.

122. Gruber, C.M., *et al.* A toxicological and pharmacological investigation of sodium secbutyl ethyl barbituric acid (butisol sodium). *J. Pharmacol. Exp. Ther.* 81: 254-268, 1944.

123. MacFarlane, A.W. and J.S. McKenzie. The pharmacology of a new central nervous system stimulant, ßß methyl isopropyl glutarimide. *Arch. Int. Pharmacodyn.* 127: 379-401, 1960.

124. Kuhn, W.L. and E.F. Von Maanen. Central nervous system effects of thalidomide. *J. Pharmacol. Exp. Ther.* 134: 60-68, 1961.

Bibliography

125. Eddy, N.B. Studies of morphine, codeine and their derivatives. IX. Methyl ethers of the morphine and codeine series. *J. Pharmacol. Exp. Ther.* 55: 127-135, 1935.

126. Underhill, F.P. and O.R. Johnson. A comparative study of new ether derivatives of barbituric acid. *J. Pharmacol. Exp. Ther.* 35: 441-448, 1929.

127. Lendle, L. Investigation on the different points of attack of some narcotics in the central nervous system. *Arch. Exp. Path. Pharmakol.* 143: 108-116, 1929.

128. Jones, I. and E.V. Lynn. The toxicity of barbital derivatives. *J. Amer. Pharm. Ass.* 25: 597-601, 1936.

129. Fitch, R.H. and E.E. McCandless. A comparison of the intraperitoneal and oral effects of the barbituric acid derivatives. *J. Pharmacol. Exp. Ther.* 42: 266-267, 1931.

130. Elliott, K.A.C. and N.M. von Golder. The state of factor I in rat brain: The effects of metabolic conditions and drugs. *J. Physiol. (Lond.)* 153: 423-432, 1960.

131. Schuster, R., *et al.* Pharmacological data on the analeptic bemegride. *Latvijas PSR Zinatnu Akad.* 8: 105-110, 1961.

132. Denisenko, P.P. The effect of certain esters of R,R'-aminoethanol and diphenylacetic acid on the central nervous system. *Farmakol. i Toksikol.* 23: 206-215, 1960.

133. Dobkin, A.B. Drugs which stimulate affective behavior. *Anesthesia* 15: 273-279, 1961.

134. Oberdorf, A. and H.J. Meyer. On the pharmacology of megimide. *Arch. Exp. Path. Pharmak.* 238: 128-129, 1960.

135. Larsen, V. The general pharmacology of benzilic acid diethylaminoester hydrochloride (benactyzine NFN, Suavitil, Parasan). *Acta Pharmacol. (Kbh.)* 11: 405-420, 1955.

136. Farquharson, M.E. and R.G. Johnston. Antagonism of the effects of tremorine by tropine derivatives. *Brit. J. Pharmacol.* 14: 559-566, 1960.

137. Boissier, J.R., *et al.* A new simple method for exploring "tranquilizing" action: The chimney test. *Med. Exptl.* 3: 81-84, 1960.

138. Bonta, I.L. New application of the motility test in screening tranquilizing drugs. *Acta Physiol. Pharmacol. Neerl.* 7: 519-522, 1958.

139. McColl, J.D. and W.B. Rice. Antagonism of tremorine by benactyzine and dioxolane analogs. *Toxicol. Appl. Pharmacol.* 4: 263- 268, 1962.

Bibliography

140.   Chen, G. The anti-tremorine effect of some drugs as determined by Haffner's method of testing analgesia in mice. *J. Pharmacol. Exp. Ther.* 124: 73-76, 1958.

141.   Denisenko, P.P. Potentiation of hypnotics and anesthetics by central cholinolytics. *Bull. Exp. Biol. Med.* 49: 593-597, 1960.

142.   Frommel, E., *et al.* On the differential pharmacodynamics of thymoanaleptics and some "neuroleptic" substances in animal experimentation. *Therapie* 15: 1175-1198, 1960.

143.   Navarro, M.G. Conditioned emotional responses and psychotropic drugs. *Acta Physiol. Lat.-Amer.* 10: 122-128, 1960.

144.   Hanson, H.M. and D.A. Brodie. Use of the restrained rat technique for study of the antiulcer effect of drugs. *J. Appl. Physiol.* 15: 291-294, 1960.

145.   Sacra, P., *et al.* A cat and mouse test for studying changes in conflict behavior. *Canad. J. Biochem.* 35: 1151-1152, 1957.

146.   Rose, C.L., *et al.* Toxicity of 3, 3'-methylenebis (4-hydroxycoumarin). *Proc. Soc. Exp. Biol. (N.Y.)* 50: 228-232, 1942.

147.   Lupton, A.M. The effect of perfusion through the isolated liver on the prothrombin activity of blood from normal and dicumarol treated rats. *J. Pharmacol. Exp. Ther.* 89: 306-312, 1947.

148.   Boura, A.L.A. and A.F. Green. The actions of bretylium: Adrenergic neurone blocking and other effects. *Brit. J. Pharmacol.* 14: 536-548, 1959.

149.   Burroughs Wellcome & Co. (U.S.A.), Inc. Personal Communication.

150.   Bhagat, B. and F.E. Shideman. Mechanism of the positive inotropic responses to bretylium and guanethidine. *Brit. J. Pharmacol.* 20: 56-62, 1963.

151.   Green, A.F. and M.F. Sim. Diuresis in rats: Effects of sympathomimetic and sympathetic blocking agents. *Brit. J. Pharmacol.* 17: 237-242, 1960.

152.   Ryd, G. Protective effect of bretylium on noradrenaline stores in organs. *Acta Physiol. Scand.* 56: 90-93, 1962.

153.   Matsumoto, C. and A. Horita. Antagonism of bretylium by sympathomimetic amines. *Nature* 195: 1212-1213, 1962.

154.   Mantegazza, P., *et al.* The peripheral action of hexamethonium and of pentolinium. *Brit. J. Pharmacol.* 13: 480-484, 1958.

155.   Gessner, P.K. The relationship between the metabolic fate and pharmacological action of serotonin, bufotenine and psilocybin. *J. Pharmacol. Exp. Ther.* 130: 126-133, 1960.

Bibliography

156. Marczynski, T. and J. Vetulani. Further investigations on the pharmacological properties of 5-methoxy-*N*-methyltryptamine. *Diss. Pharm. (Krakow)* 12: 67-84, 1960.

157. Monnier, M. and P. Krupp. Electrophysiological action of central nervous system stimulants. I. The adrenergic, cholinergic and neurohumoral serotonic systems. *Arch. Int. Pharmacodyn.* 127: 337-360, 1960.

158. Bunag, R.D. and E.J. Walaszek. Differential antagonism by RAS-Phenol of responses to the indolealkylamines. *J. Pharmacol. Exp. Ther.* 136: 59-67, 1962.

159. Beck, R., *et al.* Stimulatory effect of psychotropic drugs demonstrated by quantitative EEG. *Pharmacologist* 5: 238, 1963.

160. Himwich, W.A. and E. Costa. Behavioral changes associated with changes in concentrations of brain serotonin. *Fed. Proc.* 19: 838-845, 1960.

161. Chen, B.M. and J.K. Weston. The analgesic and anesthetic effect of 1-(1-phenylcyclohexyl) piperidine HCl on monkeys. *Anesth. Analg. Curr. Res.* 39: 132-137, 1960.

162. Molitor, H. The use of bulbocapnine in pre-anesthetic medication. *J. Pharmacol. Exp. Ther.* 56: 85-96, 1936.

163. Grieg, M.E., *et al.* Bulbocapnine catatonia in mice. *Fed. Proc.* 17: 373, 1958.

164. Zetler, G., *et al.* Pharmacological properties of antidepressive drugs. *Arch. Exp. Path. Pharmakol.* 238: 486-501, 1960.

165. Glow, P.H. The antagonism of methyl phenidate and iproniazid to bulbocapnine catatonia in the rat. *Aust. J. Exp. Biol. Med. Sci.* 40: 499-504, 1962.

166. Farris, E.J. and J.Q. Griffith, Jr. *The rat in laboratory investigation.* J.B. Lippincott Co., Philadelphia, 1949.

167. Walaszek, E.J. and J.E. Chapman. Bulbocapnine: An adrenergic and serotonin blocking agent. *J. Pharmacol. Exp. Ther.* 137: 285-290, 1962.

168. Walaszek, E.J. and J.E. Chapman. Bulbocapnine: An adrenergic and serotonin blocking agent. *Fed. Proc.* 20: 314, 1961.

169. Gantt, W.H. Cardiac conditioning. *Trans. 4th Res. Conf. Chermotherap. in Psychiat., Vet. Admin.* 4: 57-73, 1960.

170. Buchman, E.F. and C.P. Richter. Abolition of bulbocapnine catatonia by cocaine. *Arch. Neurol. Psychiat. (Chic.)* 29: 499, 1933.

171. Boura, A. and A. Green. Adrenergic neurone blockade and other acute effects caused by *N*-benzyl-*N'N''*-dimethylguanidine and its ortho-chloro derivative. *Brit. J. Pharmacol.* 20: 36-55, 1963.

Bibliography

172.   Scott, C.C. and K.K. Chen. Comparison of the action of 1-ethyl theobromine and caffeine in animals and man. *J. Pharmacol. Exp. Ther.* 82: 89-97, 1944.

173.   Funderburk, W.H., *et al.* EEG and biochemical findings with MAO inhibitors. *Ann. N.Y. Acad. Sci.* 96: 289-302, 1962.

174.   Holm, T., *et al.* Pharmacology of a series of nuclear substituted phenyl-tertiary-butylamines with particular reference to anorexigenic and central stimulating properties. *Acta Pharmacol. Toxicol.* 17: 121-136, 1960.

175.   Akiyama, T. Studies on whirling syndromes caused by iminodipropionitrile. II. The effect of several drugs on the activity and light reaction of circling mice. *Nippon Yakurigaku Zasshi* 56: 473-486, 1960.

176.   Tripod, J., *et al.* Characterization of central effects of Serpasil (reserpine, a new alkaloid of rauwolfia serpentina B.) and of their antagonistic reactions. *Arch. Int. Pharmacodyn.* 96: 406-425, 1954.

177.   Dews, P.B. The measurement of the influence of drugs on voluntary activity in mice. *Brit. J. Pharmacol.* 8: 46, 1953.

178.   Kreitmair, H. Antagonism between barbiturates and convulsants. *Arch. Exp. Path. Pharmakol.* 187: 607-617, 1937.

179.   Nelson, F. New apparatus for experimental methods using psychoactive substances. *Wiss. Z. Friedrich-Schiller-Univ. Jena, Math,-Naturwiss. Reihe* 9: 549-553, 1960.

180.   Scott, C.C., *et al.* Further study of some 1-substituted theobromine compounds. *J. Pharmacol. Exp. Ther.* 86: 113-119, 1946.

181.   Verhave, T., *et al.* Effects of various drugs on escape and avoidance behavior. *Progr. Neurobiol.* 3: 267-279, 1958.

182.   Salant, W. and J.B. Rieger. The toxicity of caffein. *J. Pharmacol. Exp. Ther.* 1: 572-574, 1910.

183.   Sollmann, T. and J.B. Pilcher. The actions of caffeine on the mammalian circulation. I. The persistent effects of caffeine on the circulation. *J. Pharmacol. Exp. Ther.* 3: 19-92, 1911.

184.   Schallek, W. and A. Kuehn. Effects of drugs on spontaneous and activated EEG of cat. *Arch. Int. Pharmacodyn.* 120: 319-333, 1959.

185.   Malis, J.L., *et al.* Drug effects on the behavior of self stimulation in monkeys. *Fed. Proc.* 19: 23, 1960.

186.   Cole, V.V., *et al.* The toxicity of strontium and calcium. *J. Pharmacol. Exp. Ther.* 71: 1-5, 1941.

Bibliography

187.   Ulrich, J.L. and V.A. Shternov. The comparative action of hypertonic solutions of the chlorates and chlorides of potassium, sodium, calcium and magnesium. *J. Pharmacol. Exp. Ther.* 35: 441-448, 1929.

188.   Main, R.J. Mineral salts as factors in urinary prolan concentrates. *Endocrinology* 24: 523-525, 1939.

189.   La Barre, J. Pharmacological properties of carbamyl-ß-methylcholine. I. Effects on blood pressure and pancreas. *Arch. Int. Pharmacodyn.* 106: 245-259, 1956.

190.   Kreitmair, H. A new class of cholinester. *Arch. Exp. Path. Pharmakol.* 164: 346-356, 1932.

191.   O'Dell, T.B. Experimental parameters in the evaluation of analgesics. *Arch. Int. Pharmacodyn.* 134: 154-174, 1961.

192.   Frommel, E., *et al*. Analgesic potency of chlorpromazine in comparison with morphine and so-called morphinic compounds. *Helv. Physiol. Pharmacol. Acta* 18: C24, 1960.

193.   Castillo, J. del and T.E. Nelson, Jr. The mode of action of carisoprodol. *Ann. N.Y. Acad. Sci.* 86: 1960.

194.   Franklin, K.J. The pharmacology of some compounds allied to chloral and to urethane. *J. Pharmacol. Exp. Ther.* 42: 1-7, 1931.

195.   Fühner, H. Contributions to comparative pharmacology. *Arch. Exp. Path. Pharmakol.* 166: 437-471, 1932.

196.   Gros, O. and H.T.A. Haas. The antagonism of narcotics against cardiazol. *Arch. Exp. Path. Pharmakol.* 192: 348-362, 1936.

197.   Lehman, G. and P.K. Knoeffel. Trichlorethanol, tribromethanol, chloral hydrate and bromal hydrate. *J. Pharmacol. Exp. Ther.* 63: 453-465, 1938.

198.   Lewin, R. Scopolamine-chloralhydrate narcosis. *Z. Exp. Path. Ther.* 18: 61-66, 1916.

199.   Lendle, L. A contribution to the general pharmacology of narcosis: On the narcotic latitudes. *Arch. Exp. Path. Pharmakol.* 132: 214-245, 1928.

200.   Wolf, A. and E.F. von Haxthausen. Toward the analysis of the effects of some centrally-acting sedative substances. *Arzneimittelforsch.* 10: 50-52, 1960.

201.   Sollmann, T. A comparative study of the dosage and effects of chloral hydrate, isopral and bromural on cats. *J. Am. Med. Assoc.* 51: 492, 1908.

202.   Sigg, E.B., *et al*. The influence of some nonbarbiturate depressants on central polysynaptic mechanisms. *Arch. Int. Pharmacodyn.* 116: 450-463, 1958.

Bibliography

203. Adams, W.D. The comparative toxicity of chloral hydrate. *J. Pharmacol. Exp. Ther.* 78: 340-345, 1943.

204. Brown, B.B. CNS drug actions and interaction in mice. *Arch. Int. Pharmacodyn.* 128: 391-414, 1960.

205. Dybing, O. and F. Dybing. Antagonism between chloralose and metrazole. *Arch. Exp. Path. Pharmakol.* 199: 435-437, 1942.

206. Heffter, A. Chloralglucose and its action. *Berl. Klin. Wschr.* 20: 475, 1893.

207. Hanroit, M.M. and C. Richet. The chloraloses. *Arch. Int. Pharmacodyn.* 3: 191-211, 1897.

208. Elliott, K.A.C. and F. Hobbigero. Gamma aminobutyric acid: Circulatory and respiratory effects in different species; re-investigation of the anti-strychnine action in mice. *J. Physiol. (Lond.)* 146: 70-84, 1959.

209. Daly, M. de B. and C.P. Luck. The effects of adrenaline and noradrenalin on pulmonary haemodynamics with special reference to the role of reflexes from the carotid sinus baroreceptors. *J. Physiol. (Lond.)* 145: 108-123, 1959.

210. Hoffman La Roche, Inc. Personal communication.

211. Randall, L.O., *et al.* The psychosedative properties of methaminodiazepoxide. *J. Pharmacol. Exp. Ther.* 129: 163-171, 1960.

212. Gershon, S. and W.J. Lang. A psycho-pharmacological study of some indole alkaloids. *Arch. Int. Pharmacodyn.* 135: 31-56, 1962.

213. Zbinder, G., *et al.* Experimental and clinical toxicology of chlordiazepoxide (Librium). *Toxicol. Appl. Pharmacol.* 3: 619-637, 1961.

214. Stone, C.A., *et al.* Ganglionic blocking properties of 3-methylamino-isocomphane hydrochloride (mecamylamine); a secondary amine. *J. Pharmacol. Exp. Ther.* 117: 169-183, 1956.

215. Plummer, A.J., *et al.* Ganglionic blockade by a new bisquaternary series including chlorisondamine dimethochloride. *J. Pharmacol. Exp. Ther.* 115: 172-184, 1955.

216. Maxwell, R.A., *et al.* Factors affecting the blood pressure response of mammals to the ganglionic blocking agent, chlorisondamine chloride. *J. Pharmacol. Exp. Ther.* 123: 238-246, 1958.

217. Nickerson, M. and G.M. Nomaguchi. Adrenergic blocking action of phenoxyethyl analogues of dibenzamine. *J. Pharmacol. Exp. Ther.* 101: 379-396, 1951.

218. Garattini, S. The pressor effect of reserpine after monoamine-oxidase inhibitors. *Med. Exp. (Basel)* 2: 252-259, 1960.

Bibliography

219. Raab, W. and R.J. Humphreys. Protective effect of adrenolytic drugs against fatal myocardial epinephrine concentrations. *J. Pharmacol. Exp. Ther.* 88: 268-276, 1946.

220. Harvey, S.C., *et al.* Blockade of epinephrine-induced hyperglycemia. *J. Pharmacol. Exp. Ther.* 104: 363-376, 1952.

221. Labelle, A. and R. Tislow. Studies on prophenpyridamine (Timeton) and chlorprophen-pyridamine (Chlortrimeton). *J. Pharmacol. Exp. Ther.* 113: 72-88, 1955.

222. Roth F.E. and W.M. Govier. Comparative pharmacology of chlorpheniramine (Chlortrimeton) and its optical isomers. *J. Pharmacol. Exp. Ther.* 124: 347-349, 1958.

223. Schering Corporation. Personal Communication.

224. Hanson, H.M., *et al.* Drug modification of runway behavior of mice as influenced by an aversive stimulus. *Fed. Proc.* 17: 375, 1958.

225. Burton, R.M., *et al.* Interaction of nicotinamide with reserpine and chlorpromazine. II. Some effects on the central nervous system of the mouse. *Arch. Int. Pharmacodyn.* 128: 253-259, 1960.

226. Fink, G.B. and E. Swinyard. Modification of maximal audiogenic and electroshock seizures in mice by psychopharmacologic drugs. *J. Pharmacol. Exp. Ther.* 127: 318-324, 1959.

227. Boissier, J.R. Neuroleptics and experimental catatonia. *Therapie* 15: 73-77, 1960.

228. Irwin, S. *Symposia on the use of tranquilizers in veterinary practice.* Schering Corp., Bloomfield, N.J., 1958.

229. Weiss, B. and V.G. Laties. Effects of amphetamine, chlorpromazine and pentobarbital on behavioral thermoregulation. *J. Pharmacol. Exp. Ther.* 140: 1-7, 1963.

230. Ito, S. The effect of several tranquilizers on the conditioned avoidance reaction of white rats. *Nippon Yakurigaku Zasshi* 56: 377-386, 1960.

231. Ishikawa, S. A pharmacological study of phenothiazine derivatives. *Nippon Yakurigaku Zasshi* 56: 498-513, 1960.

232. Jewett, R. and S. Norton. Drug effects on behavior of the rat under chronic isolation. *Pharmacologist* 5: 240, 1963.

233. Buchel, L. and J. Levy. Contribution to the study of the mechanism of sedative action of reserpine. *J. Physiol. (Paris)* 52: 727-733, 1960.

234. Yagi, K., *et al.* The effect of flavin adenine dinucleotide on the electroencephalogram modified by chlorpromazine. *J. Neurochem.* 5: 304-306, 1960.

Bibliography

235.   Domenjoz, R. and W. Theobald. The pharmacology of tofranil (N-(3-dimethyl-amino-propyl)-iminodibenzylhydrochloride). *Arch. Int. Pharmacodyn.* 120: 450-489, 1959.

236.   Komendantova, M.V. The meaning of the ion component in the pharmacodynamics of aminazine. *Farmakol. i Toksikol.* 23: 99-105, 1960.

237.   Enge, S. and H. Lechner. An experimental contribution to the mode of drug action in animals. *Wien. Z. Nervenheilk. u. Grenzg.* 17: 309-323, 1960.

238.   Barkov, N.K. Analgetic properties of phenothiazine derivatives. *Farmakol. i Toksikol.* 23: 311-315, 1960.

239.   Adey, W.R. and C.W. Dunlop. Amygdaloid and peripheral influences on caudate and palidal units in the cat and effects of chlorpromazine. *Exp. Neurol.* 2: 348-363, 1960.

240.   Kaada, B.R. and H. Bruland. Blocking of the cortically induced behavioral attention (orienting) response by chlorpromazine. *Psychopharmacologia* 1: 372-388, 1960.

241.   Feldman, S. and M. Eliakim. Observations on the mechanism of blood pressure changes following chlorpromazine administration in the cat. *Arch. Int. Pharmacodyn.* 141: 340-356, 1958.

242.   Leutova, F.A. The problem of the mechanisms of the action of aminazine and physical cooling on the therapeutic reflexes. *Zh. Nevropat. Psikhiat.* 60: 210-219, 1960.

243.   Polezhayev, E.F. Action of aminazine and adrenaline in small doses on the formation of cortical coordination. *Zh. Nevropat. Psikhiat.* 60: 568-576, 1960.

244.   Agangants, E.K. Effects of chlorpromazine and ethylene on conditioned reflexes in dogs. *Pavlov J. Higher Nerv. Activ.* 10: 899-908, 1960.

245.   Khananashbili, M.M. The mechanism of action of chlorpromazine on higher nervous activity. *Farmako. i Toksikol.* 23: 295-299, 1960.

246.   Fuller, J.L., Effects of chlorpromazine upon psychological development in the puppy. *Psychopharmacologia* 1: 393-407, 1960.

247.   Domino, E.F. and S. Ueki. An analysis of the electrical burst phenomenon in some rhinencephalic structures of the dog and monkey. *Electroenceph. Clin. Neurophysiol.* 12: 635-648, 1960.

248.   Weitzman, E. and G. Ross. Behavioral method for study of pain perception in monkeys. *Neurology(Minneap.)* 12: 264-272, 1962.

249.   Browning, H.C., *et al.* Weights of thymus and seminal vesicle in castrate mice as altered by intraperitoneal and subcutaneous injections of testcrone. *Tox. Rep. Biol. Med.* 19: 753-760, 1961.

Bibliography

250.   Stone, G.C., *et al.* Behavioral and pharmacological studies on thiopropazate, a potent tranquilizing agent. *Arch. Int. Pharmacodyn.* 127: 85-103, 1960.

251.   Chen, G. and B. Bohner. A study of certain CNS depressants. *Arch. Int. Pharmacodyn.* 125: 1-20, 1960.

252.   Tanaka, K. and Y. Kawasaki. A group of compounds possessing anticonvulsant activity in the maximal electroshock seizure test. *Jap. J. Pharmacol.* 6: 115-121, 1957.

253.   Luduena, F.P., *et al.* Effect of adrenergic blockers and related compounds on the toxicity of epinephrine in rats. *Arch. Int. Pharmacodyn.* 122: 111-122, 1959.

254.   Busch, V.G., *et al.* Electrophysiological analysis of the action of neuroleptic and tranquilizing substances (phenothiazine, meprobamate) on the spinal motor system. *Arzneimittel-Forsch.* 10: 217-223, 1960.

255.   Piala, J.J., *et al.* Pharmacology of benzhydroflumethazide (naturetin). *J. Pharmacol. Exp. Ther.* 134: 273-280, 1961.

256.   Bacharach, A.L. The effect of ingested vitamin E (tocopherol) on vitamin A storage in the liver of the albino rat. *Quart. J. Pharm.* 14: 138-149, 1940.

257.   Fromherz, K. Larocain, a new local anesthetic. *Arch. Exp. Path. Pharmakol.* 158: 368-380, 1930.

258.   Hooper, C.W. and E. Becker. A quantitative comparison of toxicity of alkamine esters of aromatic acids used as local anesthetics. *Am. J. Physiol.* 68: 120, 1924.

259.   Rose, C.L., *et al.* Studies in the pharmacology of local anesthetics. III. Comparison of gamma-(2-methyl piperidine) propyl benzoate hydrochloride with cocaine and procaine on experimental animals. *J. Lab. Clin. Med.* 15: 731-735, 1930.

260.   Eicholtz, F. and C. Hoppe. The convulsive action of local anesthetics and the effect of mineral salts and adrenaline. *Arch. Exp. Path. Pharmakol.* 173: 687-696, 1933.

261.   Rhee, H.M., *et al.* Suppression of renal nerve activity by methionine enkephalin in anesthetized rabbits. *J. Pharmacol. Exp. Ther.* 234: 534-537, 1985.

262.   Bogdanski, D. and S. Spector. Comparison of central actions of cocaine and LSD. *Fed. Proc.* 16: 284, 1957.

263.   Wingard, C. and R.S. Teague. Potentiation of the pressor response to epinephrine and sympathomimetic aldehydes. *Arch. Int. Pharmacodyn.* 116: 54-64, 1958.

264.   Chen, G. and B. Bohner. the anti-reserpine effects of certain centrally-acting agents. *J. Pharmacol. Exp. Ther.* 131: 179-184, 1961.

265.   MacMillan, W.H. A hypothesis concerning the effect of cocaine on the action of sympathomimetic amines. *Brit. J. Pharmacol.* 14: 385-391, 1959.

Bibliography

266.   Gurd, M.R. The Physiological action of dihydroxyphenylethylamine and sympatol. *Quart. J. and Year Book of Pharm.* 10: 188-211, 1937.

267.   Kissel, J.W., *et al.* The pharmacology of prodilidine hydrochloride, a new analgetic agent. *J. Pharmacol. Exp. Ther.* 134: 332-340, 1961.

268.   Poe, C.F. and J.G. Strong. The toxicity of certain compounds for male and female rats of different ages. *J. Pharmacol. Exp. Ther.* 58: 239-242, 1936.

269.   Ercoli, N. and M.N. Lewis. Studies on analgesics. *J. Pharmacol. Exp. Ther.* 84: 301-317, 1945.

270.   Eddy, N.B. and M. Sumwalt. Studies of morphine, codeine and their derivatives. IV. 2,4-dinitrophenylmorphine. *J. Pharmacol. Exp. Ther.* 67: 127-141, 1939.

271.   O'Dell, T.B., *et al.* Pharmacology of a series of new 2-substituted pyridine derivatives with emphasis on their analgesic and interneuronal blocking properties. *J. Pharmacol. Exp. Ther.* 128: 65-74, 1960.

272.   Goldberg, B., *et al.* Colchicine derivatives. I. Toxicity in mice and effects on mouse sarcoma 180. *Cancer* 3: 124-129, 1950.

273.   Streicher, E. Toxicity of colchicine, di-isopropyl fluorophosphate, intocostrin, and potassium cyanide in mice at 4°C. *Proc. Soc. Exp. Biol. (N.Y.)* 76: 536-538, 1951.

274.   Sollmann, T. *A Manual of Pharmacology and its Application to Therapeutics and Toxicology.* W.B. Saunders Co. (7th ed.), Philadelphia. 1948.

275.   Ferguson, F.C., Jr. Colchicine. I. General pharmacology. *J. Pharmacol. Exp. Ther.* 106: 261-270, 1952.

276.   Santav, F., *et al.* Mitolytic action and toxicity of new substances isolated from colchicine. *Arch. Int. Pharmacodyn.* 84: 257-268, 1950.

277.   Maurel, M. Influence of route of administration on the production of colchicine-diarrhea in the rabbit. *C.R. Soc. Biol. (Paris)* 67: 768-769, 1909.

278.   Dixon, W.E. and W. Malden. Colchicine with special reference to its mode of action and effect on bone marrow. *J. Physiol (Lond.)* 37: 50-76, 1908.

279.   Fernandez, E. and A. Cerletti. Studies on the hypotensive mechanism of protoveratrine. *Arch. Int. Pharmacodyn.* 100: 425-435, 1955.

280.   Castillo, J.C. and E.J. de Beer. The neuromuscular blocking action of succinylcholine (diacetylcholine). *J. Pharmacol. Exp. Ther.* 99: 458-464, 1950.

281.   Bovet, D., *et al.* Studies on synthetic curare-like poisons. *Arch. Int. Pharmacodyn.* 88: 1-50, 1951.

Bibliography

282.   Walton, R.P., *et al*. Inotropic activity of catechol isomers and a series of related compounds. *J. Pharmacol. Exp. Ther.* 125: 202-207, 1959.

283.   Paton, W.D.M. and E.J. Zamis. Clinical potentialities of certain bisquaternary salts causing neuromuscular and ganglionic block. *Nature (Lond.)* 162: 810, 1948.

284.   Setniker, I., *et al*. Amino-methylchromes. Brain stem stimulants and pentobarbital antagonists. *J. Pharmacol. Exp. Ther.* 128: 176-181, 1960.

285.   Day, M. and M. Rand. Evidence for a competitive antagonism of guanethidine by dexamphetamine. *Brit. J. Pharmacol.* 20: 17-28, 1963.

286.   Buchel, L., *et al*. A contribution to the study of the effects of hydrazine-2-phenyl-3-propane (PIH) on the central nervous system, compared with those of 1-isonicotinyl-2-isopropylhydrazide (Iproniazid). IV. Influence on analgesia induced by 1-methadone. *Agressologie* 1: 389-396, 1960.

287.   Hamilton, C.L. Effects of LSD-25 and amphetamine on a running response in the rat. *Arch. Gen. Psychiat.* 2: 104-109, 1960.

288.   Sergio, C. Effects of bulbocapnine in some decorticated rabbits. *Riv. Neurobiol.* 6: 51-53, 1960.

289.   Jarvik, M.E. and S. Chorover. Impairment by lysergic acid diethylamide of accuracy in performance of a delayed alternation test in monkeys. *Psychopharmacologia* 1: 221-230, 1960.

290.   Kleindorf, G.B. and J.T. Halsey. A study of the relative efficiency as "basal anesthetics" of avertin, amytal, chloral, dial, and isopropyl allyl barbituric acid. *J. Pharmacol. Exp. Ther.* 43: 449-456, 1931.

291.   Peterson, I. and E. Bohm. Differences in sensitivity to dial of motor effects elicited by stimulation of fore- and hindlimb areas of the cat's motor cortex. *Acta Physiol. Scand.* 29: 143-146, 1953.

292.   Schneider, J.A. and F.F. Yonkman. Action of serotonin (5-hydroxytryptamine) on vagal afferent impulses in the cat. *Am. J. Physiol.* 174: 127-134, 1953.

293.   O'Leary, J.F. Cardiovascular actions of 1,4-Bis (1,4-benzodioxan-2-yl-methyl) piperazine (McN-181, Dibozane), a new adrenergic blocking agent. *Fed. Proc.* 12: 355, 1953.

294.   Yelnosky, L. and L.C. Mortimer. A brief study of the sympathomimetic cardiovascular effects of bretylium. *Arch. Int. Pharmacodyn.* 130: 200-206, 1961.

295.   Rapela, C.E. and H.D. Green. Adrenergic blockade by Dibozane. *J. Pharmacol. Exp. Ther.* 132: 29-41, 1961.

296.   Powell, C.E. and I.H. Slater. Blocking of inhibitory adrenergic receptors by a dichloro analog of isoproterenol. *J. Pharmacol. Exp. Ther.* 122: 480-488, 1958.

Bibliography

297.   Eli Lilly and Company. Personal Communication.

298.   Goldstein, L. and C. Munoz. Influence of adrenergic stimulant and blocking drugs on cerebral electrical activity in curarized animals. *J. Pharmacol. Exp. Ther.* 132: 345-353, 1961.

299.   Levy, B. Adrenergic blockade produced by the dichloro analogs of epinephrine. Arterenol and isproterenol. *J. Pharmacol. Exp. Ther.* 127: 150-156, 1959.

300.   Ahlquist, R.P. and B. Levy. Adrenergic receptive mechanism of canine ileum. *J. Pharmacol. Exp. Ther.* 127: 146-149, 1959.

301.   Hall, W.J. The action of tyramine on the dog isolated atrium. *Brit. J. Pharmacol.* 20: 245-253, 1963.

302.   Fleming, W.W. and D.G. Hawkins. The actions of dichloroisoproterenol in the dog heart-lung preparation and isolated guinea pig atrium. *J. Pharmacol. Exp. Ther.* 129: 1-10, 1960.

303.   Lendle, L. Digitalis substances and related glycosides working on the heart (digitaloids). *Heffter's Hdb. E.* 1: 11-265, 1935.

304.   Röthlin, E. On the pharmacology of the hydrated natural mother seed alkaloids. *Helv. Physiol. Pharmacol. Acta* 2: C48, 1944.

305.   Naranjo, P. and E.B. de Naranjo. Pressor effect of histamine in the rabbit. *J. Pharmacol. Exp. Ther.* 123: 16-21, 1958.

306.   West, T.C. and J.M. Dille. Reversal of depressor effect of TEA. *J. Pharmacol. Exp. Ther.* 108: 233-239, 1953.

307.   Buchwald, M.E. and G.S. Eadie. The toxicology of dilaudid injected intravenously into mice. *J. Pharmacol. Exp. Ther.* 71: 197-202, 1941.

308.   Eddy, N.B. and J.G. Reid. Studies of morphine, codeine and their derivatives. VII. Dihydromorphine (paramorphan), dihydromorphinone (Dilaudid), and dihydrocodeinone (Dicodid). *J. Pharmacol. Exp. Ther.* 52: 468-493, 1934.

309.   Friebel, H. and C. Reichle. Analgesia and analgesia-enhancing effects of chlorpromazine. *Arch. Exp. Path. Pharmakol.* 226: 551-573, 1955.

310.   Eddy, N.B. and H.A. Howes. Studies of morphine, codeine and their derivatives. *J. Pharmacol. Exp. Ther.* 53: 430-439, 1935.

311.   Horton, R.G., *et al.* The acute toxicity of di-isopropyl fluorophosphate. *J. Pharmacol. Exp. Ther.* 87: 414-429, 1946.

312.   Koelle, G.B. and A. Gilman. The relationship between cholinesterase inhibition and the pharmacological action of di-isopropyl fluorophosphate (DFP). *J. Pharmacol. Exp. Ther.* 87: 421-434, 1946.

Bibliography

313. Cook, D.L., *et al.* Pharmacology of a new autonomic ganglion blocking agent, 2,6-di-methyl-1,1-diethyl piperidinium bromide (SC-1950). *J. Pharmacol. Exp. Ther.* 99: 435-443, 1950.

314. Chen, G., *et al.* Pharmacology of 1,1-di-methyl-4-phenylpiperazinium iodide, a ganglionic stimulating agent. *J. Pharmacol. Exp. Ther.* 103: 330-336, 1951.

315. Tainter, M.L. and W.C. Cutting. Miscellaneous action of dinitrophenol. Repeated administrations, antidotes, fatal doses, antiseptic tests and actions of some isomers. *J. Pharmacol. Exp. Ther.* 49: 187-208, 1933.

316. Spencer, H.C., *et al.* Toxicological studies on laboratory animals of certain alkyldinitrophenols used in agriculture. *J. Industr. Hyg.* 30: 10-25, 1948.

317. Tainter, M.L., *et al.* Metabolic activity of compounds related to dinitrophenol. *J. Pharmacol. Exp. Ther.* 53: 58-66, 1935.

318. Magne, H., *et al.* Pharmacodynamic action of the nitrated phenols: An agent increasing cellular oxidations, 2,4-dinitrophenol. *Ann. Physiol. Physiochim. Biol.* 8: 1-50, 1932.

319. Tainter, M.L. and W.C. Cutting. Febrile, respiratory and some other actions of dinitrophenol. *J. Pharmacol. Exp. Ther.* 48: 410-429, 1933.

320. Way, E.L. and W.C. Herbert. The effect of sodium pentobarbital on the toxicity of certain antihistamines. *J. Pharmacol. Exp. Ther.* 104: 115-121, 1952.

321. Gruhzit, O.M. and R.A. Fisken. A toxicological study of two histamine antagonists of the benzhydryl alkamine ether group. *J. Pharmacol. Exp. Ther.* 89: 227-233, 1947.

322. De Salva, S. and R. Evans. Anticonvulsive character of styramate and other depressant drugs. *Toxicol. Appl. Pharmacol.* 2: 397-402, 1960.

323. Chen, G. and B. Bohner. A study of central nervous system stimulants. *J. Pharmacol. Exp. Ther.* 123: 212-215, 1958.

324. Loew, E.R. Pharmacology of antihistamine compounds. *Physiol. Rev.* 27: 542-573, 1947.

325. Sachs, B.A. The toxicity of benadryl: Report of a case and review of the literature. *Ann. Intern. Med.* 29: 135-144, 1948.

326. De Salva, S. and R. Evans. Continuous intravenous infusion of strychnine in rats. II. Antagonism by various drugs. *Arch. Int. Pharmacodyn.* 125: 355-361, 1960.

327. Blaschko, H. and T.L. Chrusciel. The Decarboxylation of amino acids related to tyrosine and their awakening action in reserpine-treated mice. *J. Physiol. (Lond.)* 151: 272-284, 1960.

328. Page, I.H. and R. Reed. Hypertensive effect of L-dopa and related compounds in the rat. *Am. J. Physiol.* 143: 122-125, 1945.

Bibliography

329. Kato, R. Effects of pre-electroshock treatment on the duration of tranquilizer effect, and on the contents of brain serotonin. *Nippon Yakurigaku Zasshi* 56: 1046-1053, 1960.

330. Burn, J.H. and M.J. Rand. The depressor action of dopamine and adrenaline. *Brit. J. Pharmacol.* 13: 471-479, 1958.

331. Costa, E., *et al.* Brain concentration of biogenic amines and EEG patterns of rabbits. *J. Pharmacol. Exp. Ther.* 130: 81-88, 1960.

332. Rowe, L.W. The comparative pharmacologic action of ephedrine and adrenalin. *J. Am. Pharm. Ass.* 16: 912-918, 1927.

333. Chen, K.K. and C.F. Schmidt. The action and clinical use of ephedrine. *J. Amer. Med. Ass.* 87: 836-842, 1926.

334. Chen, K.K. The acute toxicity of Ephedrine. *J. Pharmacol. Exp. Ther.* 27: 61-76, 1926.

335. Hauschild, F. On the pharmacology of 1-phenyl-2-methylaminopropane (Pervitin). *Arch. Exp. Path. Pharm.* 191: 465-481, 1939.

336. Watson, R.H.J. Constitutional differences between two strains of rats with different behavioral characteristics. *Advanc. Psychosomatic Med.* 1: 160-165, 1960.

337. Grishina, V.M. Antihypnotic action of ephedrine. *Farmakol. i Toksiko.* 23: 287-295, 1960.

338. Axelrod, J. and R. Tomchick. Increased rate of metabolism of epinephrine and norepinephrine by sympathomimetic amines. *J. Pharmacol. Exp. Ther.* 130: 367-369, 1960.

339. Burn, J.H. and M.J. Rand. The action of sympathetic amines in animals treated with reserpine. *J. Physiol. (Lond.)* 144: 314-336, 1958.

340. Lands, A.M., *et al.* The pharmacology of N-alkyl homologues of epinephrine. *J. Pharmacol. Exp. Ther.* 90: 110-119, 1947.

341. Bovet, D. and G. Bovet-Nitti. *Medications of the Autonomic Nervous System.* S. Karger, New York, 1948.

342. Levy, J. and E. Michel-Ber. A hypothesis about the mechanisms of action of monamine oxidase inhibitors at the central nervous system level. *C.R. Acad. Sci. (Paris)* 250: 415-417, 1960.

343. Raab, W. and R.J. Humphreys. Protective effect of adrenolytic drugs against fatal myocardial epinephrine concentrations. *J. Pharmacol. Exp. Ther.* 88: 268-276, 1946.

344. Smythies, J.R. and C.K. Levy. The comparative pharmacology of some mescaline analogues. *J. Ment. Sci.* 106: 531-536, 1960.

Bibliography

345. Savoldi, F., *et al.* Action of a water-soluble derivative of theobromine on the cerebral circulation and cortical electrical activity of the rabbit. *Arch. Ital. Sci. Farmacol.* 10: 231-240, 1960.

346. Spector, W.S. *Handbook of Toxicology.* Vol. I. WADC Technical Report 55-16, 1955.

347. Kostos, V.J. and J.J. Kocsis. Tissue serotonin (5-HT) levels in colchicine treated rats and rabbits. *Pharmacologist* 5: 247, 1963.

348. Röthlin, E. Investigation of ergotamine, a specific alkaloid of ergot. *Arch. Int. Pharmacodyn.* 27: 459-479, 1923.

349. Röthlin, E. The pharmacological properties of a new alkaloid of ergot, ergobasine. *C.R. Soc. Biol. (Paris)* 119: 1302-1304, 1935.

350. Laurence, D.R. and R.S. Stacey. Mechanism of the prevention of nicotine convulsions by hexamethonium and by adrenaline blocking agents. *Brit. J. Pharmacol.* 8: 62-65, 1953.

351. Barger, G. The alkaloids of ergot. *Heffter's Hdb. E.* 6: 84-222, 1938.

352. Sandoz Pharmaceuticals. Personal Communication.

353. Ginzel, K.H. The effect of *d*-lysergic acid diethylamide and other drugs on the carotid sinus reflex. *Brit. J. Pharmacol.* 13: 250-259, 1958.

354. Mayer, S., *et al.* The effect of adrenergic blocking agents on some metabolic actions of catecholamines. *J. Pharmacol. Exp. Ther.* 134: 18-27, 1961.

355. Graham, G., *et al.* Influence of fluoroacetate on renal acid secretion. *Fed. Proc.* 12: 325, 1953.

356. Furchgott, R.F. The effect of sodium fluoroacetate on the contractility and metabolism of intestinal smooth muscle. *J. Pharmacol. Exp. Ther.* 99: 1-15, 1950.

357. Matthews, R.J. and B.J. Roberts. The effect of gamma-aminobutyric acid on synaptic transmission in autonomic ganglia. *J. Pharmacol. Exp. Ther.* 132: 19-22, 1961.

358. Rech, R.H. and E.F. Domino. Effects of gamma-aminobutyric acid on chemical and electrically evoked activity in the isolated cerebral cortex of the dog. *J. Pharmacol. Exp. Ther.* 130: 59-67, 1960.

359. Gulati, O.D. and H.C. Stanton. Some effects on the central nervous system of gamma-amino-n-butyric acid (GABA) and certain related amino acids administered systemically and intracerebrally to mice. *J. Pharmacol. Exp. Ther.* 129: 175-185, 1960.

360. Winter, C.A. and J.T. Lehman. Studies on synthetic curarizing agents. *J. Pharmacol. Exp. Ther.* 100: 489-501, 1950.

Bibliography

361.   Bovet, D., *et al*. Studies on synthetic curare-like poisons. *Arch. Int. Pharmacodyn*. 80: 172-188, 1949.

362.   Longo, V.G. Effects of scopolamine and atropine on electroencephalographic and behavioral reaction due to hypothalamic stimulation. *J. Pharmacol. Exp. Ther*. 116: 198-208, 1956.

363.   Maxwell, R.A., *et al*. Pharmacology of (2(octahydro-1-azocinyl)-ethyl)-guanidine sulfate (SU-5864). *J. Pharmacol. Exp. Ther*. 128: 22-29, 1960.

364.   Bogaert, M., *et al*. On the pharmacology of guanethidine. *Arch. Int. Pharmacodyn*. 134: 224-236, 1961.

365.   Cass, R. and T. Spriggs. Tissue amine levels and sympathetic blockade after guanethidine and bretylium. *Brit. J. Pharmacol*. 17: 442-450, 1961.

366.   Cass, R., *et al*. Norepinephrine depletion as a possible mechanism of action of guanethidine (SU-5864), a new hypotensive agent. *Proc. Soc. Exp. Biol. (N.Y.)* 103: 871-872, 1960.

367.   Dagirmanjian, R. The effects of guanethidine on the noradrenaline content of the hypothalamus in the cat and rat. *J. Pharm. Pharmacol*. 15: 518-521, 1963.

368.   Gunn, J.A. The pharmacological action of harmaline. *Trans. Roy. Soc. Edin*. 47: 245-272, 1909.

369.   Ahmed, A. and N.R.W. Taylor. The analysis of drug-induced tremor in mice. *Brit. J. Pharmacol*. 14: 350-354, 1959.

370.   Pellmont, B. and F.A. Steiner. Influence on a conditioned reflex by drugs with effects on monamine metabolism in the central nervous system. *Psychiat. et Neurol. (Basel)* 140: 216-219, 1960.

371.   Spector, S., *et al*. Evidence for release of brain amines by reserpine in presence of monoamine oxidase inhibitors: Implication of monoamine oxidase in norepinephrine metabolism in brain. *J. Pharmacol. Exp. Ther*. 130: 256-261, 1960.

372.   Goldberg, L.I. and A. Sjoerdsma. Effects of several monoamine oxidase inhibitors on the cardiovascular actions of naturally occurring amines in the dog. *J. Pharmacol. Exp. Ther*. 127: 212-218, 1959.

373.   Hara, S. and I. Mori. Investigation of poisons of the extrapyramidal paths. II. Pharmacological contribution to harmine. *Jap. J. Med. Sc. IV Pharm*. 7: 78-79, 1933.

374.   Gunn, J.A. and R.C. MacKeith. The pharmacological actions of harmol. *Quart. J. Pharm*. 4: 33-51, 1931.

375.   Lewin, L. Chemistry and pharmacological action of Banisteria caapi spr. *Arch. Exp. Path. Pharmakol*. 129: 133-149, 1928.

Bibliography

376. Goldberg, L.I. and F.M. DeCosta. Selective depression of sympathetic transmission by intravenous administration of iproniazid and harmine. *Proc. Soc. Exp. Biol. (N.Y.)* 105: 223-227, 1960.

377. Marshall, F.N. and J.P. Long. Pharmacologic studies on some compounds structurally related to the hemicholinium HC-3. *J. Pharmacol. Exp. Ther.* 127: 236-240, 1959.

378. Kase, Y. and H.L. Borison. Central respiratory depressant effect of "hemicholinium." *Fed. Proc.* 16: 311, 1957.

379. Zablocka, B. and D. Esplin. Evidence for a cholinergic link in "direct" spinal inhibition. *Pharmacologist* 5: 237, 1963.

380. Seifter, J. and A.J. Begany. Studies on the action of a synthetic heparinoid. *Am. J. Med. Sci.* 216: 234-235, 1948.

381. Montague, D., *et al.* Bradykinin: vascular relaxant, cardiac stimulant. *Science* 141: 907-908, 1963.

382. Wenke, M. Relation between the heparin dose and the esterolytic activity level in the blood serum of rats. *Arch. Int. Pharmacodyn.* 134: 417-425, 1961.

383. Gillis, C.N. and C.W. Nash. The initial pressor action of bretylium tosylate and guanethidine sulfate and their relation to release of catecholamines. *J. Pharmacol. Exp. Ther.* 134: 1-7, 1961.

384. Wolff, R. and J.J. Brignon. A study of the serum-clearing activity of several herparin-like substances *in vitro*. *Arch. Int. Pharmacodyn.* 121: 255-267, 1959.

385. Davey, M.J., *et al.* The effects of nialamide on adrenergic function. *Brit. J. Pharmacol.* 20: 121-134, 1963.

386. Salmoiraghi, G.C., *et al.* Effects of *d*-lysergic acid diethylamine and its brom derivative on cardiovascular responses to serotonin and on arterial pressure. *J. Pharmacol. Exp. Ther.* 119: 240-247, 1957.

387. Grollman, A. The effect of various hypotensive agents on the arterial blood pressure of hypertensive rats and dogs. *J. Pharmacol. Exp. Ther.* 14: 263-270, 1955.

388. Della Bella, D. and F. Rognoni. Neurovegetative control of gastric motility in the isolated nerve-stomach preparation of the rat. *J. Pharmacol. Exp. Ther.* 134: 184-189, 1961.

389. Kennedy, W.P. Sodium salt of *C-C*-Cyclohexenylmethyl-*N*-methyl barbituric acid (Evipan) anaesthesia in laboratory animals. *J. Pharmacol. Exp. Ther.* 50: 347-353, 1934.

390. Buller, R.H., *et al.* The potentiating effect of 4,5-dihydro-6-methyl-2[2-4(4-Pyridyl)-Ethyl]-3-pyridazinone (U-320) on hexobarbital hypnosis. *J. Pharmacol. Exp. Ther.* 134: 95-99, 1961.

Bibliography

391.   Reinhard, J.F., *et al.* Pharmacologic characteristics of
         1-(ortho-toluoxy)-2,3-bis-(2,2,2-trichloro-1 hydroxyethoxy)-propane. *J.*
         Pharmacol. Exp. Ther. 106: 444-452, 1952.

392.   Bush, M.T., *et al.* The metabolic fate of Evipal (hexobarbital) and of
         "nor-Evipal." *J. Pharmacol. Exp. Ther.* 108: 104-111, 1953.

393.   Maloney, A.H. and R. Hertz. Sodium N-methyl-cyclohexenyl-
         methyl-barbituric acid (Evipal): Hypnosis, anesthesia and toxicity. *J.*
         Pharmacol. Exp. Ther. 54: 77-83, 1935.

394.   Werner, H.W., *et al.* A comparative study of several ultrashortacting
         barbiturates, Nembutal, and tribromethanol. *J. Pharmacol. Exp. Ther.* 60:
         189-197, 1937.

395.   Shimamoto, K., *et al.* Peripheral action of the ganglion blocking agents. *Jap. J.*
         Pharmacol. 5: 66-76, 1955.

396.   Takagi, H. and T. Ban. Effect of psychotropic drugs on the limbic system of
         the cat. *Jap. J. Pharmacol.* 10: 7-14, 1960.

397.   Lin, T.M., *et al.* 3-ß-aminoethyl-1,2,4-triazole, a potent stimulant of gastric
         secretion. *J. Pharmacol. Exp. Ther.* 134: 88-94, 1961.

398.   Lands, A.M., *et al.* The pharmacological properties of three new antihistaminic
         drugs. *J. Pharmacol. Exp. Ther.* 95: 45-52, 1949.

399.   Schmidt, G.W. and A. Stahelin. Histamine sensitivity and anaphylaxis reaction.
         Z. Innunitatstorsch. 60: 222-238, 1929.

400.   Parrot, J.L., *et al.* Acute intoxication of the cobaye through gastric
         administration of histamine alone or associated with putrescence. *17th Int.*
         Physiol. Cong. p. 378, 1947.

401.   Camus, L. Hordenine, the degree of the toxic symptoms of intoxication. *C. R.*
         Acad. Sci. (Paris) 142: 110-113, 1906.

402.   Barger, G. and H.H. Dale. Chemical structure and sympathomimetic action of
         amines. *J. Physiol. (Lond.)* 41: 19-59, 1910.

403.   Craver, N. The activities of 1-hydrazin-ophthalazine (Ba-5968), a hypotensive
         agent. *J. Amer. Pharm. Ass., Sci. Ed.* 40: 559-564, 1961.

404.   Schmitt, H. Adrenolytic, noradrenolytic and sympatholytic action of dibenzyline
         (SKF 688A). *Arch. Int. Pharmacodyn.* 109: 263-270, 1957.

405.   Rocha e Silva, M., *et al.* Potentiation of duration of the vasodilator effect of
         bradykinin by sympatholytic drugs and reserpine. *J. Pharmacol. Exp. Ther.* 128:
         217-226, 1960.

Bibliography

406. Kuschinsky, G. Investigation of sympathol, an adrenergic compound. *Arch. Exp. Path. Pharmakol.* 156: 290-308, 1930.

407. Mancini, M.A. The pharmacology of the autonomous system. *Boll. Soc. Ital. Biol. Sper.* 4: 224-225, 1929.

408. Maxwell, R.A., *et al.* Concerning a possible action of guanethidine (SU-5864) in smooth muscle. *J. Pharmacol. Exp. Ther.* 129: 24-30, 1960.

409. Randall, L.O. and G. Lehmann. Analgesic action of 3-hydroxy-*N*-methyl morphinan hydrobromide (dromoran). *J. Pharmacol. Exp. Ther.* 99: 163-170, 1950.

410. Bogdanski, D.F., *et al.* Pharmacological studies with the serotonin precursor, 5-hydroxytryptophan. *J. Pharmacol. Exp. Ther.* 122: 182-194, 1958.

411. Buchel, L. and J. Levy. Contribution to the study of the effects on the central nervous system of monoamine oxidase inhibitors, hydrazine-2-phenyl-3 propane (P.I.H.), isopropylhydrazide of isonicotinic acid (iproniazid). II. Influence on potentiation of experimental sleep by reserpine. *Anesth. et Analg.* 17: 313-328, 1960.

412. Anderson. E.G. The effects of harmaline and 5-hydroxytryptamine on spinal synaptic transmission. *Pharmacologist* 5: 238, 1963.

413. Cronhein, G.E. and J.T. Gourzis. Cardiovascular and behavioral effects of serotonin and related substances in dogs without and with reserpine premedications. *J. Pharmacol. Exp. Ther.* 130: 444-449, 1960.

414. Haas, H. On 3-piperidino-1-phyenyl-1-bi-cycloheptenylpropanol-(1) (akineton). Second Report. *Arch. Int. Pharmacodyn.* 128: 204-238, 1960.

415. Read, G.W., *et al.* Comparison of excited phases after sedatives and tranquilizers. *Psychopharmacologia.* 1: 346-350, 1960.

416. Hughes, F.W. and E. Kopman. Influence of pentobarbital, hydroxyzine, chlorpromazine, reserpine, and meprobamate on choice-discrimination behavior in the rat. *Arch. Int. Pharmacodyn.* 126: 158-170, 1960.

417. Hotovy, R. and J. Kepff-Walter. On the pharmacological properties of perphenazin-sulfoxide. *Arzneimittel-Forsch.* 10: 638-650, 1960.

418. Lynes, T.E. and F.M. Berger. Some pharmacological properties of hydroxyzine (1-(p-chlorobenzhydryl-4-(2-(2-hydroxyethoxy)-ethyl) diethylenediamine dihydrochloride). *J. Pharmacol. Exp. Ther.* 119: 163, 1957.

419. Hutcheon, E., *et al.* Cardiovascular action of hydroxyzine (Atarax). *J. Pharmacol. Exp. Ther.* 118: 451-460, 1956.

420. Blackmore, W.P. Effect of hydroxyzine on urine flow in the dog. *Proc. Soc. Exp. Biol. (N.Y.)* 103: 518-520, 1960.

Bibliography

421. Randall, L.O. and T.H. Smith. The adrenergic blocking action of some dibenzazepine derivatives. *J. Pharmacol. Exp. Ther.* 103: 10-23, 1951.

422. Cotton, M., *et al.* A comparison of the effectiveness of adrenergic blocking drugs in inhibiting the cardiac actions of sympathomimetic amines. *J. Pharmacol. Exp. Ther.* 121: 183-190, 1957.

423. Frommel, E., *et al.* On the pharmacology of a new neuroleptic: The alpha-isomer of 2-chloro-9 (3-dimethylaminopropylidene)-thioxanthene or taractan: Action on sleep centers, on motor excitation due to nikethamide on Pentetrazol, electroshock and psychomotor excitation due to amphetamine. *C.R. Soc. Biol. (Paris)* 154: 1182-1185, 1960.

424. Oberholzer, R.J.H. Experimental data on iminodibenzyl derivative: Tofranil. *J. Med. (Porto.)* 42: 602-605, 1960.

425. Dobkin, A.B. Potentiation of thiopental anesthesia by derivatives and analogs of phenothiazine. *Anesthesiology* 21: 292-296, 1960.

426. Gokhale, S., *et al.* Mechanism of the initial adrenergic effects of bretylium and guanethidine. *Brit. J. Pharmacol.* 20: 362-377, 1963.

427. Gyermek, L. and C. Possemato. Potentiation of 5-hydroxytryptamine by imipramine. *Med. Exp. (Basel)* 3: 225-229, 1960.

428. Benson, W.M., *et al.* Pharmacologic and toxicologic observations of hydrazine derivatives of isonicotinic acid (Rimifon, Marsilid). *Amer. Rev. Tuberc.* 65: 376-391, 1952.

429. Randall, L.O. and R.E. Bagdon. Pharmacology of iproniazid and other amine oxidase inhibitors. *Ann. N.Y. Acad. Sci.* 80: 626-642, 1959.

430. Spector, S., *et al.* Biochemical and pharmacological effects of the monoamine oxidase inhibitors, iproniazid, 1-phenyl-2-hydrazino-propane (JB 516) and 1-phenyl-3-hydrazino-butane (JB 835). *J. Pharmacol. Exp. Ther.* 128: 15-21, 1960.

431. Bartlet, A.L. The 5-hydroxytryptamine content of mouse brain and whole mice after treatment with some drugs affecting the central nervous system. *Brit. J. Pharmacol.* 15: 140-146, 1960.

432. Wirth, W., *et al.* On testing stimulating substances (hydrazine derivatives) on "annoyed" animals. *Arch. Exp. Path. Pharmakol.* 238: 62-66, 1960.

433. Green, H. and R.W. Erickson. Effect of trans-2-phenylcyclopropylamine upon norepinephrine concentration and monoamine oxidase activity of rat brain. *J. Pharmacol. Exp. Ther.* 129: 237-242, 1960.

434. Spector, S. Effect of iproniazid on brain levels of norepinephrine and serotonin. *Science* 127: 704, 1958.

Bibliography

435.   Benson, W.M., *et al.* Comparative pharmacology of levorphan, racemorphan and dextrorphan and related methyl ethers. *J. Pharmacol. Exp. Ther.* 109: 189-200, 1953.

436.   Hunter, A.R. The toxicity of xylocaine. *Brit. J. Anaesth.* 23: 153-161, 1951.

437.   Goldberg, L. Studies on local anesthetics. Pharmacological properties of homologues and isomers of xylocaine (alkyl amino-acid derivatives). *Acta Physiol. Scand.* 18: 1-18, 1949.

438.   Sorel, L. and R. Lejeune. EEG changes in the rabbit following intravenous injection of cocaine. *Arch. Int. Pharmacodyn.* 102: 314-334, 1955.

439.   Kovalev, I.E. On the influence of mezocaine and zylocaine on the central nervous system. *Famikol. i Toksikol.* 23: 385-390, 1960.

440.   Bernard, C.G., *et al.* On the evaluation of the anticonvulsive effect of different local anesthetics. *Arch. Int. Pharmacodyn.* 108: 392-401, 1956

441.   Wagers, P.W. and C.M. Smith. Responses in dental nerves of dogs to tooth stimulation and the effects of systemically administered procaine, lidocaine and morphine. *J. Pharmacol. Exp. Ther.* 130: 89-105, 1960.

442.   Bernhard, C.G., *et al.* The difference in action on normal and convulsive cortical activity between a local anesthetic (lidocaine) and barbiturate. *Arch. Int. Pharmacodyn.* 108: 408-419, 1956.

443.   Gogerty, J. and J. Dille. Pharmacology of *d*-lysergic-acid morpholide (LSM). *J. Pharmacol. Exp. Ther.* 120: 340-348, 1957.

444.   Delphant, J. and M. Lanza. Comparative action of mescaline, LSD 25, and yajeine on the central temperature of the rat. *J. Physiol. (Paris)* 52: 70-71, 1960.

445.   Weltman, A.S., *et al.* Endocrine effects of lysergic acid diethylamide on male rats. *Fed. Proc.* 22: 165, 1963.

446.   Yui, T. and Y. Takeo. Neuropharmacological studies on a new series of ergot alkaloids. *Jap. J. Pharmacol.* 7: 157-161, 1958.

447.   Key, B.J. and P.B. Bradley. The effects of drugs on conditioning and habituation to arousal stimuli in animals. *Psychopharmacologia* 1: 450-462, 1960.

448.   Passonant, P., *et al.* The action of LSD-25 on the behavior and on the cortical and rhinencephalic rhythms of the chronic cat. *Electroenceph. Clin. Neurophysiol.* 8: 702, 1956.

449.   Apter, J.T. LSD-25 versus pentobarbital sodium. *Fed. Proc.* 17: 5, 1958.

450.   Elder, J.T. Phenoxybenzamine (PBA) antogonism of lysergic acid diethylamide (LSD)-induced hyperglycemia. *Pharmacologist* 5: 261, 1963.

451. Dobkin, A.B. and J.H. Havland. Drugs which stimulate affective behavior. I. Action of lysergic acid diethylamide (LSD-25) against thiopentone anesthesia in dogs. *Anaesthesia* 15: 48-54, 1960.

452. Murray, E.J. and S. Chorover. Effects of lysergic acid diethylamine upon certain aspects of memory (delayed alternation) in monkeys. *Fed. Proc.* 17: 381, 1958.

453. Weidmann, H. and A. Cerletti. Investigation of the pressor activity of 5-hydroyxtryptamine (serotonin). *Arch. Int. Pharmacodyn.* 111: 98-107, 1957.

454. Meltzer, S.J. and J. Auer. Physiological and pharmacological studies of magnesium salts. I. General anesthesia by subcutaneous injections. *Amer. J. Physiol.* 14: 366-388, 1905.

455. Gylus, J.A., *et al*. Pharmacological and toxicological properties of 2-methyl-3-piperidinopyrazine, a new antidepressant. *Ann. N.Y. Acad. Sci.* 107: 899-912, 1963.

456. Heise, G.A. and E. Boff. Behavioral determination of time and dose parameters of monoamine oxidase inhibitors. *J. Pharmacol. Exp. Ther.* 129: 155-162, 1960.

457. Berger, F.M., *et al*. The pharmacological properties of 2-methyl-2-sec-butyl-1,3-propanediol dicarbamate (mebutamate, W-583), a new centrally acting blood pressure lowering agent. *J. Pharmacol. Exp. Ther.* 134: 356-365, 1961.

458. Rowe, G.G., *et al*. The effect of mecamylamine on coronary flow, cardiac work and cardiac efficiency in normotensive dogs. *J. Lab. Clin. Med.* 52: 883-887, 1958.

459. Lum, B.K.B. and P.L. Rushleigh. Potentiation of vasoactive durgs by ganglionic blocking agents. *J. Pharmacol. Exp. Ther.* 132: 13-18, 1961.

460. Lakeside Laboratories. Personal communication.

461. Roszkowski, A.P. A pharmacological comparison of therapeutically useful centrally acting skeletal muscle relaxants. *J. Pharmacol. Exp. Ther.* 129: 75-81, 1960.

462. Burke, J.C., *et al*. The muscle relaxant properties of 2,2-dichloro-1-(p-chlorophenyl)-1,3-propanediol-O^3-carbamate. *Arch. Int. Pharmacodyn.* 134: 216-223, 1961.

463. Della Bella, D. and F. Rognoni. Pharmacologic properties of a new synthetic derivative with central depressant activity: 2-2-bis-chloromethyl-1,3-propanediol (dispranol). *Boll. Chim. Farm.* 99: 67-78, 1960.

464. Seifter, J., *et al*. Pharmacology of N-methyl-ω-phenyl-tert-butylamine. *116th Meeting Am. Chem. Soc.* 17L, 1949.

465. Day, M.D. Effect of sympathomimetic amines on the blocking action of guanethidine, bretylium and xylocholine. *Brit. J. Pharmacol.* 18: 421-439, 1962.

Bibliography

466.   Covino, B.G. Antifibrillary effect of mephentermine sulfate (Wyamine) in general hypothermia. *J. Pharmacol. Exp. Ther.* 122: 418-422, 1958.

467.   Brofman, B.L., *et al.* Treatment of hypotension accompanying myocardial infarction: Use of a pressor substance. *J. Lab. Clin. Med.* 36: 802, 1950.

468.   Fawaz, G. The effect of mephentermine on isolate dog hearts, normal and pretreated with reserpine. *Brit. J. Pharmacol.* 16: 309-314, 1961.

469.   Aston, R. and H. Cullumbine. The effects of combinations of ataraxics with hypnotics, LSD and iproniazid in the mouse. *Arch. Int. Pharmacodyn.* 126: 219-227, 1960.

470.   Geller, I. and J. Seifter. The effects of meprobamate, barbiturates, d-amphetamine and promazine on experimentally induced conflict in the rat. *Psychopharmacologia (Berl.)* 1: 482-492, 1960.

471.   Takeda, Y. Pharmacological and toxicological studies on tranquilizers. *Yakugaku Kenkya* 32: 585-616, 1960.

472.   Ledebur, I.V., *et al.* Nalorphine antagonism of the narcotic action of chlorpromazine, meprobamate, and methaminodiazepoxide (Librium) *Med. Exptl.* 7: 177-179, 1962.

473.   Hendley, C.D., *et al.* Effects of meprobamate (Milltown), chlorpromazine, and reserpine on behavior in the monkey. *Fed. Proc.* 15: 436, 1956.

474.   Barnes, T.C. Effects of tranquilizers and antiepileptic drugs on EEG-flicker response and on convulsive behavior. *Fed. Proc.* 17: 347, 1958.

475.   Orth, O.S., *et al.* Subacute toxicity of "Thiomerin" compared to other mercurial diuretics. *Fed. Proc.* 9: 305-306, 1950.

476.   Ernst, A.M. Experiments with an o-methylated product of dopamine on cats. *Acta Physiol. Pharmacol. Neerl.* 11: 48-53, 1962.

477.   Parker, J.M. and N. Hildebrand. Mescaline blocking effects of dibenamine. *Fed. Proc.* 21: 419, 1962.

478.   Hosko, M.J., Jr. and R. Tislow. Acute tolerance to mescaline in the dog. *Fed. Proc.* 15: 440, 1956.

479.   Bridger, W.H. and W.H. Gantt. The effect of mescaline on differentiated conditional reflexes. *Amer. J. Psychiat.* 113: 352-360, 1956.

480.   Chen, K.K. Pharmacology of methadone and related compounds. *Ann. N.Y. Acad. Sci.* 51: 83-97, 1948.

Bibliography

481. Finnegan, J.K, *et al*. Observations on the comparative pharmacologic action of 6-di-methylamino-4,4-diphenyl-3-heptanone (amidone) and morphine. *J. Pharmacol. Exp. Ther.* 92: 269-276, 1948.

482. Eddy, N.B. and D. Leimbach. Synthetic analgesics. II. Dithienylbutenyl and dithienylbutylamines, *J. Pharmacol. Exp. Ther.* 107: 385-393, 1953.

483. Holten, C.H. and E. Sonne. Action of a series of benactyzine-derivatives and other compounds on stress-induced behavior in the rat. *Acta Pharmacol. (Kbh.)* 11: 148-155, 1955.

484. Somers, G.F. Pharmacological properties of thalidomide (α-phthalimido glutarimide), a new sedative hypnotic drug. *Brit. J. Pharmacol.* 15: 111-116, 1960.

485. Hauschild, F. The pharmacology of phenylalkylamine. *Arch. Exp. Path. Pharmakol.* 195: 647-680, 1940.

486. Owen, J.E., Jr. The influence of dl, d- and l-amphetamine and d-methamphetamine on a fixed-ratio schedule. *J. Exp. Anal. Behav.* 3: 293-310, 1960.

487. John, E.R., *et al*. Differential effects on various conditioned responses in cats caused by intraventricular and intramuscular injection of reserpine and other substances. *J. Pharmacol. Exp. Ther.* 123: 193-205, 1958.

488. Hjort, A.M., *et al*. The pharmacology of compounds related to ß-2,5-dimethoxy, phenethyl amine. *J. Pharmacol. Exp. Ther.* 92: 283-290, 1948.

489. De Beer, E.J., *et al*. The restoration of arterial pressure from various hypotensive states by methoxamine. *Arch. Int. Pharmacodyn.* 104: 487-498, 1956.

490. Stormorken, H., *et al*. Mechanism of bradycardia by methoxamine. *Arch. Int. Pharmacodyn.* 120: 386-401, 1959.

491. Visscher, F.E., *et al*. Pharmacology of pamine bromide. *J. Pharmacol. Exp. Ther.* 110: 188-204, 1954.

492. Smith, S.E. The pharmacological actions of 3-4-dihydroxyphenyl-α-methylamine (α-methyldopa), an inhibitor of 5-hydroxytryptophan decarboxylase. *Brit. J. Pharmacol.* 15: 319-327, 1960.

493. Dangler, H. and G. Reichel. Inhibition of dopa decarboxylase by 2-methyl-3-(3,4-dihydroxyphenyl) alanine (α-methyl dopa) *in vivo*. *Arch. Exp. Path. Pharmakol.* 234: 275-281, 1958.

494. Westermann, E., *et al*. Inhibition of serotonin formation by α-methyl-3,4-dihydroxy-phenyl-L-alanine. *Arch. Exp. Path. Pharmakol.* 234: 194-205, 1958.

495. Sergio, C. and V.G. Longo. Action of several drugs on EEG and behavior of decorticate rabbits. *Arch. Int. Pharmacodyn.* 125: 65-82, 1960.

Bibliography

496. Maxwell, R.A., *et al.* Differential potentiation of norephinephrine and epinephrine by cardiovascular and CNS-active agents. *J. Pharmacol. Exp. Ther.* 128: 140-144, 1960.

497. Maxwell, R.A., *et al.* Studies concerning the cardiovascular action of the central nervous stimulant, methyphenidate. *J. Pharmacol. Exp. Ther.* 123: 22-27, 1958.

498. Maxwell, R.A., *et al.* A comparison of some of the cardiovascular action of methylphenidate and cocaine. *J. Pharmacol. Exp. Ther.* 126: 250-257, 1959.

499. Eddy, N.B. Pharmacology of metopon and other new analgesic opium derivatives. *Ann. N.Y. Acad. Sci.* 51: 51-58, 1948.

500. Chesler, A., *et al.* A study of the comparative toxic effects of morphine on the fetal newborn and adult rat. *J. Pharmacol. Exp. Ther.* 75: 363-366, 1942.

501. Haag, H.B., *et al.* Pharmacologic observation on 1,1-diphenyl-1-(dimethylaminoisopropyl)-butanone-2. *Fed. Proc.* 6: 334, 1947.

502. Hatcher, R.A. and C. Eggleston. Studies on the absorption of drugs. *J. Amer. Med. Ass.* 63: 469-473, 1914.

503. Himmelsbach, C.K., *et al.* A method for testing addiction, tolerance and abstinence in the rat. *J. Pharmacol. Exp. Ther.* 53: 179-188, 1935.

504. Blozovski, M. and J. Jacob. The effect of morphine on the behavior of mice trained to run through an elevated maze. *Arch. Int. Pharmacodyn.* 124: 422-435, 1960.

505. Olds, H. and R.P. Travis. Effects of chlorpromazine, meprobamate, pentobarbital and morphine on self-stimulation. *J. Pharmacol. Exp. Ther.* 128: 397-404, 1960.

506. Tedeschi, D.H., *et al.* Analgesic and other neuropharmacologic effects of phenazocine (NIH 7519, Prinadol) compared with morphine. *J. Pharmacol. Exp. Ther.* 130: 431-435, 1960.

507. Zirm, K.L. and A. Pongratz. The analgetic action of the pyridin-3-carbonic acid bis ester of morphine. *Arzneimittel-Forsch.* 10: 137-139, 1960.

508. Wright, C.I. and F.A. Barbour. The respiratory effects of morphine, codeine and related substances. *J. Pharmacol. Exp. Ther.* 53: 34-45, 1935.

509. Longo, V.G. *Electroencephalographic atlas for pharmacological research.* Elsevier Publ. Co., New York and Amsterdam, 1962.

510. Takagi, H., *et al.* The effect of analgesics of the spinal reflex activity of the cat. *Jap. J. Pharmacol.* 4: 176-187, 1955.

511. Fühner, H. Pharmacological actions of muscarine derivatives. *Arch Exp. Path. Pharm.* 61: 283-296, 1909.

Bibliography

512. Mattila, M. and P. Lavikainen. The mouse tail reaction induced by morphine and the sedative action after reserpine and nalorphine. *Ann. Med. Exp. Fenn.* 38: 115-120, 1960.

513. Hart. E.R. and E.L. McCawley. The pharmacology of *N*-allylnormorphine as compared with morphine. *J. Pharmacol. Exp. Ther.* 182: 339-348, 1944.

514. Kirvoy, W.A. and R.A. Huggins. The action of morphine, methadone, merperidine and nalorphine on dorsal root potentials of cat spinal cord. *J. Pharmacol. Exp. Ther.* 134: 210-213, 1961.

515. Unna, K. Antagonistic effect of *N*-allyl-normorphine upon morphine. *J. Pharmacol. Exp. Ther.* 79: 27-31, 1943.

516. Goldstein, L. and J. Aldunate. Quantitative electroencephalographic studies of the effects of morphine and nalorphine on rabbit brain. *J. Pharmacol. Exp. Ther.* 130: 204-211, 1960.

517. Brown, B.B., *et al.* A comparative study of tetramethoquin, a new parasympathetic stimulant, neostigmine and physostigmine. *Arch. Int. Pharmacodyn.* 81: 276-289, 1950.

518. Haley, T.J. and B.M. Rhodes. A note on the acute toxicity of neostigmine methyl bromide in the rat. *J. Am. Pharm. Ass.* 39: 701, 1950.

519. Aeschlimann, J.A. and M. Reinert. The pharmacological action of some analogues of physostigmine. *J. Pharmacol. Exp. Ther.* 43: 413-444, 1931.

520. Heathcote, R. St. A. The pharmacological action of eseridine. *J. Pharmacol. Exp. Ther.* 46: 375-385, 1932.

521. Polonovski, M. and M. Polonovski. Alkaloidal derivatives with attenuated toxicity. *C.R. Acad. Sci. (Paris)* 181: 887-88, 1925.

522. Carlsson, A. and N. Hillarp. Formation of phenolic acids in brain after administration of 3,4-dihydroxyphenylalanine. *Acta Physiol. Scand.* 55: 95-100, 1962.

523. P'an, S.Y., *et al.* Anticonvulsant effect of nialamide and diphenylhydantoin. *Proc. Soc. Exp. Biol. & Med.* 108: 680-683, 1961.

524. Larson, P.S., *et al.* Studies on the fate of nicotine in the body. VI. Observations on the relative rate of elimination of nicotine by the dog, cat, rabbit and mouse. *J. Pharmacol. Exp. Ther.* 95: 506-508, 1949.

525. Heubner, W. and J. Papierkowski. On the toxicity of nicotine in mice. *Arch. Exp. Path. Pharmakol.* 188: 605-610, 1938.

526. Behrend, A. and C.H. Thienes. The development of tolerance to nicotine by rats. *J. Pharmacol. Exp. Ther.* 48: 317-325, 1933.

Bibliography

527. Chen, K.K., *et al*. Toxicity of nicotinic acid. *Proc. Soc. Exp. Biol. (N.Y.)* 38: 241-245, 1938.

528. Hatcher, R.A. Nicotine tolerance in rabbits and the difference in the total dose in adult and young guinea pigs. *Amer. J. Physiol.* 11: 17-27, 1904.

529. Bonta, I.L., *et al*. A newly developed motility apparatus and its applicability in two pharmacological designs. *Arch. Int. Pharmacodyn.* 129: 381-394, 1960.

530. Hardt, A. and R. Hotovy. Methods of testing for compounds with curare-like action. *Arch. Exp. Path. Pharmakol.* 209: 264-278, 1950.

531. Smith, C. S., *et al*. Study of the effect of nicotinism in the albino rat. *J. Pharmacol. Exp. Ther.* 55: 274-287, 1935.

532. Kuschinsky, G. and R. Hotovy. On the central stimulative action of nicotine. *Klin. Wschr.* 22: 649-650, 1943.

533. Knapp, D.E. and E.F. Comino. Evidence for a nicotinic receptor in the central nervous system related to EEG arousal. *Fed. Proc.* 20: 307, 1961.

534. Novikova, A.A. Influence of nicotine upon reflex activity. *Bull. Eksp. Biol. Med. S.S.S.R.* 9: 38-42, 1940.

535. Schaepdryver, A.F. de. Hypertensive responses in reserpinized dogs. *Arch. Int. Pharmacodyn.* 124: 45-52, 1960.

536. Behrens, B. and E. Reichelt. A comparison of cardiazol and coramin in an animal experiment. *Klin. Wschr.* 12: 1860-1862, 1933.

537. Hildebrandt, F. Pentamethylentetrazol (Cardiazol). *Heffter's Hdb. E.* 5: 151-183, 1937.

538. Albus, G. Animal experiments with commercial stimulants with particular consideration of cardiazole and coramine. *Arch. Int. Path. Pharmakol.* 182: 471-476, 1936.

539. Eichholtz, F. and T. Kirsch. The effect of depressor substances on cocaine convulsions. *Arch Exp. Path. Pharmakol.* 184: 674-679, 1937.

540. Heubner, W. and A.V. Nyary. Cumulation of the digitalis glucosides. *Arch. Exp. Path. Pharmakol.* 177: 60-73, 1934.

541. White, A.C. The pharmacological and toxic action of digoxin. *J. Pharmacol. Exp. Ther.* 52: 1-22, 1934.

542. Boyajy, L.D. and C.B. Nash. Influence of reserpine on fibrillatory and positive inotropic responses to ouabain. *Fed. Proc.* 22: 185, 1963.

Bibliography

543. Henderson, F.G., *et al.* Pharmacologic studies of 6,7-Dimethoxy, 1-(4'-ethoxy-3'-methoxybenzyl)3-methyl-isoquinoline. *J. Amer. Pharm. Ass.* 40: 207, 1951.

544. Macht, D.I. An pharmacologic and clinical study of papaverin. *Arch. Intern. Med.* 17: 786-805, 1916.

545. Leopold-Lowenthal, H. On the pharmacological properties of 1-methyl-butyl-2-phenyl-2-hydroxypropionate (spasmol). *Wien Med. Wschr.* 101: 61, 1951.

546. Drommond, F.G., *et al.* Toxicity of some opium alkaloids. *Acta Pharmacol. (Kbh.)* 6: 235-249, 1950.

547. Tunger, H. The duration of narcosis and the narcotic range of nonspecific narcotics in different methods of administration. *Arch. Exp. Path. Pharmakol.* 160: 74-91, 1931.

548. Figot, P.P., *et al.* The estimation and significance of paraldehyde levels in blood and brain. *Acta Pharmacol. (Kbh.)* 8: 290-304, 1952.

549. Kay, F.A., *et al.* Studies on paraldehyde I. The median lethal dose, LD_{50}, of paraldehyde for guinea pigs. *Anesthesiology* 5: 182-185, 1944.

550. Jenney, E.H. and C.C. Pfeiffer. The convulsant effect of hydrazides and the antidotal effect of anticonvulsants and metabolites. *J. Pharmacol. Exp. Ther.* 122: 110-123, 1958.

551. Everett, G.M. Pharmacologic studies of some nonhydrazine MAO inhibitors. *Ann. N.Y. Acad. Sci.* 107: 1068-1077, 1963.

552. Spector, S. Monoamine oxidase in control of brain serotonin and norepinephrine content. *Ann. N.Y. Acad. Sci.* 107: 856-861, 1963.

553. Schoepke, H.G. and R.G. Wiegand. Relation between norepinephrine accumulation or depletion and blood pressure responses in the cat and rat following pargyline administration. *Ann. N.Y. Acad. Sci.* 107: 924-934, 1963.

554. Taylor, J.D., *et al.* A new non-hydrazide monoamine oxidase inhibitor (A 19120) (*N*-methyl-*N*-benzyl-2-propynylamine hydrochloride). *Fed. Proc.* 19: 278, 1960.

555. Calesnick, B., *et al.* Combined action of cardiotoxic drugs: A study on the acute toxicity of combined quinidine, meperidine, pentobarbital, procaine, and procaine amide. *J. Pharmacol. Exp. Ther.* 102: 138-143, 1951.

556. Carmichael, E.B. and L.C. Posey. Toxicity of nembutal for guinea pigs. *Proc. Soc. Exp. Biol. (N.Y)* 33: 527-528, 1936.

557. Westhues, M. and R. Fritsch. *The Narcosis of Animals.* Paul Parcy, Berlin, 1961.

558. Krop, S. and H. Gold. Comparative study of several barbiturates with observations on irreversible neurological distrubances. *J. Pharmacol. Exp. Ther.* 88: 260-267, 1946.

559. White, R.P. and L.D. Boyajy. Comparison of physostigmine and amphetamine in antagonizing the electroencephalogram (EEG) effects of central nervous system depressants. *Proc. Soc. Exp. Biol. (N.Y.)* 102: 479-483, 1959.

560. Schallek, W., *et al.* Central depressant effects of methyprylon. *J. Pharmacol. Exp. Ther.* 118: 139-147, 1956.

561. Kneip, P. Climbing impulse and climbing test. *Arch. Int. Pharmacodyn.* 126: 238-245, 1960.

562. Tsobkallo, G.I. and M.K. Kalinina. Effect of barbamyl, nembutal and thiopental on the higher nervous activity of rabbits. *Pavlov J. High. Nerv. Act.* 10: 644-652, 1960.

563. Bradley, P.B. and B.J. Key. The effect of drugs on arousal responses produced by electrical stimulation of the reticular formation. *Electroenceph. Clin. Neurophysiol.* 10: 97-110, 1958.

564. Pfeiffer, C.C., *et al.* Comparative study of the effect of meprobamate on the conditoned response, on strychnine and pentylenetetrazol thresholds, on the normal electroencephalogram, and on polysynaptic reflexes. *Ann. N.Y. Acad. Sci.* 67: 734-743, 1957.

565. Martin, W.R. and C.G. Eades. A comparative study of the effect of drugs on activation and vasomotor responses evoked by midbrain stimulation: atropine, pentobarbital, chlorpromazine and chlorpromazine sulfoxide. *Psychopharmacologia* 1: 303-335, 1960.

566. Abdulian, D.H., *et al.* Effects of central nervous system depressants on inhibition and facilitation of the patellar reflex. *Arch. Int. Pharmacodyn.* 128: 169-186, 1960.

567. Mitchell, J.C. and F.A. King. The effects of chlorpromazine on water maze learning retention, and stereotyped behavior in the rat. *Psychopharmacologia.* 1: 463-468, 1960.

568. Domer, F.R. and W. Feldberg. The effect of administration of drugs into the cerebral ventricles. *Brit. J. Pharmacol.* 15: 578-587, 1960.

569. McOmie, W.A. Local and systemic effects of 2-methyl 2,4-pentanedial (hexylene glycol). *Fed. Proc.* 6: 357, 1947.

570. Hildebrandt, F. Pyridin-ß-carboxylic acid diethylamide (coramin). *Heffter's Hdb. E.* 5: 128-150.

Bibliography

571. Gross, E.G. and R.M. Featherstone. Studies with tetrazole derivatives. I. Some pharmacologic properties of aliphatic substitutes pentamethylene tetrazole derivatives. *J. Pharmacol. Exp. Ther.* 87: 291-305, 1946.

572. Werner, H.W. and A.L. Tatum A comparative study of the stimulant analeptics picrotoxin, metrazol and coramine. *J. Pharmacol. Exp. Ther.* 66: 260-278, 1939.

573. Ziph, K., *et al.* The antagonistic action of cardiazole, coramine, hexetone, strychnine and icoral to narcotics. *Arch. Exp. Path. Pharmakol.* 185: 113-124, 1937.

574. Hildebrandt, F. and J. Voss. Absorption of cardiazol following oral administration. *Munchen Med. Wchnschr.* 73: 862, 1926.

575. Chusid, J. and L. Kopeloff. Chlordiazepoxide as an anticonvulsant in monkeys. *Proc. Soc. Exp. Biol. (N.Y.)* 109: 546-548, 1962.

576. Wallace, G.D., *et al.* Restraint of chimpanzees with perphenazine. *J. Am. Vet. Med. Ass.* 136: 222-224, 1960.

577. High, J.P., *et al.* Pharmacology of fluphenazine (Prolixin). *Toxicol. Appl. Pharmacol.* 2: 540-552, 1960.

578. Taeschler, M., *et al.* On the significance of various pharmacodynamic properties of phenothiazine derivatives for their clinical effectiveness. *Psychiat. et Neurol. (Basel)* 139: 85-104, 1960.

579. Scott, C.C., *et al.* Comparison of the pharmacologic properties of some new analgesic substances. *Curr. Res. Anesth.* 26: 12-17, 1947.

580. Gruber, C.M. and E.R. Hart. The pharmacology and toxicology of the ethyl ester of 1-methyl-4-phenyl-piperidine-4-carboxylic acid (demerol). *J. Pharmacol. Exp. Ther.* 73: 319-334, 1941.

581. Foster, R.H.K. and A.L. Carman. Studies in analgesia: Piperidine derivatives with morphine-like activity. *J. Pharmacol. Exp. Ther.* 91: 195-209, 1947.

582. Emele, J.F., *et al.* The analgesic activity of phenelzine and other compounds. *J. Pharmacol. Exp. Ther.* 134: 206-209, 1961.

583. Ben, M., *et al.* Cardiovascular activity of ß-phenylethylhydrazine (phenelzine). *Angiology* 11: 62-66, 1960.

584. Eltherington, L.G. and A. Horita. Some pharmacological actions of beta-phenylisopropylhydrazine (PIH). *J. Pharmacol. Exp. Ther.* 128: 7-14, 1960.

585. Buchel, L. and J. Levy. Contribution to the study of the effects of hydrazine-2-phenyl-3-propane (PIH) on the central nervous system, compared with those of 1-isonicotinyl-2-isopropylhydrazine (iproniazid). I. Influence on experimental hypnosis. *Anesth. et Analg.* 17: 289-312, 1960.

Bibliography

586.   Buckley, J.P., *et al*. The pharmacology of beta-phenylisopropylhydrazine. *Fed. Proc.* 19: 278, 1960.

587.   Schaffarsick, R.W. and B.J. Brown. The anticonvulsant activity and toxicity of methylparafynol (Dormison) and some other alcohols. *Science* 116: 663-665, 1952.

588.   Fitch, R.H. and A.L. Tatum. The duration of action of the barbituric acid hypnotics as a basis of classification. *J. Pharmacol. Exp. Ther.* 44: 325-335, 1932.

589.   Anderson, E.G. and D.D. Bonnycastle. A study of the central depressant action of pentobarbital, phenobarbital and diethyl ether in relationship to increases in brain 5-hydroxytryptamine. *J. Pharmacol. Exp. Ther.* 130: 138-143, 1960.

590.   Wilson, J. and J.P. Long. The effect of hemicholinium (HC-3) at various peripheral cholinergic transmitting sites. *Arch. Int. Pharmacodyn.* 120: 343-352, 1959.

591.   Bodo, R.C. de and K.F. Prescott. The antidiuretic action of barbiturates (phenobarbital, amytal, pentobarbital) and the mechanism involved in this action. *J. Pharmacol. Exp. Ther.* 85: 222-233, 1945.

592.   Truitt, E.B., Jr., *et al*. Measurement of brain excitability by use of hexafluorodiethyl ether (Indoklon). *J. Pharmacol. Exp. Ther.* 129: 445-453, 1960.

593.   De Salva, S. Continuous intravenous infusion of strychnine in rats. III. Endocrine influences. *Arch. Int. Pharmacodyn.* 125: 355-361, 1960.

594.   Weaver, L.C., *et al*. Central nervous system effects of a local anesthetic, dyclonine. *Toxicol. Appl. Pharmacol.* 2: 616-627, 1960.

595.   Delgado, J.M.R., *et al*. Effect of amphenidone on the brain of the conscious monkey. *Arch. Int. Pharmacodyn.* 125: 161-171, 1960.

596.   Vogel, G. and L. Ther. The behavior of the cotton rat as determinant of neuroleptic ratio of central-depressing compounds. *Arzneimittel-Forsch.* 10: 806-808, 1960.

597.   Domino, E.F., *et al*. Differential effects of some CNS depressants on a quantitative shock avoidance response in the dog. *J. Pharmacol. Exp. Ther.* 122: 20A, 1958.

598.   Scheer, E. The depressant effect of sodium ethylcrotyl barbiturate on the central nervous system and influences on blood pressure and blood sugar. *Acta Biol. et Med. Ger.* 5: 545-560, 1960.

599.   Sobek, V. Effects of barbiturates on reflex peristaltic inhibition. *Farmakol. i. Toksikol.* 23: 17-20, 1960.

600.   Schapiro, S. Effect of a catechol amine blocking agent (dibenzyline) on organ content and urine excretion of noradrenaline and adrenaline. *Acta Physiol. Scand.* 42: 371-375, 1958.

Bibliography

601.   Quinn, G.P., *et al.* Biochemical and pharmacological studies of RO1-9569 (tetrabenazine), a non-indole tranquilizing agent with reserpine-like effects. *J. Pharmacol. Exp. Ther.* 127: 103-109, 1959.

602.   Innes, I.R. Identification of the smooth muscle excitatory receptors for ergot alkaloids. *Brit. J. Pharmacol.* 19: 120-128, 1962.

603.   Meier, R., *et al.* A new imidazoline derivative with marked adrenolytic properties. *Proc. Soc. Exp. Biol. (N.Y.)* 71: 70-72, 1949.

604.   Furchgott, R.F. In: *Ciba Foundation Symposium*, eds. Vane, J.R., *et al.* Little Brown, Boston, 1960, p. 246.

605.   Hazleton, L.W., *et al.* Toxicity of phenylbutazone (Butazolidin). *Fed. Proc.* 12: 330, 1962.

606.   Kuschinsky, G. and K. Oberdisse. Circulatory effects of meta-sympatole. *Arch. Exp. Path. Pharm.* 162: 46-55, 1931.

607.   Warren, M.R. and H.W. Werner. The central stimulant action of some vasopressor amines. *J. Pharmacol. Exp. Ther.* 85: 119-121, 1945.

608.   Chessin, M., *et al.* Biochemical and pharmacological studies of ß-phenylhydrazine and selected related compounds. *Ann. N.Y. Acad. Sci.* 80: 597-608, 1959.

609.   Way, E.L. Barbiturate antagonism of isonipecaine convulsions and isonipecaine potentiation of barbiturate depression. *J. Pharmacol. Exp. Ther.* 87: 265-272, 1946.

610.   Gruhzit, O.M. Sodium diphenyl hydantoinate: Pharmacologic and histopathologic studies. *Arch. Path.* 28: 761-762, 1939.

611.   Knoefel, P.K. and G. Lehmann. The anticonvulsive action of diphenyl hydantoin and some related compounds. *J. Pharmacol. Exp. Ther.* 72: 194-201, 1942.

612.   Everett, G.M. and R.K. Richards. Comparative anti-convulsive action of 3,5,5-trimethyloxazolidine-2, 4-dione (Tridione), Dilantin and phenobarbital. *J. Pharmacol. Exp. Ther.* 81: 402-407, 1944.

613.   Esplin, D.W. and J.W. Freston. Physiological and pharmacological analysis of spinal cord convulsions. *J. Pharmacol. Exp. Ther.* 130: 68-80, 1960.

614.   Heubner, W. Pharmacological and chemical investigation of physostigmine. *Arch. Exp. Path. Pharmakol.* 53: 313-330, 1905.

615.   Zetler, G., *et al.* Research toward a pharmacological differentiation of cataleptic effects. *Arch. Exp. Path. Pharmakol.* 238: 468-501, 1960.

616.   Hjort, A.M. and E.J. deBeer. The effect of the diet upon the anesthetic qualities of some hypnotics. *J. Pharmacol. Exp. Ther.* 65: 79-88, 1939.

Bibliography

617. Swanson, E.E. and K.K. Chen. The pharmacological action of coriamyrtin. *J. Pharmacol. Exp. Ther.* 57: 410-418, 1936.

618. Apter, J.T. Analeptic action of lysergic acid diethylamide (LSD-25) against pentobarbital. *Arch. Neurol. Psychiat. (Chic.)* 79: 711-715, 1958.

619. Holck, H.G.O. and P.R. Cannon. On the cause of the delayed death in the rat by isopropyl betabromallyl barbituric acid (Nostal) and some related barbiturates. *J. Pharmacol. Exp. Ther.* 57: 289-309, 1936.

620. Zablocka, B. and D.W. Esplin. Central excitatory and depressant effect of pilocarpine in rats and mice. *J. Pharmacol. Exp. Ther.* 140: 162-169, 1963.

621. Singh, S.D. and H.J. Eysenck. Conditioned emotional response in the rat. III. Drug antagonism. *J. Gen. Psychol.* 63: 275-285, 1960.

622. Stone, G.C. Effects of some centrally acting drugs upon learning of escape and avoidance habits. *J. Comp. Physiol. Psychol.* 53: 33-37, 1960.

623. Larson, R.E. and G.L. Plaa. Effect of spinal cord transection on CCl_4 hepatotoxicity. *Fed. Proc.* 22: 189, 1963.

624. Gettler, A.O. and J. Baine. The toxicology of cyanide. *Amer. J. Med. Sci.* 195: 182-188, 1938.

625. Lindgren, P. and A. Sundwall. Parasympatholytic effects of TMB-4 (1, 1-trimethylenebis (4-formylpyridinium bromide)-dioxime) and some related oximes in the cat. *Acta Pharmacol. (Kbh.)* 17: 69-83, 1960.

626. Santi, R., *et al*. Pharmacological action of N, N-Diisorpropylammonium dichloroacetate (DIEDI). *Minerva Med.* 51, Suppl. 71: 2909-2919, 1960.

627. McKinney, S.E., *et al*. Benemid, p-(D1-n-propylsulamyl)-Benzoic acid: toxicologic properties. *J. Pharmacol. Exp. Ther.* 102: 208-214, 1951.

628. Seiffer, J., *et al*. The toxicity of N, N'-Dibenzylethylenediamine (DBED) and DBED dipinecillin. *Antibiot. et Chemother. (Basel)* 1: 504-508, 1951.

629. Naranjo, P. and E.B. de Naranjo. Local anesthetic activity of some antihistamines and its relationship with the antihistaminic and anticholinergic activities. *Arch. Int. Pharmacodyn.* 113: 313-335, 1958.

630. Richards, R.K. and K.E. Kueter. Competitive inhibition of procaine convulsions in guinea pigs. *J. Pharmacol. Exp. Ther.* 87: 42-52, 1946.

631. Schneider, J.A. and F.F. Yonkman. Species differences in the respiratory and cardiovascular response to serotonin (5-hydroxytryptamine). *J. Pharmacol. Exp. Ther.* 111: 84-98, 1954.

Bibliography

632. Ilyuchenok, R.Y. Comparative study of the influence of chlorpromazine and propazine of the bioelectric activity of the cerebrum. *Zh. Nevopat. Psikhiat.* 60: 202-209, 1960.

633. Ekstron, N. and F. Sandberg. A method for quantitative determination of the inhibitory action on C.A.R. of mice. *Arzneimittel-Forsch.* 12: 1208-1209, 1962.

634. Schneider, J.A. Further characterization of central effects of reserpine (Serpasil). *Am. J. Physiol.* 181: 64-68, 1955.

635. Innes, I.R. Sensitization of the heart and nictitating membrane of the cat to sympathomimetic amines by antihistamine drugs. *Brit. J. Pharmacol.* 13: 6-10, 1958.

636. Black, J.W. and J.S. Stephenson. Pharmacology of a new adrenergic beta-receptor blocking compound (nethalide). *Lancet* 2: 311-314, 18 Aug., 1962.

637. Goldberg, M.E. and G.V. Rossi. The effect of anticholinergic compounds on several components of gastric secretion in pylorus-ligated rats. *J. Amer. Pharm. Ass.* 49: 543-547, 1960.

638. Abbott, C.E.B., *et al.* Effect of propantheline bromide (Pro-Banthine) on fluid and electrolyte loss in dogs with pyloric obstruction. *Canad. Med. Ass. J.* 76: 176-180, 1957.

639. Krayer, O., *et al.* Studies on veratrum alkaloids. VI. Protoveratrine: its comparative toxicity and its circulatory action. *J. Pharmacol. Exp. Ther.* 82: 167-186, 1944.

640. Swiss, E.D. and R.O. Bauer. Acute toxicity of veratrum derivatives. *Proc. Soc. Exp. Biol. (N.Y.)* 76: 847-849, 1951.

641. Haas, H.T.A. Pharmacology of germerine and its degradation products. I. *Arch. Exp. Path. Pharmakol.* 189: 397-410, 1938.

642. Martini, L. and L. Calliauw. On the pharmacology of protoveratrine in dogs. *Arch. Int. Pharmacodyn.* 101: 49-67, 1955.

643. Mosey, L. and A. Kaplan. Respiratory effects of potent hypotensive derivatives of veratrum. *J. Pharmacol. Exp. Ther.* 104: 67-75, 1952.

644. Woolley, D.W. and N.K. Campbell. Serotonin-like and antiserotonin properties of psilocybin and psilocin. *Science* 136: 777-778, 1962.

645. Maxwell, G.M., *et al.* The effect of psilocybin upon the systemic, pulmonary and coronary circulation of the intact dog. *Arch. Int. Pharmacodyn.* 137: 108-115, 1962.

646. Castillo, J.C., *et al.* A pharmacological study of *N*-methyl-N'-(4-chlorobenzhydryl) piperazine dihydrochloride--a new antihistamine. *J. Pharmacol. Exp. Ther.* 96: 388-395, 1949.

Bibliography

647. Halpern, B.N. and M. Briot. Comparison of the acute toxicity of several synthetic antihistaminics in the rat. *C.R. Soc. Biol (Paris)* 144: 887-890, 1950.

648. Swift, J.G. A study of sustained ionic release antihistamine. *Arch. Int. Pharmacodyn.* 124: 341-348, 1960.

649. Virno, M., *et al*. Action of histamine on the jugular venous pressure and cerebral circulation of the dog. Effects of antihistaminic drugs (pyrilamine and chlorpheniramine) and a histamine liberating agent (48/80 B.W). *J. Pharmacol. Exp. Ther.* 118: 63-76, 1956.

650. Binet, D. The study of polyuria in convalescence from acute sickness. *Rev. Med. Suisse Rom.* 15: 329-341, 1885.

651. Gibbs, W. and H.A. Hare. Systematic investigation of related chemicals on animal organisms. *Arch. F. Physiol. (Leipz.)* 1: 344-359, 1890.

652. Gatgounis, J. and R.P. Walton. Resorcinol isomers and pentylenetetrazol; their centrally mediated sympathetic circulatory effects. *J. Pharmacol. Exp. Ther.* 127: 363-371, 1959.

653. Yoshi, N., *et al*. Studies on the unit discharge of brainstem reticular formation in the cat. II. Effect of catechol, amphetamine, Nembutal and Megimide. *Med. J. Osaka Univ.* 11: 19-33, 1960.

654. Neisser A. Clinical and experimental findings on the action of pyrogallus acid. *Z. Klin. Med.* 1: 88-108, 1880.

655. Wylie, D.W. Augmentation of the processor response to guanethedine by inhibition of catechol-o-methyltransferase. *Nature* 189: 490-491, 1961.

656. Udenfriend, S., *et al*. Inhibitors of norepinephrine metabolism *in vivo*. *Arch. Biochem.* 84: 249-251, 1959.

657. Bonsmann, M.R. The pharmacology of the quinine alkaloids. *Arch. Exp. Path. Pharmakol.* 205: 129-136, 1948.

658. Kirchmann, L.L. Detoxification of quinidine by synephrine. *Arch. Exp. Path. Pharmakol.* 192: 639-644, 1939.

659. Scott, C.C., *et al*. Comparison of the pharmacologic action of quinidine and dihydroquinidine. *J. Pharmacol. Exp. Ther.* 84: 184-188, 1945.

660. Cole, J. and D. Dearnaley. Contrasting tail and other responses to morphine and reserpine in rats and mice. *Experientia (Basel)* 16: 78-80, 1960.

661. Brodie, B.B. and P.A. Shore. A concept for a role of serotonin and norepinephrine as chemical mediators in the brain. *Ann. N.Y. Acad. Sci.* 66: 631-642, 1957.

Bibliography

662. Burn, J.H. and D.B. McDougal, Jr. The effect of reserpine on gangrene produced by thiopental in the mouse tail. *J. Pharmacol. Exp. Ther.* 131: 167-170, 1961.

663. Paasonen, M.K. and O. Krayer. Effect of reserpine upon the mammalian heart. *Fed. Proc.* 16: 326-327, 1957.

664. Canal, N. and A. Maffei-Faccioli. Reversal of the reserpine-induced depletion of brain serotonin by a monoamine oxidase inhibitor. *J. Neurochem.* 5: 99-100, 1959.

665. Muscholl, E. and M. Vogt. The action of reserpine on the peripheral sympathetic system. *J. Physiol. (Lond.)* 141: 132-155, 1958.

666. Sheppard, H. and J.H. Zimmerman. Reserpine and the levels of serotonin and norepinephrine in the brain. *Nature* 185: 40-41, 1960.

667. Shore, P.A., *et al.* Release of brain norepinephrine by reserpine. *Fed. Proc.* 16: 335-336, 1957.

668. Wilson, C.W.M., *et al.* The effects of reserpine on uptake of epinephrine in brain and certain areas outside the blood-brain barrier. *J. Pharmacol. Exp. Ther.* 135: 11-16, 1961.

669. Trendelenburg, U. and J.S. Gravenstein. Effect of reserpine pretreatment on stimulation of the accelerans nerve of the dog. *Science* 128: 901-902, 1958.

670. Brady, J.V. Animal experimental evaluation of drug effects upon behavior. *Fed. Proc.* 17: 1031-1043, 1958.

671. Weiskrantz, L. and W.A. Wilson, Jr. The effects of reserpine on emotional behavior of normal and brain-operated monkeys. *Ann. N.Y. Acad. Sci.* 61: 36-55, 1955.

672. Tui, C. and C. Debruille. The comparative toxicity and effectiveness of scopolamine hydrobromide ($C_{17}H_{21}O_4N \cdot HBr$) and scopolamine aminoxide hydrobromide ($C_{17}H_{21}O_5N \cdot HBr$). *Am. J. Pharm.* 117: 319-326, 1945.

673. Frommel, E., *et al.* On the pharmacodynamic action of a new tranquilizer: methaminodiazepoxide, or Librium. An experimental study. *Therapie* 15: 1233-1244, 1960.

674. Gruhzit, O.M. and A.W. Dox. A pharmacologic study of certain thiobarbiturates. *J. Pharmacol. Exp. Ther.* 60: 125-142, 1937.

675. Silvestrini, B., *et al.* Action of synchronizing and desynchronizing drugs on strychnine induced convulsive cortical activity. *Fed. Proc.* 16: 336, 1957.

676. Costa, E. and G. Zetler. Interactions between epinephrine and psychotomimetic drugs on cat nictitating membrane. *Fed. Proc.* 17: 360, 1958.

677. Winter D. and M. Timar. Experimental studies on the rehypnosis of animals just awakened from barbiturate anesthesia. *Pharmazie* 17: 454-455, 1962.

Bibliography

678. Revzin, A.M. and E. Costa. Effects of exogenous serotonin on paleocortical excitability. *Am. J. Physiol.* 198: 959-961, 1960.

679. Zilberstein, R. Effects of reserpine, serotonin and vasopressin on the survival of cold-stressed rats. *Nature* 185: 249, 1960.

680. Soulairac, A. and M.L. Soulairac. Action of reserpine, serotonin and iproniazid on the feeding behavior of the rat. *C.R. Soc. Biol. (Paris)* 154: 510-513, 1960.

681. Laroche, M.J. and B.B. Brodie. Lack of relationship between inhibition of monoamine oxidase and potentiation of hexobarbital hypnosis. *J. Pharmacol. Exp. Ther.* 130: 134-137, 1960.

682. Smith, P.K. and W.E. Hambourger. Antipyretic and toxic effects of combinations of acetanilid with sodium bromide and with caffein. *J. Pharmacol. Exp. Ther.* 55: 200-205, 1935.

683. Roholm, K. Fluorine and fluorine compounds. *Heffter's Hdb. E.* 7: 1-62, 1938.

684. Muehlberger, C.W. Toxicity studies of fluorine insecticides. *J. Pharmacol. Exp. Ther.* 39: 246-248, 1930.

685. Lehman, A.J. Chemicals in food: A report to the association of food and drug officials on current developments. *Assoc. Food & Drug Officials U.S. Quart. Bull.* 15: 122-133, 1951.

686. Ambard, L. and M.S. Trautmann. Demonstration of the existence of different invertases. *C.R. Soc. Biol. (Paris)* 125: 133-135, 1937.

687. Leake, C.D. The toxicity of sodium fluoride in intravenous injection in rabbits. *J. Pharmacol. Exp. Ther.* 33: 279-280, 1928.

688. Becker, T., *et al.* A theory of chlorate poisoning. *Arch. Exp. Path. Pharmakol.* 201: 197-209, 1943.

689. Oltman, T.V. and L.A. Crandal, Jr. The acute toxicity of glyceryl trinitrate and sodium nitrite in rabbits. *J. Pharmacol. Exp. Ther.* 41: 121-126, 1931.

690. Hesse, E. Detoxification of nitrites. *Arch. Exp. Path. Pharmakol.* 126: 209-221, 1927.

691. Dossin, F. Contribution to the experimental study of hypotensive medication. *Arch. Int. Pharmacodyn.* 21: 425-465, 1911.

692. Zipf, H.F. and G. Triller. α-Isosparteine and α-Didehydrosparteine. *Arch. Exp. Path. Pharmakol.* 200: 536-550, 1943.

693. Lu, G. Sparteine on mammalian circulations. *Arch. Int. Pharmacodyn.* 89: 209-222, 1963.

Bibliography

694. Lu, G. Dual vasomotor actions of sparteine. *Arch. Int. Pharmacodyn.* 89: 129-144, 1952.

695. Amann, A., *et al.* A comparative study of strychnine and strychnine derivatives. *Arch. Exp. Path. Pharmakol.* 201: 161-171, 1943.

696. Ward, J.C. and D.G. Crabtree. Strychnine X. Comparative accuracies of stomach tube and intraperitoneal injection methods of bioassay. *J. Amer. Pharm. Ass., Sci. Ed.* 31: 113-115, 1942.

697. Poe, C.F., *et al.* Toxicity of strychnine for male and female rats of different ages. *J. Pharmacol. Exp. Ther.* 58: 239-242, 1936.

698. Leroy, J.G. and A.F. de Schaepdryver. Catecholamine levels of brain and heart in mice after iproniazid, syrosingopine and 10-methoxydeserpidine. *Arch. Int. Pharmacodyn.* 130: 231-234, 1961.

699. Garattini, S., *et al.* Reserpine derivatives with specific hypotensive or sedative activity. *Nature (Lond.)* 183: 1273-1274, 1959.

700. Orlans, F.G.H., *et al.* Pharmacological consequences of the selective release of peripheral norepinephrine by syrosingopine (SU 3119). *J. Pharmacol. Exp. Ther.* 128: 131-139, 1960.

701. Cook, L. and E. Weidley. Effects of a series of psychopharmacological agents on isolated induced attack behavior in mice. *Fed. Proc.* 19: 22, 1960.

702. Heise, G.A. Behavioral analysis of tetrabenazine in animals. *Dis. Nerv. Syst. (Suppl.)* 21: 111-114, 1960.

703. Pletscher, A. Release of 5-hydroxytryptamine by benzoquinolizine derivatives with sedative action. *Science* 126: 507, 1957.

704. Astrom, A. and N.H. Persson. The toxicity of some local anesthetics after application on different mucous membranes and its relation to anesthetic action on the nasal mucosa of the rabbit. *J. Pharmacol. Exp. Ther.* 132: 87-90, 1961.

705. Eichholtz, F. and G. Hoppe. The convulsive action of local anesthetics and the effect of mineral salts and adrenaline. *Arch. Exp. Path. Pharmakol.* 173: 687-696, 1933.

706. Randall, L.O., *et al.* The ganglionic blocking action of thiophanium derivatives. *J. Pharmacol. Exp. Ther.* 97: 48-59, 1949.

707. Hunt, R. and R.R. Renshaw. On some effects of arsonium, stibonium, phosphonium and sulfonium compounds on the autonomic nervous system. *J. Pharmacol. Exp. Ther.* 25: 315-355, 1925.

708. Acheson, G.H. and G.K. Moe. The action of tetraethylammonium ion on the mammalian circulation. *J. Pharmacol. Exp. Ther.* 87: 220-236, 1946.

Bibliography

709. Acheson, G.H. and G.K. Moe. Some effects of tetraethylammonium on the mammalian heart. *J. Pharmacol. Exp. Ther.* 84: 189-195, 1945.

710. Jodlbauer, A. The action of tetramethylammonium chloride. *Arch. Int. Pharmacodyn.* 7: 183-202, 1900.

711. Kuhn, W.L. and E.F. Van Maanen. Effects of thalidomide on central nervous system drugs. *Fed. Proc.* 19: 264, 1960.

712. Martindale, K., *et al.* The effect of thalidomide in experimental gastric ulcers. *J. Pharm. and Pharmacol.* 12: 153T-158T, 1960.

713. Robinson, M.H. The effect of different intravenous injection rates upon the AD_{50}, LD_{50} and anesthetic duration of pentothal in mice, and strength-duration curves of depression. *J. Pharmacol. Exp. Ther.* 85: 176-191, 1945.

714. Carmichael, E.B. The median lethal dose (LD_{50}) of pentothal sodium for both young and old guinea pigs and rats. *Anesthesiology* 8: 589-593, 1947.

715. Hart, R. The toxicity and analgetic potency of salicylamide and certain of its derivatives as compared with established analgetic-antipyretic drugs. *J. Pharmacol. Exp. Ther.* 89: 205-209, 1947.

716. Irwin, R.L., *et al.* The activity of certain lycoramine derivatives on muscle. *J. Pharmacol. Exp. Ther.* 134: 53-59, 1961.

717. Somjen, G.G. and M. Gill. The mechanism of the blockade of synaptic transmission in the mammalian spinal cord by diethyl ether and by thiopental. *J. Pharmacol. Exp. Ther.* 140: 19-30, 1963.

718. Hey, P. and G.L. Willey. Choline 2: 6-xylyl ether bromide; an active quaternary local anesthetic. *Brit. J. Pharmacol.* 9: 471-475, 1954.

719. Nasmyth, P.A. and W.H.H. Andrews. The antagonism of cocaine to the action of choline 2,6-xylyl ether bromide at sympathetic nerve endings. *Brit. J. Pharmacol.* 14: 477-483, 1959.

720. McLean, R.A., *et al.* A series of 2,6-di-substituted phenoxylethyl ammonium bromides with true sympathomimetic properties. *J. Pharmacol. Exp. Ther.* 129: 11-16, 1960.

721. Coupland, R.E. and K.A. Exley. Effects of choline 2:6 xylyl ether bromide upon the suprarenal medulla of the rat. *Brit. J. Pharmacol.* 12: 306-311, 1957.

722. McLean, R.A., *et al.* Pharmacology of trimethyl (2-(2,6-dimethylphenoxy) propyl)-trimethylammonium chloride, monohydrate; compound 6890 or ß-TM10. *J. Pharmacol. Exp. Ther.* 129: 17-23, 1960.

723. Everett, G.M., *et al.* Tremor induced by tremorine and its antagonism by anti-Parkinson drugs. *Science* 124: 79, 1956.

Bibliography

724.   Everett, G.M., *et al.* Production of tremor and a Parkinson-like syndrome by 1-4 dipyrrolidino-2-butyne, "tremorine." *Fed. Proc.* 15: 420-421, 1956.

725.   Kaelber, W.W. and R.E. Correll. Cortical and subcortical electrical effects of psychopharmacologic and tremor-producing compounds. *Arch. Neurol. Psychiat. (Chic.)* 80: 544-553, 1958.

726.   Korol, B. and L. Soffer. Cardiovascular activity of *D*- and *L*-octopamine. *Pharmacologist* 5: 247, 1963.

727.   Barlow, O.W. Reactions of the rat to avertin crystals, avertin fluid and amylene hydrate. *Arch. Surg.* 26: 689-695, 1933.

728.   Burtner, R.R. and G. Lehmann. The hypnotic properties of some derivatives of trihalogenated alcohols. *J. Pharmacol. Exp. Ther.* 63: 183-192, 1938.

729.   Barnes, T.C. Relationship of chemical structure to central nervous system effects of tranquilizing and anticonvulsant drugs. *J. Amer. Pharm. Ass., Sci. Ed.* 49: 415-417, 1960.

730.   Tedeschi, D.H., *et al.* The neuropharmacology of trifluoperazine: a potent psychotherapeutic agent. *Arch. Int. Pharmacodyn.* 122: 129-143, 1957.

731.   Richards, R.K. and G.M. Everett. Tridione: a new anticonvulsant drug. *J. Lab. Clin. Med.* 31: 1330-1336, 1946.

732.   Hoppe, J.O. and A.M. Lands. The toxicologic properties of N,N-dimethyl-N'(3-thenyl-N' (2-pyridyl) ethylenediamine hydrochloride (Thenfadil): A new antihistamine drug. *J. Pharmacol. Exp. Ther.* 97: 371-378, 1949.

733.   Macri, F.V. Curare-like activity of some bis-fluorenyl-bis-quaternary ammonium compounds. *Proc. Soc. Exp. Biol. (N.Y.)* 85: 603-606, 1954.

734.   Berger, F.M. and R.P. Schwartz. The toxicity and muscular effect of d-tubocurarine combined with ß-erythroidine, myanesin or Evipal. *J. Pharmacol. Exp. Ther.* 93: 362-367, 1948.

735.   Marsh, D.F. and M.H. Pelletier. Curariform activity of quaternary ammonium iodides derived from cinchona alkaloids. *J. Pharmacol. Exp. Ther.* 92: 127-130, 1948.

736.   Everett, G.M. Pharmacological studies of d-tubocurarine and other curare fractions. *J. Pharmacol. Exp. Ther.* 92: 236-248, 1948.

737.   Barbour, H.G. and L.L. Maurer. Tyramine as a morphine antagonist. *J. Pharmacol. Exp. Ther.* 15: 305-330, 1920.

738.   Kuntzman, R. and M. Jacobson. Depletion of heart norepinephrine by tyramine. *Pharmacologist.* 5: 258, 1963.

739.   Nasmyth, P.A. In: *Ciba Foundation Symposium*, eds. Vane, J.R., *et al.* Little Brown, Boston, p. 337, 1960.

740.   Egami, M. A pharmacological study of afferent impulse from the small intestine. *Jap. J. Pharmacol.* 4: 160-167, 1955.

741.   Barer, G.R. and E. Nusser. Cardiac output during excitation of chemo-reflexes in the cat. *Brit. J. Pharmacol.* 13: 372-377, 1958.

742.   Benforado, J.M., *et al.* Studies on veratrum alkaloids. XXIX. The action of some germine esters and of veratridine upon blood pressure, heart rate and femoral blood flow in the dog. *J. Pharmacol. Exp. Ther.* 130: 311-320, 1960.

743.   Hagen, E.C. and J.L. Radomski. The toxicity of 3-(acetonylbenzyl)-4-hydroxycoumarin (warfarin) to laboratory animals. *J. Am. Pharm. Ass.* 42: 379-382, 1953.

744.   Preziosi, P., *et al.* On the pulmonary and cardiovascular effects of warfarin sodium. *Arch. Int. Pharmacodyn.* 123: 227-238, 1959.

745.   Röthlin, E. and R. Hamet. On the toxicity and adrenolytic activity of pseudocorynanthine compared with that of corynanthine and yohimbine. *Arch. Int. Pharmacodyn.* 50: 241-250, 1935.

746.   Barrett, E., *et al.* A comparison of the activity of various adrenolytic agents in antagonizing the epinephrine potentiation induced by ganglionic blockage. *J. Pharmacol. Exp. Ther.* 110: 3-4, 1954.

747.   McCubbin, J.W. and I. Page. Do ganglionic blocking agents and reserpine affect central vasomotor activity? *Circ. Res.* 6: 816-824, 1958.

748.   Nasmyth, P.A. An investigation of the action of tyramine and its interrelationship with the effects of other sympathomimetic amines. *Brit. J. Pharmacol.* 18: 65-75, 1962.

749.   György, L. and M. Doda. Adrenaline tachyphylaxis after dibenamine. *Arch. Int. Pharmacodyn.* 124: 66-75, 1960.

750.   Riker, W.K. and A. Komalahiranya. Observations on the frequency dependence of sympathetic ganglionic blockade. *J. Pharmacol. Exp. Ther.* 137: 267-274, 1962.

751.   Melville, K.I. Studies on the cardiovascular actions of chlorpromazine. I. Antiadrenergic and antifibrillatory actions. *Arch. Int. Pharmacodyn.* 115: 278-305, 1958.

752.   Ross, J., Jr., *et al.* The influence of intracardiac baroreceptors on venous return, systemic vascular volume and peripheral resistance. *J. Clin. Inves.* 40: 563-572, 1961.

753.   Byck, R. The effect of C_6 on the carotid chemoreceptor response to nicotine and cyanide. *Brit. J. Pharmacol.* 16: 15-22, 1961.

Bibliography

754. Lamond, D.R. and C.W. Emmens. The effect of hypophysectomy on the mouse uterine response to gonadotrophins. *J. Endocrin.* 18: 251-261, 1959.

755. Boccabella, A.V. Reinitiation and restoration of spermatogenesis with testosterone propionate and other hormones after a longterm post-hypophysectomy regression period. *Endocrinology* 72: 787-798, 1963.

756. Smith, B.D. and J.T. Bradburg. Ovarian weight response to varying doses of estrogens in intact and hypophysectomized rats. *Proc. Sec. Exp. Biol. (N.Y.)* 107: 946-949, 1961.

757. Fain, J.N. and A.E. Wilhelmi. Effects of adrenalectomy, hypophysectomy, growth hormone and thyroxine on fatty acid synthesis *in vivo*. *Endocrinology* 71: 541-548, 1962.

758. Nejad, N.S., *et al.* Hormonal repair of defective lipogenesis from glucose in the liver of the hypophysectomized rat. *Endocrinology* 71: 107-112, 1962.

759. Meineke, H.A. and R.C. Crafts. Correlation between oxygen consumption and erythropoiesis in hypophysectomized rats treated with various doses of thyroxine. *Proc. Soc. Exp. Biol. (N.Y.)* 102: 121-124, 1959.

760. Evans, E.S., *et al.* Erythropoietic response to calorigenic hormones. *Endocrinology* 68: 517-532, 1961.

761. Baker, B.L. Elevation of proteolytic activity in the pancreas of hypophysectomized rats by hormonal therapy. *Proc. Soc. Biol. (N.Y.)* 108: 238-242, 1961.

762. De Bodo, R.C. and M.W. Sinkoff. The role of growth hormone in carbohydrate metabolism. *Ann. N.Y. Acad. Sci.* 57: 23-60, 1953.

763. Wick, A.N., *et al.* Effect of 11-desoxycorticosterone acetate upon carbohydrate utilization by the depancreatized rat. *Proc. Soc. Exp. Biol. (N.Y.)* 71: 445-446, 1949.

764. Scow, R.O., *et al.* Effect of hypophysectomy on the insulin requirement and response to fasting of "totally" pancreatectomized rats. *Endocrinology* 61: 380-391, 1957.

765. Allegretti, N. Gamma-globulin concentration in normal and depancreatized rats subjected to formalin stress. *Arch. Int. Pharmacodyn.* 93: 367-372, 1953.

766. Ingle, D.J., *et al.* Comparison of the effect of 11-ketoprogesterone, 11α-hydroxyprogesterone and 11ß-hydroxyprogesterone upon the glycosuria of the partially depancreatized rat. *Endocrinology* 53: 221-225, 1953.

767. Ingle, D.J. Effect of 11-desoxycorticosterone acetate on the glycosuria of partially depancreatized rats. *Proc. Soc. Exp. Biol. (N.Y.)* 69: 329-330, 1948.

768. Greeley, P.O. The action of insulin as indicated by depancreatized herbivora. *Am. J. Physiol.* 150: 46-51, 1947.

Bibliography

769. Gastaldi, F. Glycemic changes caused by testosterone propionate in normal and pancreatectomized dogs. *Studi Sassaresi* 25: 601-606, 1947.

770. Gillman, J. The relationship of hyperglycemia to hyperlipemia and ketonaemia in depancreatized baboons *(Papio ursinus)*. *J. Endocrin.* 17: 349-362, 1958.

771. Glasser, S.R. and J.L. Izzo. The influence of adrenalectomy on the metabolic actions of glucagon in the fasting rat. *Endocrinology* 70: 54-61, 1962.

772. Gross, F. and P. Lichtlen. Experimental renal hypertension: renal content of kidneys in intact and adrenalectomzied rats given cortexone. *Am. J. Physiol.* 195: 543-548, 1958.

773. Smith, S., *et al.* Some metabolic effects of diethylstilbestrol and deoxycorticosterone acetate in adrenalectomized and intact male rats. *Proc. West. Va. Acad. Sci.* 32: 22-25, 1960.

774. Pores, G. Effects of aldosterone on carbohydrate metabolism of normal and adrenalectomized rats. *C.R. Soc. Biol. (Paris)* 155: 790-792, 1961.

775. Hungerford, G.F. Effect of adrenalectomy and hydrocortisone on lymph glucose in rats. *Proc. Soc. Exp. Biol. (N.Y.)* 100: 754-756, 1959.

776. Pederson-Bjergaard, K. and M. Tonnesen. The effects of steroid hormones on muscular activity in rats. *Acta Endocrinol.* 17: 329-337, 1954.

777. Aterman, K. Cortisol and spermiogenesis. *Acta Endocrinol.* 22: 371-378, 1956.

778. Fain, J.N. Effects of dexamethasone and growth hormone on fatty acid mobilization and glucose utilization in adrenalectomized rats. *Endocrinology* 71: 633-635, 1962.

779. Peres, G. and G. Zwingelstein. Action of aldosterone on the blood proteins of the normal and adrenalectomized rat. *J. Physiol. (Paris)* 53: 444-446, 1961.

780. Peters, G. Distribution of water and electrolytes in the organism in normal and adrenalectomzied, untreated rats or such rats treated with adrenocortical hormone, and the influence of large oral water loads. *Arch. Exp. Pathol. Pharmakol.* 237: 119-150, 1959.

781. Winter, H., *et al.* Antibody formation in the adrenalectomized rat and the effect of cortisone. *Inter. Arch. Allergy Appl. Immunol.* 19: 360-376, 1961.

782. Kahlson, G. and S. Renvall. Atrophy of salivary gland following adrenalectomy or hypophysectomy and the effect of deoxycorticosterone in cats. *Acta Physiol. Scand.* 37: 150-158, 1956.

783. Sesso, A. and R. Migliorini. Nucleic acid content and amylase activity in the pancreas of the rat following adrenalectomy and cortisone administration. *Acta Physiol. Lat. Amer.* 9: 5-12, 1959.

Bibliography

784. Gross, F. and H. Haefeli. The activity of deoxycorticosterone, cortisone, and antihistamine substances on the anaphylactic shock of adrenalectomized guinea pigs. *Intern. Arch. Allergy Appl. Immunol.* 3: 44-53, 1952.

785. Berlin, R.D., *et al.* Abrupt changes of water and sodium excretion in normal and adrenalectomized dogs. *Am. J. Physiol.* 199: 275-280, 1960.

786. Daane, T.A. and W.R. Lyons. Effect of estrone, progesterone, and pituitary mammotropin on the mammary glands of castrated C$_3$H male mice. *Endocrinology* 55: 191-199, 1954.

787. Kitay, J.T. Pituitary-adrenal function in the rat after gonadectomy and gonadal hormone replacement. *Endocrinology* 73: 253-260, 1963.

788. Meli, A. Route of administration as a factor influencing the biological activity of certain androgens and their corresponding 3-cyclopentyl enol ethers. *Endocrinology* 72: 715-719, 1963.

789. Rudolph, G.G. and W.R. Starnes. Effect of castration and testosterone administration on seminal vesicles and prostates of rats. *A. J. Physiol.* 179: 415-418, 1954.

790. Mandel, P., *et al.* Effect of testosterone on the calcium balance in the rat. *C.R. Acad. Sci. (Paris)* 148: 713-715, 1954.

791. Kanai, T. Effect of androgen on fine structure of the prostate of castrated rats. II. The effect of administration of small doses of testosterone 3 days after castration. *Tohoku J. Exptl. Med.* 75: 309-318, 1961.

792. Levey, H.A. and C.M. Szego. Effects of castration and androgen administration on metabolic characteristics of the guinea pig seminal vesicle. *Am. J. Physiol.* 183: 371-376, 1955.

793. Dagradi, A. and G. Peronato. Influence of the gonads on carbohydrate metabolism. *Patol. Sper. Chir.* 1: 420-429, 1953.

794. Grunt, J.A. Exogenous androgen and nondirected hyperexcitability in castrated male guinea pigs. *Proc. Soc. Exp. Biol. (N.Y.)* 85: 540-542, 1954.

795. Munford, R.E. The effect of cortisol acetate on estrone-induced mammary gland growth in immature ovariectomized albino mice. *J. Endocrin.* 16: 72-79, 1957.

796. Grosvenor, C.E. Effects of estrogen upon thyroidal I[131] release and excretion of thyroxine in ovariectomized rats. *Endocrinology* 70: 673-678, 1962.

797. Lerner, J., *et al.* Pregnancy maintenance in ovariectomized rats with 16α, 17α Di-hydroxyprogesterone derivatives and other progestogens. *Endocrinology* 70: 283-287, 1962.

Bibliography

798.   Woolley, D.E. and P.S. Timiras.   The gonad-brain relationship: Effects of female sex hormones on electroshock convulsions in the rat. *Endocrinology* 72: 196-209, 1963.

799.   Escobar del Rey, R. and G. Morreale de Escobar.   Studies on the peripheral disappearance of thyroid hormone. *Acta Endocrin.* 29: 161-175, 1958.

800.   Barker, S.B., *et al.* Metabolic effects of thyroxine injected into normal, thiouracil-treated, and thyroidectomized rats. *Endocrinology* 45: 624-627, 1949.

801.   Halmi, N.S., *et al.* Improved intravenous glucose tolerance in thyroidectomized or hypophysectomized rats treated with triiodothyronine. *Endocrinology* 64: 618-621, 1959.

802.   De Bastiani, G., *et al.* Significance of the thyrotropic hormone of the hypophysis in the syndrome resulting from thyroidectomy. *Boll. Soc. Ital. Biol. Sper.* 32: 200-204, 1956.

803.   Von Berswordt-Wallrabe, R. and C.W. Turner.   Successful replacement theraphy in lactating thyro-parathyroidectomized rats. *Proc. Soc. Exp. Biol. (N.Y.)* 104: 113-116, 1960.

804.   Harrison, R.G. and T.J. Barnett.   Production of arthritis in thyroparathyroidectomized rat by injection of deoxycorticosterone acetate. *Ann. Rheum. Dis.* 12: 275-282, 1953.

805.   Cramer, C.F.   Participation of parathyroid glands in control of calcium absorption in dogs. *Endocrinology* 72: 192-196, 1963.

806.   Gordon, A.H.   The parathyroid hormone. *Congr. Intern. Biochim., Resumes Commmuns, 2e Congr. Paris.* pp. 53-54, 1952.

807.   Talmage, R.V., *et al.* Effect of parathyroid extract and phosphate salts on renal calcium and phosphate excretion after parathyroidectomy. *Proc. Soc. Exp. Biol. (N.Y.)* 88: 600-604, 1955.

808.   Laron, Z., *et al.* Phosphaturic effect of cortisone in normal and parathyroidectomized rats. *Proc. Soc. Exp. Biol. (N.Y.)* 96: 649-651, 1957.

809.   Page, I.H. and J.W. McCubbin.   Effect of pentobarbital and atropine on arterial pressure response to ganglion blocking agents. *Am. J. Physiol.* 194: 597-600, 1958.

810.   Costa, E., *et al.* Interactions between reserpine, chlorpromazine, and imipramine. *Experientia* (Basel) 16: 461-463, 1960.

811.   Crout, J.R.   Inhibition of catechol-o-methyl transferase by pyrogallol in the rat. *Biochem. Pharmacol.* 6: 47-50, 1961.

812.   Finkleman, B.   On the nature of inhibition in the intestines. *J. Physiol. (Lond.)* 70: 145-157, 1930.

Bibliography

813.   Chorover, S.L.   Effects of mescaline and chlorpromazine on two aspects of locomotor activity in rats. *Fed. Proc.* 19: 22, 1960.

814.   Freyburger, W.A., *et al.*   The pharmacology of 5-hydroxytryptamine (serotonin). *J. Pharmacol. Exp. Ther.* 105: 80-86, 1952.

815.   Gutman, J. and M. Chaimovitz.   The effect of anesthetics on blood pressure response to pain. *Arch. Int. Pharmacodyn.* 137: 40-48, 1962.

816.   Millar, R.A., *et al.*   Plasma adrenaline and noradrenaline after phenoxybenzamine administration and during haemorrhagic hypotension, in normal and adrenalectomized dogs. *Brit. J. Pharmacol.* 14: 9-13, 1959.

817.   Walker, H.A., *et al.*   The effect of 1-hydrazinophthalazine (C-5968) and related compounds on the cardiovascular system of dogs. *J. Pharmacol. Exp. Ther.* 101: 368-378, 1951.

818.   Haury, V.G. and M.E. Drake.   The effect of intravenous injections of sodium diphenyl hydantoinate (Dilantin) on respiration, blood pressure, and the vagus nerve. *J. Pharmacol. Exp. Ther.* 68: 36-40, 1940.

819.   Drake, M.E., V.G. Haury and C.M. Gruber.   The action of sodium diphenyl hydantoinate (Dilantin) on the excised and intact uterus. *Arch. Int. Pharmacodyn.* 43: 288-291, 1939.

820.   Belenky, M.L. and M. Vitolina.   The pharmacological analysis of the hyperthermia caused by phenamine (amphetamine). *Int. J. Neuropharmacol.* 1: 1-7, 1962.

821.   Benfey, B.G. and D.R. Varma.   Studies on the cardiovascular actions of antisympathomimetic drugs. *Int. J. Neuropharmacol.* 1: 9-12, 1962.

822.   Campos, H.A. and F.E. Shideman.   Subcellular distribution of catecholamines in the dog heart. *Int. J. Neuropharmacol.* 1: 13-22, 1962.

823.   Kido, R. and K. Yamamoto.   An analysis of tranquilizers in chronically electrode implanted cat. *Int. J. Neuropharmacol.* 1: 49-53, 1962.

824.   White, R.P. and E.J. Westerbeke.   Relationship between central anticholinergic actions and antiparkinson efficacy of phenothiazine derivatives. *Int. J. Neuropharmacol.* 1: 213-216, 1962.

825.   Knapp, D.E. and E.F. Domino.   Action of nicotine on the ascending reticular activating system. *Int. J. Neuropharmacol.* 1: 333-351, 1962.

826.   Riehl, J.L., *et al.*   Comparison of the effects of arecoline and muscarine on the central nervous system. *Int. J. Neuropharmacol.* 1: 393-401, 1962.

827.   Knapp, D.E. and E.F. Domino.   Species differences in the EEG response to epinephrine, 5-hydroxytryptamine and nicotine in brainstem transected animals. *Int. J. Neuropharmacol.* 2: 51-55, 1963.

Bibliography

828. Koll, W., *et al.* The predilective action of small doses of morphine on nociceptive spinal reflexes of low spinal cats. *Int. J. Neuropharmacol.* 2: 57-65, 1963.

829. Liberson, W.I., *et al.* Effects of chlorodiazepoxide (Librium) on fixated behavior in rats. *Int. J. Neuropharmacol.* 2: 67-78, 1963.

830. Spector, S., *et al.* Association of behavioral effects of pargyline, a non-hydrazide MAO inhibitor with increase in brain norepinephrine. *Int. J. Neuropharmacol.* 2: 81-93, 1963.

831. Herz, A. Excitation and inhibition of cholinoceptive brain structures and its relationship to pharmacological induced behavior changes. *Int. J. Neuropharmacol.* 2: 205-216, 1963.

832. White, R.P. and C.B. Nash. Catechol antagonism to the EEG effects of reserpine, chlorpromazine, pentobarbital and atropine. *Int. J. Neuropharmacol.* 2: 249-254, 1963.

833. Liberson, W.T., *et al.* Synaptic transmission in the hippocampus and psychopharmacological agents. *Int. J. Neuropharmacol.* 2: 291-302, 1964.

834. Olds, M.E. and J. Olds. Pharmacological patterns in subcortical reinforcement behavior. *Int. J. Neuropharmacol.* 2: 309-325, 1964.

835. Steiner, W.G., *et al.* An electroencephalographic study of some structural aspects of *d*-amphetamine antagonism in phenothiazine and related compounds. *Int. J. Neuropharmacol.* 2: 327-335, 1964.

836. Sigg, E.B. and T.D. Sigg. Sympathetic stimulation and blockade of the urinary bladder in cat. *Int. J. Neuropharmacol.* 3: 241-251, 1964.

837. Stille, G. and A. Sayers. The effect of antidepressant drugs on the convulsive excitability of brain structures. *Int. J. Neuropharmacol.* 3: 605-609, 1964.

838. Metysova, J. and J. Metys. Pharmacological properties of the desmethyl derivatives of some antidepressants of imipramine type. *Int. J. Neuropharmacol.* 4: 111-124, 1965.

839. Herz, A., *et al.* The importance of lipidsolubility for the central action of cholinolytic drugs. *Int. J. Neuropharmacol.* 4: 207-218, 1965.

840. Dungan, K.M., *et al.* Amidephrine - I: Pharmacologic characterization of a sympathomimetic alkylsulfonamidophenethanolamine. *Int. J. Neuropharmacol.* 4: 219-234, 1965.

841. Jurna, I. Depression of facilitatory influences on spinal motor activity by carisoprodol. *Int. J. Neuropharmacol.* 4: 245-254, 1965.

842. Eidelberg, E., *et al.* Spectrum analysis of EEG changes induced by psychotomimetic agents. *Int. J. Neuropharmacol.* 4: 255-264, 1965.

Bibliography

843. Schalleck, W., *et al.* Effects of mogadon on responses to stimulation of sciatic nerve, amygdala and hypothalamus of cat. *Int. J. Neuropharmacol.* 4: 317-326, 1965.

844. Stille, G., *et al.* The pharmacological properties of a potent neurotropic compound from the dibenzothiazepine group. *Int. J. Neuropharmacol.* 4: 375-391, 1965.

845. Diamantis, W. and M. Kletzkin. Evaluation of muscle relaxant drugs by head-drop and by decerebrate rigidity. *Int. J. Neuropharmacol.* 5: 305-310, 1966.

846. Straw, R.N. and C.L. Mitchell. Effect of phenobarbital on cortical afterdischarge and overt seizure patterns in the cat. *Int. J. Neuropharmacol.* 5: 323-330, 1966.

847. Jurna, I. Depression of the dorsal root potential of the cat spinal cord by amidopyrine. *Int. J. Neuropharmacol.* 5: 361-365, 1966.

848. Horovitz, Z.P., *et al.* Effects of drugs on the mouse-killing (muricide) test and its relationship to amygdaloid function. *Int. J. Neuropharmacol.* 5: 405-411, 1966.

849. McClane, T.K. and W.R. Martin. Effects of morphine, nalorphine, cyclazocine, and naloxone on the flexor reflex. *Int. J. Neuropharmacol.* 6: 89-98, 1967.

850. Brimblecombe, R.W. and D.M. Green. Central effects of imipramine-like anti-depressants in relation to their peripheral anticholinergic activity. *Int. J. Neuropharmacol.* 6: 133-142, 1967.

851. Stille, G. and A. Sayers. Motor convulsions and EEG during maximal electroshock in the rat. *Int. J. Neuropharmacol.* 6: 169-174, 1967.

852. Bohdanecky, Z. and M.E. Jarvik. Impairment of one-trial passive avoidance learning in mice by scopolamine, scopolamine methyl-bromide, and physostigmine. *Int. J. Neuropharmacol.* 6: 217-222, 1967.

853. Norton, S. An analysis of cat behavior using chlorpromazine and amphetamine. *Int. J. Neuropharmacol.* 6: 307-316, 1967.

854. Collins, R.J. and V.R. Simonton. Inhibition of evoked potentials by caudate stimulation and its antagonism by centrally acting drugs. *Int. J. Neuropharmacol.* 6: 349-356, 1967.

855. Cummings, J.R., *et al.* Cardiovascular actions of guancydine in normotensive and hypertensive animals. *J. Pharmacol. Exp. Ther.* 161: 88-97, 1968.

856. Dilts, S.L. and C.A. Berry. Effect of cholinergic drugs on passive avoidance in the mouse. *J. Pharmacol. Exp. Ther.* 158: 278-285, 1967.

857. King, A.B. and J.A. Thomas. Effect of exogenous dopamine on rat adrenal ascorbic acid. *J. Pharmacol. Exp. Ther.* 159: 18-21, 1968.

858. Lawson, J.W. Anti-arrhythmic activity of some isoquinoline derivatives determined by a rapid screening procedure in the mouse. *J. Pharmacol. Exp. Ther.* 160: 22-31, 1968.

Bibliography

859. Schumacher, H., *et al*. A comparison of the teratogenic activity of thalidomide in rabbits and rats. *J. Pharmacol. Exp. Ther*. 160: 189-200, 1968.

860. Goldberg, S.J., *et al*. The pulmonary and systemic hemodynamic effects produced by meperidine and hydroxyzine. *J. Pharmacol. Exp. Ther*. 159: 306-313, 1968.

861. Creveling, C.R., *et al*. The depletion of cardiac norepinephrine by 3,5-dihydroxy-4-methoxyphenethylamine and related compounds. *J. Pharmacol. Exp. Ther*. 158: 46-54, 1967.

862. Lehr, D., *et al*. Copious drinking and simultaneous inhibition of urine flow elicited by beta-adrenergic stimulation and contrary effect of alpha-adrenergic stimulation. *J. Pharmacol. Exp. Ther*. 158: 150-163, 1967.

863. McChesney, E.W., *et al*. The hyperglycemic action of some analogs of epinephrine. *Soc. Exptl. Biol. Med*. 71: 220-223, 1949.

864. Pratesi, P., *et al*. Chemical structure and biologic activity of the catecholamines. I. Influence of the N-alkyl substitution. *Farmaco. Ed. Sci*. 18: 920-931, 1963.

865. McCutcheon, R.S. Canine blood sugar and lactic acid responses to adrenergic amines after adrenergic block. *J. Pharmacol. Exp. Ther*. 136: 209-212, 1962.

866. Mayer, S., *et al*. The effect of adrenergic blocking agents on some metabolic actions of catecholamines. *J. Pharmacol. Exp. Ther*. 134: 18-27, 1961.

867. Bhagat, B. The influence of sympathetic nervous activity on cardiac catecholamine levels. *J. Pharmacol. Exp. Ther*. 157: 74-80. 1967.

868. Maitre, L. Monoamine oxidase inhibiting properties of SU-11,739 in the rat. Comparison with pargyline, tranylcypromine and iproniazid. *J. Pharmacol. Exp. Ther*. 157: 81-88, 1967.

869. Saito, S. and Y. Tokunaga. Some correlations between picrotoxin-induced seizures and γ-amino-butyric acid in animal brain. *J. Pharmacol. Exp. Ther*. 157: 546-554, 1967.

870. Lorenzo, A.V. and C.F. Barlow. Effect of strychnine convulsions upon the entry of S^{35} sulfate into the cat central nervous system. *J. Pharmacol. Exp. Ther*. 157: 555-564, 1967.

871. Vaillant, G.E. A comparison of antagonists of physostigmine-induced suppression of behavior. *J. Pharmacol. Exp. Ther*. 157: 636-648, 1967.

872. Long, J.P., *et al*. A pharmacologic evaluation of hemicholinium analogs. *J. Pharmacol. Exp. Ther*. 155: 223-230, 1967.

873. Herman, E.H. and C.D. Barnes. Drug modification of the Schiff-Sherrington phenomenon. *J. Pharmacol. Exp. Ther*. 156: 48-54, 1967.

Bibliography

874. Latz., A., *et al.* Maze learning after the administration of antidepressant drugs. *J. Pharmacol. Exp. Ther.* 156: 76-84, 1967.

875. Chai, C.Y. and S.C. Wang. Cardiovascular actions of diazepam in the cat. *J. Pharmacol. Exp. Ther.* 154: 271-280, 1966.

876. Oliverio, A. Effects of mecamylamine on avoidance conditioning and maze learning in mice. *J. Pharmacol. Exp. Ther.* 154: 350-356, 1966.

877. Bainbridge, J.G. and D.T. Greenwood. Tranquilizing effects of propranolol demonstrated in rats. *Neuropharmacol.* 10: 453-458, 1971.

878. Suwandi, I.S. and J.A. Bevan. Antagonism of lobeline by ganglion-blocking agents of afferent nerve endings. *J. Pharmacol. Exp. Ther.* 153: 1-7, 1966.

879. Bhagat, B. and J. Gilliam, Jr. Factors influencing the depletion of cardiac norepinephrine by tyramine. *J. Pharmacol. Exp. Ther.* 153: 191-196, 1966.

880. Kulharni, A.S. and F.E. Shideman. Sensitivities of the brains of infant and adult rats in catecholamine-depleting actions of reserpine and tetrabenazine. *J. Pharmacol. Exp. Ther.* 153: 428-433, 1965.

881. Swinyard, E.A. and A.W. Castellion. Anticonvulsant properties of some benzodiazepines. *J. Pharmacol. Exp. Ther.* 151: 369-375, 1966.

882. Williams, B., *et al.* Electrical activity of the prepyriform cortex after reserpine in the rat. *J. Pharmacol. Exp. Ther.* 150: 10-16, 1965.

883. Eble, J.N. and A. Rudzik. The potentiation of the pressor response to tyramine by amphetamine in the anesthetized dog. *J. Pharmacol. Exp. Ther.* 150: 375-381, 1965.

884. Boshart, C.R., *et al.* The effects of reserpine, guanethidine and other automatic drugs on free fatty acid mobilization induced by phenotolamine. *J. Pharmacol. Exp. Ther.* 149: 57-64, 1965.

885. Chen, G., *et al.* An investigation on the sympathomimetic properties of phencyclidine by comparison with cocaine and desoxy-ephedrine. *J. Pharmacol. Exp. Ther.* 149: 71-78, 1965.

886. Bircher, R.P., *et al.* Effects of hexamethonium and tetraethylammonium on cardiac arrhythmias produced by pentylenetetrazol, picrotoxin and deslanoside in dogs. *J. Pharmacol. Exp. Ther.* 149: 91-97, 1965.

887. Lish, P.M., *et al.* Pharmacological and toxicological properties of two new ß-adrenergic receptor antagonists. *J. Pharmacol. Exp. Ther.* 149: 161-173, 1965.

888. Bhagat, B. Pressor responses to amphetamine in the spinal cat and its influence on tachyphylaxis to tyramine. *J. Pharmacol. Exp. Ther.* 149: 206-211, 1965.

Bibliography

889.   Norton, S. and R.E. Jewett. Effect of drugs on spontaneous slow potential
         oscillations of the cerebral cortex. *J. Pharmacol. Exp. Ther.* 149: 301-310, 1965.

890.   Gaitonde, B.B., *et al.* Central emetic action and toxic effects of digitalis in
         cats. *J. Pharmacol. Exp. Ther.* 147: 409-415, 1965.

891.   Straw, R.N. and C.L. Mitchell. The effects of morphine, pentobarbital,
         pentazocine and nalorphine bioelectrical potentials evoked in the brain stem of
         the cat by electrical stimulation of the tooth pulp. *J. Pharmacol. Exp. Ther.*
         146: 7-15, 1964.

892.   Rosenberg, F.J. and P.J. Savarie. Histamine and the reversal of
         chlorpromazine-induced depression. *J. Pharmacol. Exp. Ther.* 146: 180-185,
         1964.

893.   Lucchesi, B.R. The action of nethalide upon experimentally induced cardiac
         arrhythmias. *J. Pharmacol. Exp. Ther.* 145: 286-291, 1964.

894.   Martin, W.R., *et al.* Use of hindlimb reflexes of the chronic spinal dog for
         comparing analgesics. *J. Pharmacol. Exp. Ther.* 144: 8-11, 1964.

895.   Weiss, B. and V.G. Laties. Effects of amphetamine, chlorpromazine,
         pentobarbital, and ethanol on operant response duration. *J. Pharmacol. Exp.
         Ther.* 144: 17-23, 1964.

896.   Swinyard, E.A., *et al.* Effect of epinephrine and norepinephrine on excitability
         of central nervous system of mice. *J. Pharmacol. Exp. Ther.* 144: 52-59, 1964.

897.   Erij, D. and R. Mendez. The modification of digitalis intoxication by excluding
         adrenergic influences on the heart. *J. Pharmacol. Exp. Ther.* 144: 97-103, 1964.

898.   Nechay, B.R. Potentiation of diuretic effect of methyl xanthines and
         pyrimidines by carbonic anhydrase inhibitors. *J. Pharmacol. Exp. Ther.* 144:
         276-283, 1964.

899.   Sulser, F., *et al.* The action of desmethylimipramine in counteracting sedation
         and cholinergic effects of reserpine-like drugs. *J. Pharmacol. Exp. Ther.* 144:
         321-330, 1964.

900.   Esplin, D.W. and B. Zablocka. Pilocarpine blockade of spinal inhibition in cats.
         J. Pharmacol. Exp. Ther. 143: 174-180, 1964.

901.   Kirpekar, S.M. and P. Cervoni. Effect of cocaine, phenoxybenzamine and
         phentolamine on the catecholamine output from spleen and adrenal medulla. *J.
         Pharmacol. Exp. Ther.* 142: 59-70, 1963.

902.   Zimmerman, A.M. and L.S. Harris. Microcirculation effects of guanethidine and
         reserpine. *J. Pharmacol. Exp. Ther.* 142: 76-82, 1963.

903.   Goldberg, M.E., *et al.* Psychopharmacological effects of reversible cholinesterase
         inhibition induced by N-methyl 3-isopropyl phenyl carbamate (compound
         10854). *J. Pharmacol. Exp. Ther.* 141: 244-252, 1963.

Bibliography

904.   Eckhardt, E.T. and F.W. Schweler. The pharmacology of methane sulfonyl choline. *J. Pharmacol. Exp. Ther.* 141: 343-348, 1963.

905.   Winter, C.A., *et al.* Anti-inflammatory and anti-pyretic activities of indomethacin, (1-p-chlorbenzoyl)-5-methoxy-2-methyl-indole-3-acetic acid. *J. Pharmacol. Exp. Ther.* 141: 369-376, 1963.

906.   Brodey, J.F., *et al.* An electrographic study of psilocin and 4-methyl-α-methyltryptamine (MP-809). *J. Pharmacol. Exp. Ther.* 140: 8-18, 1963.

907.   Natoff, I.L. Influence of the route of administration on the toxicity of some cholinesterase inhibitors. *J. Pharm. Pharmacol.* 19: 612-616, 1967.

908.   Blane, G.F. Blockade of bradykinin-induced nociception in the rat as a test for analgesic drugs with particular references to morphine antagonists. *J. Pharm. Pharmacol.* 19: 367-373, 1967.

909.   Brittain, R.T. The pharmacology of 2-amino-4-methyl-6-phenylamino-1,3,5-triazine, a centrally acting muscle relaxant. *J. Pharm. Pharmac.* 18: 294-304, 1966.

910.   Ross, S.B. and A.L. Renyi. In vivo inhibition of ^{3}H-noradrenaline uptake by mouse brain slices in vitro. *J. Pharm. Pharmac.* 18: 322-323, 1966.

911.   Buckett, W.R. Some pharmacological studies with 14-cinnamoyloxycodeinone. *J. Pharm. Pharmac.* 17: 759-760, 1965.

912.   Korol, B., *et al.* Some cardiovascular studies on octopamine. *Arch. Int. Pharmacodyn.* 171: 415-424, 1968.

913.   Raines, A., *et al.* Action of phentolamine on respiratory reflexes in the rabbit. *Arch. Int. Pharmacodyn.* 170: 485-490, 1967.

914.   Sergman, F., *et al.* Action of phentolamine on respiratory reflexes in the rabbit. *Arch. Int. Pharmacodyn.* 169: 348-353, 1967.

915.   Cohen, M.A. A comparative study of anticholinergic psychotomimetic agents in mice and dogs. *Arch. Int. Pharmacodyn.* 169: 412-420, 1967.

916.   Stanton, H.C. and C.M. Cooper. Antihypertenive effects of drugs measured in unanesthetized rats with established adrenal regeneration hypertension. *Arch. Int. Pharmacodyn.* 168: 1-13, 1967.

917.   McKean, W.., Jr. In vivo antiserotonin activity in unanesthetized guinea pig. *Arch. Int. Pharmacodyn.* 168: 373-382, 1967.

918.   Straw, R.N. and C.L. Mitchell. The effect of pentylenetetrazol on biochemical activity recorded from the cat brain. *Arch. Int. Pharmacodyn.* 186: 456-466, 1967.

919.   Westfall, T.C. Accumulation of norepinephrine in rat tissue following treatment with three ß-adrenergic antagonists. *Arch. Int. Pharmacodyn.* 167: 69-79, 1967.

Bibliography

920. Banziger, R. and D. Hane. Evaluations of a new convulsant for anticonvulsant screening. *Arch. Int. Pharmacodyn.* 167: 245-249, 1967.

921. Uyeno, E.T. Effects of mescaline and psilocybin on dominant behavior of the rat. *Arch. Int. Pharmacodyn.* 166: 60-64, 1967.

922. Georges, A., *et al.* Cardiotonic properties of formiloxin, a semi-synthetic glycoside. *Arch. Int. Pharmacodyn.* 164: 47-55, 1966.

923. Coscia, L., *et al.* A new synthetic analgesic drug, p-phentidine-α-N-n-propylpropionamide (FC 379). *Arch. Int. Pharmacodyn.* 164: 331-339, 1966.

924. Coscia, L., *et al.* General pharmacological properties of p-phenetidine-α-N-n-propylpropionamide (FC 379). *Arch. Int. Pharmacodyn.* 164: 340-344, 1966.

925. Essman, W.B. Anticonvulsive properties of xylocaine in mice susceptible to audiogenic seizures. *Arch. Int. Pharmacodyn.* 164: 376-386, 1966.

926. Mitchell, C.L. The effect of drugs on the latency for an escape response elicited by electrical stimulation of the tooth pulp in cats. *Arch. Int. Pharmacodyn.* 164: 427-433, 1966.

927. Hill, H.E., *et al.* Comparative effects of methadone, meperidine and morphine on conditioned suppression. *Arch. Int. Pharmacodyn.* 163: 341-352, 1966.

928. Marazzi-Uberti, E. and C. Turba. α-isopropyl-α-(2-dimethylaminoethyl)-1-naphylacetamide (naphthpyramide, DA 992): A new anti-inflammatory agent. I. Anti-inflammatory activity and acute toxicity. *Arch. Int. Pharmacodyn.* 162: 378-397, 1966.

929. Hanson, H.M., *et al.* Estimation of relative antiavoidance activity of depressant drugs in squirrel monkeys. *Arch. Int. Pharmacodyn.* 161: 7-16, 1966.

930. Dashputra, P.G., *et al.* Modification of metrazol induced convulsions in rats by antihistamines. *Arch. Int. Pharmacodyn.* 160: 106-112, 1966.

931. Weiss, B. and V.G. Laties. Changes in pain tolerance and other behavior produced by salicylates. *J. Pharmacol. Exp. Ther.* 131: 120-129, 1961.

932. Aceto, M.D., *et al.* Effects of drugs on conditioning in the rat. *J. Pharm. Sci.* 56: 823-827, 1961.

933. Kuhn, W.I. and E.F. Van Maanen. Central nervous system affects of thalidomide. *J. Pharmacol. Exp. Ther.* 134: 60-68, 1961.

934. Kelleher, R.T., *et al.* Effects of meprobamate on operant behavior in rats. *J. Pharmacol. Exp. Ther.* 133: 271-280, 1961.

579

Bibliography

935.   Bastian, J.W.   Classification of CNS drugs by a mouse screening battery. *Arch. Int. Pharmacodyn.* 133: 347-364, 1961.

936.   Becker, B.A.   Pharmacologic activity of phentermine (phenyl-t-butylamine). *Toxicol. Appl. Pharmacol.* 3: 256-259, 1961.

937.   Cho, M.H.   Quantitation of spontaneous movements of animals given psychotropic drugs. *J. Appl. Physiol.* 16: 390-391, 1961.

938.   Dresse, A. and C. Niemengeers.   Is the stimulation of certain nervous centers by apomorphine subject to tachyphylaxis? *Comt. Rend. Soc. Biol.* 155: 1713-1715, 1961.

939.   Fischer, E. and M. Lopez Amalfara.   Effects of catecholamine on the motor behavior of lauchas (rodents) and their modification by adrenergic blocking. *Ciencia Invest. (Buenos Aires)* 17: 138-140, 1961.

940.   Kameyama, T., Studies on analgesics. VI. Analgesic activity of sympathomimetic amines and other drugs. *Yakugaku Zasshi* 81: 215-221, 1961.

941.   Linyuchev, M.N., *et al.* Restoration with phenamine (amphetamine) of conditioned reflexes deranged through the use of cholinolytics. *Farmakol. i Toksikol.* 24: 659-664, 1961.

942.   Mantegazza, P. and M. Riva.   Anorexigenic activity of L (-) DOPA in animals pretreated with monoaminoxidase inhibitor. *Med. Exptl.* 4: 367-373, 1961.

943.   Petkov, W.   The mechanism of action of *Panax ginseng* C.A. Mey. The problem of the pharmacology of response mechanism. *Arzneimittel-Forsch.* 11: 288-295, 1961.

944.   van Andel, H. and A.M. Ernst.   Tryptamine-catatonia, a cholinergic hypofunction in the central nervous system. *Psychopharmacologia* 2: 461-466, 1961.

945.   White, R.P., *et al.* Phylogenetic comparison of central actions produced by different doses of atropine and hyoscine. *Arch. Int. Pharmacodyn.* 132: 349-363, 1961.

946.   Fujimura, H., *et al.* Pharmacological action of 2-anilinoacetamide derivatives. *Yakugaku Zasshi* 81: 659-663, 1961.

947.   Vorobiova, T.M.   Effect of small doses of various pharmacological preparations on conditioned reflexes in dogs. *Fiziol. Zh. Akad. Nauk Ukr.* RSR 7: 24-31, 1961.

948.   Silvestrini, B. and C. Pozzatti.   Pharmacological properties of 3-phenyl-5-diethylamino-ethyl-1,2,4-oxadiazole. *Brit. J. Pharmacol.* 16: 209-217, 1961.

949.   Vernier, V.G.   The pharmacology of antidepressant agents. *Diseases Nervous System* 22: 7-13, 1961.

950.   Sabelli, H.C., *et al.* Cholinergic mechanisms and antidepressive agents. *Rev. Soc. Arg. Biol.* 37: 87-92, 1961.

Bibliography

951.   Kudrin, A.N. and L.P. Kokina. Effect of somniferous agents and of their combination with pentamin on the external inhibition of positive conditioned food reflexes. *Farmikol. i Toksikol.* 24: 397-403, 1961.

952.   Steinberg, H., *et al.* Modification of the effects of amphetamine-barbiturate mixture by the past experience of rats. *Nature* 192: 533-535, 1961.

953.   Muller-Calgan, H. and R. Hotovy. Behavioral changes in the cat in response to various drugs acting as stimulants of the central nervous system. *Arzneimittel-Forsch.* 11: 642-649, 1961.

954.   Vane, J.R., *et al.* Tryptamine receptors in the central nervous system. *Nature* 191: 1068-1069, 1961.

955.   Chen, G. and B. Bohner. Anticonvulsant properties of 1-(1-phenylcyclohexyl) piperidine-HCl and certain other drugs. *Proc. Soc. Exptl. Biol. Med.* 106: 632-635, 1961.

956.   Child, K.J., *et al.* Some effects of reserpine on barbitone anesthesia in mice. *Biochem. Pharmacol.* 6: 252-256, 1961.

957.   Fukushima, K. Experimental studies on the drugs of antishock. *Kagoshima Daigaku Igaku Zasshi.* 13: 416-437, 1961.

958.   Kita, T., *et al.* Studies on central depressants. I. Pharmacological activity of γ-substituted butyric acid derivatives. *Yakugaku Kenkyu* 33: 36-47, 1961.

959.   Bentley, G.A. The susceptibility of rats to audiogenic seizures following acute and prolonged medication with narcotic drugs. *Arch. Int. Pharmacodyn.* 132: 378-391, 1961.

960.   Greenblatt, E.N. and A.C. Osterberg. Correlations of activating and lethal effects of excitatory drugs in grouped and isolated mice. *J. Pharmacol. Exp. Ther.* 131: 115-119, 1961.

961.   Shuster, V., *et al.* Pharmacological data on the analeptic bemegride. *Latvijas PSR Zinatm Akad. Vestis.* No. 8: 105-110, 1961.

962.   Maffii, G., *et al.* A new analeptic: 5,5-diethyl-1,3-oxazin-2,4-dione (dioxone). *J. Pharmacol.* 13: 244-253, 1961.

963.   Nicholls, P.J. Pharmacological properties of some ß-glutarimides. *Arch. Int. Pharmacodyn.* 133: 212-235, 1961.

964.   Zbinden, G., *et al.* Experimental and clinical toxicology of chlorodiazepoxide (Librium). *Toxicol. App. Pharmacol.* 3: 619-637, 1961.

965.   Kuriyama, K. Electroencephalographic studies on the antagonism between ß,ß-methyl-ethylglutarimide and some kinds of anesthetics. *Nippon Yakurigaku Zasshi* 57: 560-565, 1961.

Bibliography

966.   Hahn, F., *et al.* The effect of bemegrid, noradrenalin and artificial respiration on thiopental anesthesia in dogs. *Arch. Exptl. Pathol. Pharmakol.* 242: 168-187, 1961.

967.   Denisenko, P.P. The effect of cholinolytics, chiefly acting on the central nervous system, on conditioned reflex activity in rabbits. *Pavlov J. Higher Nervous Activity* 11: 113-118, 1961.

968.   Ilyuchenok, R.Y. and M.D. Mashkovskii. Correlation of anticholinesterase substances (galanthamine and eserine) with choline- and adreno-lytics in the region of the reticular formation in the brain stem. *Farmakol. i Toksikol.* 24: 403-410, 1961.

969.   Denisenko, P.P. The antagonistic action of cholinomimetic and central cholinolytic agents on the EEG of the rabbit. *Seckenov Physiol. J. USSR* 47: 124-131, 1961.

970.   Sergio, C. The effect of bulbocapnine on EEG and flight reaction by hypothalmic stimulation in rabbits. *Riv. Neurobiol.* 7: 451-462, 1961.

971.   Van Harreveld, A. and J.E. Bogen. The clinging position of the bulbocapninized cat. *Exptl. Neurol.* 4: 241-261, 1961.

972.   Hughes, F.W. and R.B Forney. Alcohol and caffeine in choice-discrimination tests in rats. *Proc. Soc. Exptl. Biol. Med.* 108: 157-159, 1961.

973.   Sommer, S. and R. Hotovy. Differentiation of the central stimulating action of 2-ethyl-amino-3-phenyl-norcomphane. *Arzneimittel-Forsch.* 11: 969-972, 1961.

974.   Gerber, C.J. Effect of selected excitant and depressant agents on the cortical response to midline thalamic stimulation in the rabbit. *Electroencephalog. Clin. Neurophysiol.* 13: 354-364, 1961.

975   Carroll, M.N., Jr., *et al.* The pharmacology of a new oxazolidimon with anti-convulsant, analgetic and muscle relaxant properties. *Arch. Int. Pharmacodyn.* 130: 280-298, 1961.

976.   Baruk, H. and J. Launay. Experimental psychotropic action of chlorodiazepoxide in the monkey. Practical consequences in human therapy. *Ann. Medicopsychol.* 119: 957-962, 1961.

977.   Randall, L.O., *et al.* Pharmacological and clinical studies on Valium, a new psychotherapeutic agent of the benzodiazepine class. *Current Therap. Res.* 3: 405-425, 1961.

978.   Frommel, F., *et al.* What is the place of morphine and cocaine in the armamentarium of the so-called psychopharmacological drugs? *Schweitz. Med. Wochschr.* 91: 1102-1108, 1961.

979.   Nikitina, G.M. The effect of chlorpromazine on the interrelation of motor and autonomic components of the conditioned defense reaction in animals during ontogenesis. *Pavlov J. Higher Nervous Activity* 11: 98-104, 1961.

Bibliography

980. Khrabrova, O.P. Specific features of the animal reaction to a shock-inducing stimulus following the administration of aminazine. *Bull. Exptl. Biol. Med.* 51: 147-150, 1961.

981. Smith, M E., *et al.* Psychotherapeutic agents and ethyl alcohol. *Quart. J. Studies Alc.* 22: 241-249, 1961.

982. Faenzi, C. Effect of neuroleptic and relaxant drugs in convulsive states induced by toxic doses of local anesthetics. *Boll. Soc. Ital. Biol. Sper.* 39: 414-417, 1961.

983. Lambert, P.A., *et al.* Notes on the neuroleptic inactivity of a phenothiazine derivative with pure anti-apomorphine properties. Pharmacodynamic and clinical study of 3-dimethyl-sulfamoyl-10-[3-1-methylsulfonyl-4-piperazino)-propyl] phenothiazine (R.P. 9,260). *Psychopharmacologia* 2: 209-213, 1961.

984. Schuette, D.V. and W.L. Gulick. The effects of chlorpromazine upon the ear and the VIII cranial nerve. *Ann. Otol. Rhinol. Laryngol.* 70: 143-163, 1961.

985. Wu, Hsi-Jui. The action mechanism of reserpine compared with that of certain other tranquilizing substances. *Bull. Exptl. Biol. Med.* 51: 461-465, 1961.

986. Bienfet, V., *et al.* Pharmacologic assay of dixyrazine. *Acta Neurol. Psychiat. Belg.* 61: 669-685, 1961.

987. Knoll, J. Motimeter, a new sensitive apparatus for the quantitative measurement of hypermotility caused by psychostimulants. *Arch. Int. Pharmacodyn.* 130: 141-154, 1961.

988. Maxwell, D.R. and H.T. Palmer. Demonstration of anti-depressant or stimulant properties of imipramine in experimental animals. *Nature* 191: 84-85, 1961.

989. Cahen, R. The pharmacology of pholcodine. *Bull. Narcotics U.N. Dept. Social Affairs* 13: 19-36, 1961.

990. Pinto Corrado, A. and V.G. Longo. An electrophysiological analysis of the convulsant action of morphine, codeine and thebaine. *Arch. Int. Pharmacodyn.* 132: 255-269, 1961.

991. Frommell, E., *et al.* The pharmacodynamics of the anilide of (pyrrolidino-N)-3-N-butyric acids (WS 10), a basal neuroleptic and cortical thymoleptic drug. *Arch. Int. Pharmacodyn.* 130: 235-259, 1961.

992. Harris, L.S. and F.C. Uhle. Enhancement of amphetamine stimulation and prolongation of barbiturate depression by a substituted pyrid [3,4-6] indole derivative. *J. Pharmacol. Exp. Ther.* 132: 251-257, 1961.

993. Crampton, G.H. Habituation of vestibular nystagmus in the cat during sustained arousal produced by d-amphetamine. *U.S. Army Medical Research Lab. Ft. Knox, Kentucky, Rept.* No. 488, Aug. 18, 1961.

Bibliography

994.   McLennan, H. The effect of some catecholamines upon a monosynaptic reflex pathway in the spinal cord. *J. Physiol.* 158: 411-425, 1961.

995.   Goldstein, K. and C. Munoz. Influence of adrenergic stimulant and blocking drugs on cerebral electrical activity in curarized animals. *J. Pharmacol. Exp. Ther.* 132: 345-353, 1961.

996.   Takahashi, R., *et al.* Relationship of ammonia and acetylcholine levels to brain excitability. *J. Neurochem.* 7: 103-112, 1961.

997.   Bastian, J.W. and G.R. Clements. Pharmacology and toxicology of hydroxyphenamate (Listica). *Diseases Nervous System. Suppl.* 22: 9-16, 1961.

998.   Van Tai-An and M.G. Belekhova. The influences of the cervical sympathetic nerve and the effects of some pharmacological substances on the "recruitment reaction." *Secherov. Physiol. J. USSR* 47: 18-29, 1961.

999.   Kita, T. and H. Kamiya. Central depressant. II. Several methods of screening γ-amino-butyric acid derivatives by mouse behavior. *Yakugaku Kenkyu* 33: 758-766, 1961.

1000.   Busche, E. Test of spinal reflexes and neuromuscular transmission in decerebrate rats and the effect of muscle relaxants on them. *Arch. Int. Pharmacodyn.* 132: 139-146, 1961.

1001.   Vacek, L. A study on steroid anesthesia: 6. The effect of serotonin and its antagonists on the central inhibiting effect of hydroxypregnanedione. *Scripta Med. Fac. Med. Univ. Brun. Olomuc.* 34: 65-72, 1961.

1002.   Levis, S., *et al.* Pharmacological characteristics of a new tranquilizing agent: Dixyrazine. *Arch. Int. Pharmacodyn.* 131: 262-282, 1961.

1003.   Herr, F., *et al.* Tranquilizers and anti-depressants: a pharmacological comparison. *Arch. Int. Pharmacodyn.* 134: 328-342, 1961.

1004.   Rubio-Chevamier, H., *et al.* Potentiating action of imipramine upon "reticular arousal." *Exptl. Neurol.* 4: 214-220, 1961.

1005.   Crepax, P., *et al.* Effects of imipramine on cerebral electrical phenomena in the cat due to activation of thalamo-cortical, transcallosal and intracortical circuits. *Boll. Soc. Ital. Biol. Sper.* 37: 180-183, 1961.

1006.   Himwich, W.A. and J.C. Petersen. Effect of the combined administration of imipramine and a monoamine oxidase inhibitor. *Am. J. Psychiat.* 117: 928-929, 1961.

1007.   Muller-Calgan, H. and R. Hotovy. Behavioral changes in the cat in response to various drugs acting as stimulants of the central nervous system. *Arzneimittel-Forsch.* 11: 642-649, 1961.

Bibliography

1008. Pfeifer, A.F., *et al.* Effect of tranquilizing drugs on the pharmacological actions of diethyltryptamine. *Acta Physiol. Acad. Sci. Hung.* 19: 225-233, 1961.

1009. Schallek, W., *et al.* Effects of chlorodiazepoxide (Librium) and other psychotropic agents on the limbic system of the brain. *Ann. N.Y. Acad. Sci.* 96: 303-312, 1961.

1010. Acheson, R.M., *et al.* Attempted correlations between behavioral and biochemical changes in rats following reserpine and chronic administration of amine-oxidase inhibitors. *Psychopharmacologia* 2: 277-294, 1961.

1011. Angelucci, L. Analgesia without respiratory depression by means of association of morphine, structural antagonists and Daptazo. *Minerva Anestesiologia* 27: 216-222, 1961.

1012. Berry, C.A., *et al.* A comparison of the anticonvulsant activity of mepivacaine and lidocaine. *J. Pharmacol. Exp. Ther.* 133: 357-363, 1961.

1013. Dhawan, B.N. and G.P. Gupta. Anti-emetic activity of D-lysergic acid diethylamide. *J. Pharmacol. Exp. Ther.* 133: 137-139, 1961.

1014. Fluckiger, E. and R. Salzmann. Serotonin antagonism (observed) on the placenta. *Experientia* 17: 131, 1961.

1015. Ueki, S., *et al.* Effects of mecamylamine on the Golgi recurrent collateral-Renshaw-cell synapse in the spinal cord. *Exptl. Neurol.* 3: 141-148, 1961.

1016. Burke, J.C. The muscle relaxant properties of 2,2-dichloro-1-(p-chlorophenyl)-1,3-propanediol-O^3-carbamate. *Arch. Int. Pharmacodyn.* 134: 216-223, 1961.

1017. Gross, C.G. and L. Weiskrantz. The effect of the "tranquilizers" on auditory discrimination and delayed response performance of monkeys. *Quart. J. Exptl. Psychol.* 13: 34-39, 1961.

1018. Gray, W.D., *et al.* Neuropharmacological actions of mephenoxalone. *Arch. Int. Pharmacodyn.* 134: 198-215, 1961.

1019. Frommel, E., *et al.* Meprobamate, phenobarbital, or meprobamate plus phenobarbital. *Anais Azevedos (Lisbon)* 13: 184-207, 1961.

1020. Inoki, R., *et al.* Comparison of the action of related compounds of Soma. *Nippon Yakurigaku Zaschi* 57: 280-288, 1961.

1021. Jacob, J. and M. Blozovski. Effects of various analgesic agents on the behavior of mice subjected to a thermoalgesic stimulus. II. Learning under nociceptive stress conditions. Comparative effects of analgesic and psychoactive agents on licking and leaping reactions. *Arch. Int. Pharmacodyn.* 133: 296-309, 1961.

Bibliography

1022.   Maxwell, D.R., *et al.* A comparison of the analgesic and some other central properties of methotromeprazine and morphine. *Arch. Int. Pharmacodyn.* 132: 60-73, 1961.

1023.   Kikutomo, T. The electroencephalogram of rabbits under the influence of reserpine and the effects of methamphetamine. *Nippon Yakurigaku Zasshi* 57: 173-192, 1961.

1024.   Faidherbe, J., *et al.* Differential action of a central nervous stimulant demonstrated by a technique of "operant" conditioning in the cat. *Arch. Int. Physiol. Biochim.* 69: 52-68, 1961.

1025.   Szporny, L. and P. Gorog. Investigations into the correlations between monoamine oxidase inhibition and other effects due to methylphenidate and its stereoisomers. *Biochem. Pharmacol.* 8: 263-268, 1961.

1026.   Farner, D. Studies on the effect of drugs on animals of various ages. IV. The effect of Ritalin and Regitine on young and old rats. *Gerontologia* 5:45-54, 1961.

1027.   Shemano, I., *et al.* A pharmacological comparison of phenazocaine hydrobromide and morphine sulfate as narcotic analgesics. *J. Pharmacol. Exp. Ther.* 132: 258-263, 1961.

1028.   Martin, W.R. and C.G. Eades. Demonstration of tolerance and physical dependence in the dog following a short-term infusion of morphine. *J. Pharmacol. Exp. Ther.* 133: 262-270, 1961.

1029.   Ohnesorge, F.K. and A.L. Khan. Effects of phenmetrozine on oxygen consumption and spontaneous motor activity. *Arzneimittel-Forsch.* 11: 793-795, 1961.

1030.   Janssen, P.A.J. Pirinitramide (R3365), a potent analgesic with unusual chemical structure. *J. Pharm. Pharmac.* 13: 513-530, 1961.

1031.   Hotovy, R., *et al.* Pharmacologic properties of 2-ethyl-amino-3-phenyl-norcamphane. *Arzneimittel-Forsch* 11: 20-29, 1967.

1032.   Szegi, J., *et al.* New contributions to the antagonism of morphine and N-allylnormorphine derivatives. *Acta Physiol. Acad. Sci. Hung.* 19: 273-285, 1961.

1033.   Witkin, L.B., *et al.* Pharmacology of 2-amino-indane hydrochloride (Su-8629): a potent non-narcotic analgesic. *J. Pharmacol. Exp. Ther.* 133: 400-408, 1961.

1034.   Mashkovskii, M.D. and R.Y. Hyuchenok. The effect of galanthamine on the central nervous system. *Zh. Nevropatol. i Pskhiatr.* 51: 166-175, 1961.

1035.   P'an, S.Y., *et al.* Anticonvulsant effect of nialamide and diphenylhydantoin. *Proc. Soc. Exptl. Biol. Med.* 108: 680-683, 1961.

1036.   Cortes, J.L. and G.V. Villagran. Nialamide and anaphylactic and histamine shock in guinea pigs. *Medicine* 41: 146-163, 1961.

586

Bibliography

1037. Lebeden, V.P. Effect of nicotine on proprioceptive reflexes. *Farmakol. i Toksikol.* 24: 515-518, 1961.

1038. DaVanzo, J.P., *et al*. Anticonulsant properties of amino-oxyacetic acid. *Am. J. Physiol.* 24: 833-837, 1961.

1039. Ohashi, H. The relation between corticospinal electrical activity and convulsions produced by the intravenous injection of ammonium salts. *Seishin Shinkeigaku Zasshi* 63: 31-43, 1961.

1040. Janssen, P.A.J. Comparative pharmacological data on 6 new basic 4'-fluorobutyrophenone derivatives: haloperidol, haloanisone, triperidol, methylperidide, haloperidide, and dipiperone. *Arzneimittle-Forsch* 11: 819-824, 1961.

1041. Tislow, R. Pharmacology and Toxicity of carphenazine. *Diseases Nervous System* 22: 7-13, 1961.

1042. Alema, G., *et al*. Experimental catatonia induced by neuroleptic drugs. I. Action of phenothiazine derivatives. *Boll. Soc. Ital. Biol. Sper.* 37: 1037-1040, 1961.

1043. O'Dell, T.B. Experimental parameters in the evaluation of analgesics. *Chicago Med.* 63: 9-15, 1961.

1044. Schneider, C. Effects of morphine-like drugs in chicks. *Nature* 191: 607-608, 1961.

1045. Nilsen, P.L. Studies on algesimetry by electrical stimulation of the mouse tail. *Acta Pharmacol. Toxicol.* 18: 10-22, 1961.

1046. Bovet-Nitti, F., *et al*. A new MAO inhibitor: N'-(1,4-benzodioxane-2-methyl)-N-benzyl-hydrazine (2596 IS). *Comput. Rend.* 252: 614-616, 1961.

1047. Frommel, E., *et al*. Pharmacodynamics of a new tranquilizer with relaxant and antitremor effects and prolonged action: Go 560 or 3 (γ-butoxy, ß-carbamyl, ß-propanol-5-phenyl, 5-ethylmalonylurea. Experimental study. *Helv. Physiol. Pharmacol. Acta.* 19: 241-253, 1961.

1048. Aston, R. and E.E. Domino. Differential effects of phenobarbital, pentobarbital, and diphenylhydantoin on motor cortical and reticular thresholds in the Rhesus monkey. *Psychopharmacologia* 2: 304-317, 1961.

1049. Popova, E.N. Some data on eserine's effect on the cerebral cortex of white rats. Communication 1. The effect of eserine on conditioned reflex activity. *Bull. Exptl. Biol.* 51: 198-203, 1961.

1050. Venulet, J. Correlation between antiserotonin and depressor action of some phenothiazine derivatives. *Acta Physiol. Polan.* 12: 281-290, 1961.

Bibliography

1051. Kucherenko, T.M. changes in higher nervous activity in dogs under the influence of pirhydrol. *Pavlov J. Higher Nervous Activity* 11: 64-69, 1961.

1052. Beaulness, A. and G. Viens. Catatonia and catalepsy. *Rev. Can. Bil.* 20: 215-220, 1961.

1053. Geller, I. Behavioral procedures used in evaluation of the psychopharmacological effects of carphenazine. *Diseases Nervous System Suppl.* 22: 19-22, 1961.

1054. Logerspetz, K. and R. Tirri. The induction of physiological tolerance to promazine in mice. *Ann. Med. Exptl. Biol. Fenniae Suppl.* 5, 39: 1-24, 1961.

1055. Deesi, I. Further studies on the metabolic background of tranquilizing drug action. *Psychopharmacologia* 2: 224-242, 1961.

1056. Tedeschi, D.H., *et al.* Interaction of neuroleptics with serotonin in the central nervous system. *Rev. Can. Bio.* 20: 209-214, 1961.

1057. Hyuchenok, R.Y. and R.U. Ostrovskaia. The effect of diprazine on the bioelectric activity of the brain. *Farmakol. i Toksikol.* 24: 18-22, 1961.

1058. Laborit, H., *et al.* An experimental "excitation-hypotonic" syndrome. *Arch. Int. Pharmacodyn.* 131: 151-163, 1961.

1059. Menge, H.G. Experimental studies with animals on the central stimulating effect of a new theophilline derivative. *Arzneimittel-Forsch.* 11: 271-273, 1961.

1060. Melson, F. Pharmacological study of some derivatives of 1,3-dioxolane with special reference to their actions on the central nervous system. *Acta Biol. Med. Ger.* 6: 395-406, 1961.

1061. Herz, A. Influence of anticholinergic, nicotinolytic and antihistamine drugs on the central inhibitory and stimulating morphine effects in the rat. *Arch. Exptl. Pathol. Pharmakol.* 241: 236-253, 1961.

1062. Knoll, J., *et al.* Experimental analysis of the central effect of convulsive hydrazines. *Acta Physiol. Acad. Sci. Hung.* 9: 169-178, 1961.

1063. Voss, E., *et al.* Reduction of tetramine toxicity by sedatives and anti-convulsants. *J. Pharm. Sci.* 50: 858-860, 1961.

1064. Melander, B. and G. Gliniecke. Amphetamine, diethylpropion and tranylcypromine, a psychopharmacological study in the relation between structure and activity. *Acta Pharmacol. Toxiol.* 18: 239-248, 1961.

1065. Costa, E. and G.R. Pscheidt. Correlations between active eyelid closure and depletion of brain biogenic amines by reserpine. *Proc. Soc. Exptl. Biol. Med.* 106: 693-696, 1961.

Bibliography

1066. Decsi, L., *et al.* Tolerance to tremorine. *Acta Physiol. Acad. Sci. Hung.* 18: 353-356, 1961.

1067. Arrigo, A., *et al.* Electroencephalographic study of the central action of yohimbine and yohimbic acid. *Boll. Soc. Ital. Biol. Sper.* 37: 787-790, 1961.

1068. Baxter, B.L. The effect of selected drugs on the "emotional" behavior elicited via hypothalamic stimulation. *Int. J. Neuropharmacol.* 7: 47-54, 1968.

1069. Olds, M.E. and G. Baldrighi. Effects of meprobamate, chlorodiazepoxide, diazepam and sodium pentobarbital on visually evoked responses in the tectotegmental area of the rat. *Int. J. Neuropharmacol.* 7: 231-239, 1968.

1070. Miyasaka, M. and E.F. Domino. Neuronal mechanisms of ketamine-induced anesthesia. *Int. J. Neuropharmacol.* 7: 557-573, 1968.

1071. Barnett, A., *et al.* Activity of antihistamines in laboratory antidepressant tests. *Int. J. Neuropharmacol.* 8: 73-79, 1969.

1072. Christmas, A.J. and D.R. Maxwell. A comparison of the effects of some benzodiazepines and other drugs on aggressive and exploratory behavior in mice and rats. *Neuropharmacology* 9: 17-29, 1970.

1073. Chen, G., *et al.* The neuropharmacology of 2-(o-chlorophenyl)-2-methylaminocyclohexanone hydrochloride. *J. Pharmacol. Exp. Ther.* 152: 332-339, 1966.

1074. Tobia, A.M., *et al.* Altered reflex vasodilation in the hypertensive rat: Possible role of histamine. *J. Pharmacol. Exp. Ther.* 175: 619-626, 1970.

1075. Downes, H., *et al.* A study of the excitatory effects of barbiturates. *J. Pharmacol. Exp. Ther.* 175: 692-699, 1970.

1076. Büch, H., *et al.* Stereospecificity of anesthetic activity, distribution, inactivation, and protein binding of the optical antipodes of two N-methylated barbiturates. *J. Pharmacol. Exp. Ther.* 175: 703-716, 1970.

1077. Nigrovic, V., *et al.* Diuretic response to mercuric cysteine: Dependency on urinary pH. *J. Pharmacol. Exp. Ther.* 175: 741-748, 1970.

1078. Dren, A.T. and E.F. Domino. Effects of hemicholinium (HC-3) on EEG activation and brain acetylcholine in the dog. *J. Pharmacol. Exp. Ther.* 161: 141-154, 1968.

1079. Levin, J.A., *et al.* Active reflex vasodilation induced by intravenous epinephrine or norepinephrine in primates. *J. Pharmacol. Exp. Ther.* 161: 262-270, 1968.

1080. Pfeiffer, C.C., *et al.* Comparative study of the effect of meprobamate on the conditioned response on strychnine and pentylenetetrazol thresholds, on the normal electroencephalogram and on polysynaptic reflexes. *Ann. N.Y. Acad. Sci.* 67: 734-745, 1957.

Bibliography

1081. Lish, P.M., *et al*. Mode of the bronchodilator action of Phentolamine. *J. Pharmacol. Exp. Ther*. 163: 11-16, 1968.

1082. Brown, J.H., *et al*. Oral effectiveness of beta adrenergic antagonists in preventing epinephrine-induced metabolic responses. *J. Pharmacol. Exp. Ther*. 163: 25-35, 1968.

1083. Kvam, D.C., *et al*. Effect of some new ß-adrenergic blocking agents on certain metabolic responses to catecholamines. *J. Pharmacol. Exp. Ther*. 149: 183-192, 1965.

1084. Dungan, K.W., *et al*. Pharmacologic potency and selectivity of a new bronchodilator agent: Soterenol (MJ 1992). *J. Pharmacol. Exp. Ther*. 164: 290-301, 1968.

1085. Miranda, P.M.S., *et al*. Vasodilation of brainstem origin suppressed by neuromuscular blockade in the cat. *J. Pharmacol. Exp. Ther*. 164: 333-341, 1968.

1086. Weinstock, M. and A.S. Marshall. The influence of the sympathetic nervous system on the action of drugs on the lens. *J. Pharmacol. Exp. Ther*. 166: 8-13, 1969.

1087. Friedman, M.J. and J.H. Jaffee. A central hypothermic response to pilocarpine in the mouse. *J. Pharmacol. Exp. Ther*. 167: 34-44, 1969.

1088. McKenna, D.H., *et al*. Effect of propranolol on systemic and coronary hemodynamics at rest and during simulated exercise. *Circ. Res*. 19: 520-527, 1966.

1089. Lucchesi, B.R. The effects of pronethalol and its dextro isomer upon experimental cardiac arrhythmias. *J. Pharmacol. Exp. Ther*. 148: 94-99, 1965.

1090. Parmley, W.W. and E. Braunwald. Comparative myocardial depressant and anti-arrhythmic properties of d-propranolol, dl-propranolol and quinidine. *J. Pharmacol. Exp. Ther*. 158: 11-21, 1967.

1091. Giudicelli, J.-F., *et al*. Studies on dl-4-(2-hydroxy-3-isopropylaminopropoxy)-indole (LB 46), a new potent ß-adrenergic blocking drug. *J. Pharmacol. Exp. Ther*. 168: 116-126, 1969.

1092. Stitzer, M., *et al*. Effects of nicotine on fixed interval behavior and their modification by cholinergic antagonists. *J. Pharmacol. Exp. Ther*. 171: 166-177, 1970.

1093. Carlson, G.M., *et al*. Effects of nicotine on gastric antral and duodenal contractile activity in the dog. *J. Pharmacol. Exp. Ther*. 172: 367-376, 1970.

1094. Alexander, G.J., *et al*. Lysergic acid diethylamide intake in pregnancy: Fetal damage in rats. *J. Pharmacol. Exp. Ther*. 173: 48-59, 1970

1095. Kubena, R.K. and H. Barry, III. Interactions of Δ^1-tetrahydrocannibinol with barbiturates and methamphetamine. *J. Pharmacol. Exp. Ther*. 173: 94-100, 1970.

1096. Killam, K.F., *et al*. An animal model of light sensitive epilepsy. *Electroencephalogr. Clin. Neurophysiol*. 22: 497-513, 1967.

Bibliography

1097. Stark, I.G., *et al.* The anticonvulsant effects of phenobarbital, diphenylhydantoin and two benzodiazepines in the baboon. *Papio papio. J. Pharmacol. Exp. Ther.* 173: 125-132, 1970.

1098. Baker, R.G. and E.G. Anderson. The effects of L-3,4-dihydroxyphenylalanine on spinal reflex activity. *J. Pharmacol. Exp. Ther.* 173: 212-223, 1970.

1099. Herz, A., *et al.* Central nicotine- and muscarinelike properties of cholinomimetic drugs with regard to their lipid solubilities. *Ann. N.Y. Acad. Sci.* 142: 21-26, 1967.

1100. Vazquez, A.J. and J.E.P. Toman. Some interactions of nicotine with other drugs upon central nervous function. *Ann. N.Y. Acad. Sci.* 142: 201-215, 1967.

1001. Morrison, C.F. and A.K. Armitage. Effects of nicotine upon the free operant behavior of rats and spontaneous motor activity of mice. *Ann. N.Y. Acad. Sci.* 142: 268-276, 1967.

1102. Kadzielawa, K. and E. Widy. The influence of imipramine on the central effects of dihydroxyphenylalanine. *Neuropharmacology* 9: 467-480, 1970.

1103. Banna, N.R. and S.J. Jabbur. The action of bemegride on presynaptic inhibition. *Neuropharmacology* 9: 553-560, 1970.

1104. Kirkpatrick, W.E. and P. Lomax. Temperature changes induced by chlorpromazine and N-methyl chlorpromazine in the rat. *Neuropharmacology* 10: 61-66, 1971.

1105. Fuentes, J.A. and V.G. Longo. An investigation on the central effects of harmine, harmaline and related ß-carbolines. *Neuropharmacology* 10: 15-23, 1971.

1106. Peterson, A.E. and C.N. Gillis. Pharmacological alteration of cardiovascular changes secondary to hypothalamic stimulation in rats. *Fed. Proc.* 29: 741, 1970.

1107. Korol, B. and M.L. Brown. A behavioral and autonomic nervous system study of RO-5-3350 and diazepam in conscious dogs. *Pharmacology* 1: 115-128, 1968.

1108. Yen, H.C.Y., *et al.* Effects of some psychoactive drugs on experimental "neurotic" (conflict induced) behavior in cats. *Pharmacology* 3: 32-40, 1970.

1109. Evangelista, A.M., *et al.* Effect of amphetamine, nicotine, and hexamethonium on performance of a conditioned response during acquisition and retention trials. *Pharmacology* 3: 91-96, 1970.

1110. Schueler, F.W. The mechanisms of action of the hemicholiniums. *Int. Rev. Neurobiol.* 2: 77-97, 1960.

1111. Lomax, P. Drugs and body temperature. *Int. Rev. Neurobiol.* 12: 1-43, 1970.

1112. Singh, K.P. and M.M. Mahawar. Some inhibitory actions of catecholamines and their blockade by propranolol. *Arch. Int. Pharmacodyn.* 171: 58-67, 1968.

Bibliography

1113. Mazurkiewicz, I.M. The effects of ß-adrenergic receptor blockade on the blood pressure and heart rate changes induced by noradrenaline infusion and postinfusional hypotension. *Arch. Int. Pharmacodyn.* 171: 136-158, 1968.

1114. Rodriguez, R. and E.G. Pardo. Drug reversal of pain induced functional impairment. *Arch. Int. Pharmacodyn.* 172: 148-160, 1968.

1115. Chen, G., *et al*. Studies of drug effects on electrically induced extensor seizures and clinical implications. *Arch. Int. Pharmacodyn.* 172: 183-218, 1968.

1116. Cohen, M. and H. Wakeley. A comparative behavioral study of ditran and LSD in mice, rats, and dogs. *Arch. Int. Pharmacodyn.* 173: 316-326, 1968.

1117. Straw, R.N. The effect of certain benzodiazepines on the threshold for pentylenetetrazol-induced seizures in the cat. *Arch. Int. Pharmacodyn.* 175: 464-469, 1968.

1118. Dandiya, P.C. and L.P. Bhargava. The antiparkinsonian activity of monoamine oxidase inhibitors and other agents in rats and mice. *Arch. Int. Pharmacodyn.* 176: 157-167, 1968.

1119. Weller, C.P., *et al*. Analgesic profile of tranquilizers in multiple screening tests in mice. *Arch. Int. Pharmacodyn.* 177: 287-289, 1968.

1120. Erill, S. Persistence of the hypoglycemic effect of tolbutamide after block of ß-adrenergic receptors. *Arch. Int. Pharmacodyn.* 177: 88-91, 1969.

1121. Ganesan, D. Influence of female sex hormones on pentobarbitone sodium anesthesia in rats. *Arch. Int. Pharmacodyn.* 177: 88-91, 1969.

1122. Bernauer, W., *et al*. Comparison of the antilethal, broncholytic, and antiemphysematous activities of mepyramine in anaphylactic, histamine, and anaphylatoxin shock of guinea pigs. *Arch. Int. Pharmacodyn.* 178: 137-151, 1969.

1123. Randall, L.O., *et al*. Pharmacological studies on fluazepam hydrochloride (R05-6901), a new psychotropic agent of the benzodiazepine class. *Arch. Int. Pharmacodyn.* 178: 216-241, 1969.

1124. Marchetti, E. Pharmacological activities of a new antitussive agent: Morphethylbutyne. *Arch. Int. Pharmacodyn.* 178: 400-406, 1969.

1125. Wardell, J.R., Jr. and R.G. Staples, III. Animal studies comparing the neuropharmacological profile of a trifluoperazine HCl-amobarbital combination with that of the individual components. *Arch. Int. Pharmacodyn.* 179: 106-120, 1969.

1126. McClure, D.A. 4-Dimethyl-amino methyl-2-methyl 1,3-dioxolane--a new potent analgesic agent. *Arch. Int. Pharmacodyn.* 179: 154-160, 1969.

1127. Yamamoto, J. and A. Sekiya. On the pressor action of propanolol in the rat. *Arch. Int. Pharmacodyn.* 179: 372-380, 1969.

Bibliography

1128. Stockhaus, K und H. Wick. Toxizitätsunterschiede von pharmaka bei subcutaner, intragastraler and introduodenaler applikation bei Ratten. *Arch. Int. Pharmacodyn.* 180: 155-161, 1969.

1129. Molinengo, L. and S. Ricci Gamalero. Behavioral action and tranquilizing effects of reserpine, diazepam and hydroxyzine. *Arch. Int. Pharmacodyn.* 180: 217-231, 1969.

1130. Chopra, Y.M. and P.C. Dandiya. On the mechanism of reversal of reserpine action by pargyline hydrochloride. *Arch. Int. Pharmacodyn.* 181: 68-93, 1969.

1131. Carminati, G.M. Attivita comparata di svariatifarmaci in alcuni tests sperimentali di studio del compartamento. *Arch. Int. Pharmacodyn.* 181: 68-93, 1969.

1132. Blum, K. The effect of dopamine and other catecholamines on neuromuscular transmission. *Arch. Int. Pharmacodyn.* 181: 297-306, 1969.

1133. Parra, J. and H. Vidrio. Drug effects on the blood pressure response to postural changes in the unanesthetized rabbit. *Arch. Int. Pharmacodyn.* 181: 353-362, 1969.

1134. Barrett, W.E., *et al.* Pharmacological investigation of a new orally active anti-arrhythmic drug Su-13197. *Arch. Int. Pharmacodyn.* 182: 65-77, 1969.

1135. Isem, G.E., *et al.* A Comparison of the lethal and respiratory effects of morphine in Long-Evans and Sprague-Dawley rats. *Arch. Int. Pharmacodyn.* 182: 130-138, 1969.

1136. Voith, K. and F. Herr. Psychopharmacological evaluation of a new antidepressant: butriptyline. *Arch. Int. Pharmacodyn.* 182: 318-331, 1969.

1137. Pickering, R.W. A method for the quantitative assessment of compounds affecting respiration in conscious mice: Effect of four selected respiratory stimulants. *Arch. Int. Pharmacodyn.* 183: 12-15, 1970.

1138. Salmon, G.K. and J.D. Ireson. A correlation between the hypotensive action of methyl-dopa and its depression of peripheral sympathetic function. *Arch. Int. Pharmacodyn.* 183: 60-64, 1970.

1139. Rosenblum, W.I. Antihypertensive effect of nylidrin HCl. *Arch. Int. Pharmacodyn.* 183: 85-92, 1970.

1140. Rosic, N. Partial antagonism by cholinesterase reactivators of the effects of organophosphate compounds on shuttle-box avoidance. *Arch. Int. Pharmacodyn.* 1183: 139-147, 1970.

1141. Oliver, J.H., *et al.* Effect of reserpine and other drugs on the CNS and lethal effects of hyperbaric oxygen on mice. *Arch. Int. Pharmacodyn.* 183: 215-223, 1970.

1142. Chernov, H.I., *et al.* Pharmacological properties of Su-19789B, a unique central nervous system stimulant. *Arch. Int. Pharmacodyn.* 184: 34-44, 1970.

Bibliography

1143. Cloutier, G., *et al.* Evaluation pharmacodynamique d'un nouveau curarisant de synthese: la gallamine-acetylenique. *Arch. Int. Pharmacodyn.* 184: 75-92, 1970.

1144. Malick, J.B. and M.E. Goldberg. Effects of a choline acetyltransferase inhibitor on self-stimulatory behavior in the rat. *Arch. Int. Pharmacodyn.* 184: 254-256, 1970.

1145. Weinreich, D. and L.D. Clark. Anticonvulsant drugs and self-stimulation rates in rats. *Arch. Int. Pharmacodyn.* 185: 269-273, 1970.

1146. Lumachi, B., *et al.* Comparative pharmacological investigations on naphthypramide and some anti-inflammatory and skeletal muscle relaxant agents. *Arch. Int. Pharmacodyn.* 186: 66-83, 1970.

1147. Malick, J.B. Effects of selected drugs on stimulus-bound emotional behavior elicited by hypothalamic stimulation in the cat. *Arch. Int. Pharmacodyn.* 186: 137-141, 1970.

1148. Hudson, R.D. and M.K. Wolpert. Anticonvulsant and motor depressant effects of diazepam. *Arch. Int. Pharmacodyn.* 186: 388-401, 1970.

1149. Feinstein, M.B., *et al.* The antagonism of local anesthetic induced convulsions by the benzodiazepine derivative diazepam. *Arch. Int. Pharmacodyn.* 187: 144-154, 1970.

1150. Longo, V.G., *et al.* Effects of nicotine on the electroencephalogram of the rabbit. *Ann. N.Y. Acad. Sci.* 142: 159-169, 1967.

1151. Brown, B.B. Relationship between evoked response changes and behavior following small doses of nicotine. *Ann. N.Y. Acad. Sci.* 142: 190-200, 1967.

1152. Leszkovsky, G. and L.J. Tardos. Some effects of propranolol on the central nervous system. *J. Pharm. Pharmac.* 17: 518-519, 1965.

1153. Agarwal, S.L. and D. Bose. The role of brain catecholamines in drug induced tremor. *Br. J. Pharmac. Chemother.* 30: 349-353, 1967.

1154. Korol, B. and M.L. Brown. The role of the ß-adrenergic system in behavior: Anti-depressant effects of propranolol. *Curr. Therap. Res.* 9: 269-279, 1967.

1155. Aron, C., *et al.* Evaluation of a rapid technique for detecting minor tranquilizers. *Neuropharmacology* 10: 459-469, 1971.

1156. Nichols, R.E. and E.J. Walaszek. Antagonism of drug induced catatonia. *Fed. Proc.* 24: 390, 1965.

1157. Staff, Department of Pharmacology, University of Edinburgh. *Pharmacological Experiments on Isolated Preparations.* E. and S. Livingstone Ltd. Edinburgh and London, 1968.

1158. Bohdanecky, Z., *et al.* The effect of neocortical and hippocampal spreading depression on the slow wave EEG activity induced by atropine. *Arch. Int. Pharmacodyn.* 148: 545-556, 1964.

Bibliography

1159.   White, R.P., *et al.* Phylogenetic comparison of central actions produced by different doses of atropine and hyoscine. *Arch. Int. Pharmacodyn.* 132: 349-363, 1961.

1160.   Wikler, A. Pharmacologic dissociation of behavior and EEG "Sleep Patterns" in dogs: Morphine, N-allylnormorphine and atropine. *Proc. Soc. Exp. Biol. Med.* 79: 261-265, 1952.

1161.   McGaugh, *et al.* Electroencephalographic and behavior analysis of drug effects on an instrumental reward discrimination in rabbits. *Psychopharmacologia* 4: 126-138, 1963.

1162.   Rozhkova, E.K. Fiziologicheskaya rol atsetilkolinai izyskania novykh veshchesto in Mikhelson, M.Y. *Len. Med. Insti. in Pavlova* 230 pp 1957.

1163.   Samuel, G.K., *et al.* Effects of scopolamine and atropine and their quaternized salts on avoidance behavior in monkey. *Psychopharmacologia* 8: 205-301, 1965.

1164.   Valenstein, E.S. A note on anesthetizing rats and Guinea pigs. *J. Exp. Anal. Behav.* 4: 6, 1961.

1165.   Schallek, W. and A. Kuehn. Effects of benzodiazepines on spontaneous EEG and arousal responses of cats. *Prog. in Brain Research* 18: 231-238, 1965.

1166.   Rensch, B. and G. Ducker. Verzogerung de Vegessens erlernter visueller Aufgaben bei Tieren durch Chlorpromazin. *Pfülgers Archiv.* 289: 200-214, 1966.

1167.   Maickel, R., *et al.* Control of adipose tissue lipase activity by the sympathetic nervous system. *Life. Sci.* 3: 210-214, 1963.

1168.   Corson, S.A., *et al.* Ephedrine antagonism to behavioral and antidiuretic effects of reserpine. *Fed. Proc.* 24: 197, 1965.

1169.   Pscheidt, G.R., *et al.* Studies on norepinephrine and 5-hydroxytryptamine in various species. *Comparative Neurochemistry.* Charles Birchall and Sons, London, 1963.

1170.   Pscheidt, G.R. and H.E. Himwich. Reserpine, monoamine oxidase inhibitors and distribution of biogenic amines in monkey brain. *Biochem. Pharmacol.* 12: 65-71, 1963.

1171.   Diamantis, W. and M. Kletzkin. Evaluation of muscle relaxant drugs by head-drop and by decerebrate rigidity. *Int. J. Neuropharmicol.* 5: 305-310, 1966.

1172.   Williams, B., *et al.* Electrical activity of the prepyriform cortex after reserpine in the rat. *J. Pharmacol. Exp. Ther.* 150: 10-16, 1965.

1173.   Meyers, B., *et al.* Some effects of muscarinic cholinergic blocking drugs on behavior and the electrocorticogram. *Psychopharmacologia* 5: 289-300, 1964.

Bibliography

1174. Charney, N.H. and G.S. Reynolds. Development of behavioral compensation to the effects of scopolamine during fixed-interval reinforcement. *J. Exptl. Anal. Behavior* 8: 183-186, 1965.

1175. Motokizawa, F. and B. Fujimori. Arousal effect of afferent discharges from muscle spindles upon electroencephalograms in cats. *Jap. J. Physiol.* 14: 344-353, 1964.

1176. Marsh, D.F. Pharmacological activity of 2-amino-5-chlorobenzoxazole (zoxazolamine, Flexin). I. Duration of action. *Fed. Proc.* 16: 319, 1957.

1177. Antonaccio, M.J. Reflex responses to vertical tilting in dogs: A comparison with bilateral carotid occlusion. *Pharmacologist* 13: 192, 1971.

1178. Winger, G.D., *et al.* Patterns of barbiturate-reinforced responding in the Rhesus monkey. *Pharmacologist* 13: 206, 1971.

1179. Cumming, J.F. Development of acute tolerance to ketamine in the rat. *Pharmacologist* 13: 212, 1971.

1180. Volier, L. Effect of ethanol on adenosine 3',5'-monophosphate (cyclic AMP) in rat tissues in vivo. *Pharmacologist* 13: 213, 1971.

1181. Schleimer, R., *et al.* The anti-arrhythmic activity of dihydroergotamine (DHE). *Pharmacologist* 13: 225, 1971.

1182. Hill, H. and A. Horita. Amphetamine-induced hyperthermia in rabbits. *Pharmacologist* 12: 197, 1970.

1183. Tseng, L.F. and E.J. Walazek. Influence of alteration of catecholamine and serotonin levels on bulbocapnine-induced catatonia. *Pharmacologist* 12: 298, 1970.

1184. Gessa, A., *et al.* Essential role of testosterone in the sexual stimulation induced by p-chlorophenylalanine (PCPA) in male animals. *Pharmacologist* 12: 204, 1970.

1185. Hosko, M.J. and H.F. Hardman. Effect of Δ^9-THC on cardiovascular responses to stimulation of vasopressor loci in the neuraxis of anesthetized cats. *Pharmacologist* 13: 296, 1971.

1186. Tagliamonte, P., *et al.* Differential effect of p-chlorophenylalanine (PCPA) on the sexual behavior and on the electrocorticogram of male rabbits. *Pharmacologist* 12: 205, 1970.

1187. Gallager, D.W., *et al.* Dissociation between behavioral effects and changes in metabolism of cerebral serotonin (5HT) following Δ^9-tetrahydrocannabinol (THC). *Pharmacologist* 13: 296, 1971.

1188. Menon, M.K., *et al.* Lowering of brain histamine (Hm) by parachlorophenylalanine (PCPA) and a new histidine decarboxylase inhibitor. *Pharmacologist* 12: 205, 1970.

Bibliography

1189. Spaulding, T.C., *et al*. The pharmacological effects and the lack of Δ^9-THC blocking activity of phenitrone. *Pharmacologist* 13: 296, 1971.

1190. Hartmann, R.J. and I. Geller. Effects of para-chlorophenylalanine (p-CPA) on a conditioned emotional response (CER) in laboratory rats. *Pharmacologist* 12: 206, 1970.

1191. Thompson, G.R., *et al*. Neurotoxicity of cannabinoids in chronically-treated rats and monkeys. *Pharmacologist* 13: 296, 1971.

1192. Dewey, W.L., *et al*. Some acute and chronic interactions between Δ^9-THC and morphine in mice. *Pharmacologist* 13: 296, 1971.

1193. Mantilla-Plata, B. and R.D. Harbison. Phenobarbital and SKF 525-A effect on Δ^9-tetrahydrocannabinol (THC) toxicity and distribution in mice. *Pharmacologist* 13: 297, 1971.

1194. Gomoll, A.W. Comparative effects of propranolol (P) and sotalol (S) on myocardial contractility. *Pharmacologist* 12: 213, 1970.

1195. Joy, R.M. and K.F. Killam. A comparison of acute and chronic diazepam on the EEG. *Pharmacologist* 12: 218, 1970.

1196. Stern, W.C., *et al*. Effects of lysergic acid diethylamide (LSD) on sleep and spiking activity in the lateral geniculate nucleus (LGN) of the cat. *Pharmacologist* 13: 306, 1971.

1197. Sawyer, N. and R. Mundy. Autonomic responses in the mouse. *Pharmacologist* 12: 246, 1970.

1198. Carlini, E.A., *et al*. Effects of (-) Δ^9-trans-tetrahydrocannabinol and a synthetic derivative on maze performance of rats. *Pharmacologist* 4: 359-368, 1970.

1199. Schlosser, W., *et al*. Indications of a possible dopamine receptor at the spinal level. *Pharmacologist* 12: 287, 1970.

1200. Spratto, G.R. and J.H. Mennear. Effects of propranolol on blood glucose responses in the mouse. *Pharmacologist* 11: 253, 1969.

1201. Thut, P.D. and R.H. Rech. Electrocorticographic (ECoG) and behavioral effects of diethyldithiocarbamate (DDC) and L-DOPA. *Pharmacologist* 11: 254, 1969.

1202. Barnes, C.D. and O. Pompeiano. The interaction of brain stem adrenergic systems and VIIIth nerve stimulation on the spinal cord. *Neuropharmacology* 10: 437-446, 1971.

1203. Bhattacharya, I.C. and L. Goldstein. Influence of acute and chronic nicotine administration on the electrical activity of the rabbit brain. *Pharmacologist* 11: 254, 1969.

Bibliography

1204. Garrett, R.L. and J.H. Brown. Bradykinin-potentiated contractions induced by serotonin (5-HT), norepinephrine (NE) and potassium (K$^+$) in rabbit aortic strips. *Pharmacologist* 12: 347, 1970.

1205. Echols, S.D. and R.E. Jewett. Effects of morphine (M) on the sleep of cats. *Pharmacologist* 11: 254, 1969.

1206. Jaju, B.P. and S.C. Wang. Effects of diphenhydramine and dimenhydrinate on vestibular neuronal activity in cats. *Pharmacologist* 12: 270, 1970.

1207. Peng, Tai-Chan and C.W. Cooper. The hypocalcemic effect of ethanol in rats and dogs. *Pharmacologist* 12: 277, 1970.

1208. Chai, Kyoung and C.K. Erikson. Cholinergic modification of ethanol-induced EEG synchrony. *Pharmacologist* 12: 277, 1970.

1209. Sharkawi, M. Effects of some centrally active drugs on acetylcholine synthesis in rat brain. *Pharmacologist* 12: 294, 1970.

1210. Torchiana, M.L., *et al.* Pharmacological antagonism of the chronotropic and central manifestations of amitriptyline intoxication in unanesthetized dogs. *Pharmacologist* 11: 283, 1969.

1211. Gillis, R.A., *et al.* Effect of diphenylhydantoin on spontaneous sympathetic nerve activity. *Pharmacologist* 12: 304, 1970.

1212. Arnold, A. and J.P. McAuliff. α-adrenergic receptor mediated hyperglycemia in the laboratory rodent. *Pharmacologist* 12: 306, 1970.

1213. Proudfit, H.K. and S. Norton. The effect of morphine on the evoked potential and multiunit activity of the rat superior colliculus. *Fed. Proc.* 29: 252, 1970.

1214. Hazra, J. Disinhibition of the inhibitory effect of darkness on optic evoked potentials by lidocaine. *Fed. Proc.* 29: 252, 1970.

1215. Goridis, C. and N.H. Neff. Monoamine oxidase: Approximation of turnover rates in brain and peripheral tissues of rat. *Fed. Proc.* 30: 382, 1971.

1216. Cain, S.M. O_2 uptake during and after exercise with and without ß-adrenergic blockade. *Fed. Proc.* 29: 265, 1970.

1217. Thurman, A.E., *et al.* Altered vascular responsiveness-initial hypotensive mechanism of thiazide diuretics. *Fed. Proc.* 29: 273, 1970.

1218. O'Rourke, R.A., *et al.* Effect of amyl nitrate and nitroglycerin on cardiovascular hemodynamics in the conscious animal. *Fed. Proc.* 29: 274, 1970.

1219. Smith, C.M. and P. Luna. Effects of vasodilator drugs on ear skin temperatures in guinea pigs. *Fed. Proc.* 29: 274, 1970.

Bibliography

1220. Vernadakis, A. and P.S. Timiras. Interrelation between convulsant drugs and X-radiation on the central nervous system of rats. *Arch. Int. Pharmacodyn.* 170: 146-151, 1967.

1221. Strobel, G.E. and H. Wollman. Pharmacology of anesthetic agents. *Fed. Proc.* 28: 1386-1403, 1969.

1222. Faingold, C.L. and C.A. Berry. Studies of antihistamine-induced EEG paroxysms in the cat. *Fed. Proc.* 29: 384, 1970.

1223. Levin, P. The effect of anti-petit mal drugs on photic driving in the rabbit. *Fed. Proc.* 29: 384, 1970.

1224. Dempsey, P.J., *et al.* Evidence for a direct myocardial effect of angiotensin. II. *Fed. Proc.* 29: 389, 1970.

1225. Clark, C. and V.J. Lotti. Attenuation of the vomiting response to L-dopa after decarboxylase inhibition. *Fed. Proc.* 29: 512, 1970.

1226. Tang, A.H. Effects of L-dopa on a polysynaptic spinal reflex of the rat. *Fed. Proc.* 29: 512, 1970.

1227. Lomax, P. Animal pharmacology of marihuana. *Proc. West. Pharmacol. Soc.* 14: 10-13, 1971.

1228. Koerpel, B.J. and L.D. Davis. Effect of lidocaine (L), propranolol (P) and MJ1999 on ouabain-induced changes in membrane potential of purkinje fibers. *Fed. Proc.* 29: 517, 1970.

1229. Matsuzaki, M. and K.F. Killam. The effect of multiple doses of diphenylhydantoin on intensity discrimination in the cat. *Proc. West. Pharmacol. Soc.* 14: 145-148, 1971.

1230. Uyeno, E.T. Behavioral effects of phenothiazines and barbiturates on the squirrel monkey. *Proc. West. Pharmacol. Soc.* 14: 149-153, 1971.

1231. Marchand, C., *et al.* The effect of SKF-525A on the distribution of CCl_4 in rats. *Fed. Proc.* 29: 544, 1970.

1232. Clifford, D.H. and L.R. Soma. Feline anesthesia. *Fed. Proc.* 28: 1479-1499, 1969.

1233. Weisenthal, L. Adrenergic mechanisms in relaxation of guinea pig teniae coli. *Fed. Proc.* 29: 550, 1970.

1234. Weisse, A.B., *et al.* Prophylaxis and treatment of ventricular arrhythmias in acute myocardial infarction: A comparison of three agents. *Fed. Proc.* 29: 585, 1970.

1235. Hoar, R.M. Anesthesia in the guinea pig. *Fed. Proc.* 28: 1517-1521, 1969.

1236. Cervoni, P. and E. Reit. Angiotensin and norepinephrine (NE): Interaction on the cat nictitating membrane. *Fed. Proc.* 29: 614, 1970.

Bibliography

1237. Smith, A.A. and K. Hayashida. Blockade or reversal of propranolol of the narcotic and respiratory depression induced in mice by ethanol. *Fed. Proc.* 29: 649, 1970.

1238. Dewey, W.L., *et al.* Some autonomic gastrointestinal and metabolic effects of two constitutents of marihuana. *Fed. Proc.* 29: 650, 1970.

1239. Goldstein, M.L. Effect of LSD-25, and psilocybin on norepinephrine and 3H-norepinephrine metabolites in rat brain. *Fed. Proc.* 29: 650, 1970.

1240. Goldstein, M., *et al.* The effects of antiparkinsonian drugs (AP) on striatal dopamine. *Fed. Proc.* 29: 680, 1970.

1241. Kirkpatrick, W.E. and P. Lomax. Chlorpromazine and body temperature. *Proc. West Pharmacol. Soc.* 13: 169-172, 1970.

1242. Shaikh, M.I., *et al.* Acute and chronic effects of nicotine on rat gastric secretion. *Proc. West. Pharmacol. Soc.* 13: 178-184, 1970.

1243. Tseng, L.F. and E.J. Walazek. Blockade of the dopamine response by bulbocapnine. *Fed. Proc.* 29: 741, 1970.

1244. Lamarre, Y., *et al.* Harmaline-induced rhythmic activity of cerebellar and lower brain stem neurons. *Brain Res.* 32: 246-250, 1971.

1245. Jondorf, W.R., *et al.* Inability of newborn mice and guinea pigs to metabolize drugs. *Biochem. Pharmacol.* 1: 352-354, 1958.

1246. Davis, W.M. Day-night periodicity in pentobarbital response of mice and the influence of socio-psychological conditions. *Experentia* 18: 235-237, 1962.

1247. Lutsky, I. Preoperative evaluation and preparation of canines. *Fed. Proc.* 28: 1420-1422, 1969.

1248. Quinn, G.P., *et al.* Species, strain and sex differences in metabolism of hexabarbitone, amidopyrine, antipyrine and aniline. *Biochem. Pharmacol.* 1: 152-159, 1958.

1249. Woods, L.A. and H.E. Muehlenbeck. Urinary excretion of codeine and its metabolite(s) in the dog. *J. Pharmacol. Exp. Ther.* 110: 54, 1954.

1250. Axelrod, J. Studies on sympathomimetic amines. I. The biotransformation and physiological disposition of 1-norephedrine. *J. Pharmacol. Exp. Ther.* 109: 62-73, 1953.

1251. Fuhrman, G.J. and F.A. Fuhrman. Effects of temperature on the action of drugs. *Ann. Rev. Pharmacol.* 1: 65-78, 1961.

1252. Blair, E. Generalized hypothermia. *Fed. Proc.* 28: 1456-1462, 1969.

Bibliography

1253. Goldstein, A., *et al. Principles of Drug Action. The Basis of Pharmacology.* 2nd ed., John Wiley and Sons, Inc., New York, 1974.

1254. Usubiaga, J.E., *et al.* Interaction of intravenously administered procaine, lidocaine and succinylcholine in anesthetized subjects. *Anesth. and Analg.* 46: 39-45, 1967.

1255. Saidman, L.J. and E.I. Eger, II. The effect of thiopental metabolism on duration of anesthesia. *Anesthesiology* 27: 118-126, 1966.

1256. Gillette, J.R., *et al.* Isolation from rat brain of a metabolic product, desmethylimipramine that mediates the antidepressant activity of imipramine (Totranil). *Experentia* 17: 417-418, 1961.

1257. Gillette, J.R. Biochemistry of drug oxidation and reduction by enzymes in hepatic endoplasmic reticulum. *Adv. Pharmacol.* 4: 219-261, 1966.

1258. Conney, A. Pharmacological implications of microsomal enzyme induction. *Pharmacol. Rev.* 19: 317-366, 1967.

1259. Burns, J.J. and A.H. Conney. Enzyme stimulation and inhibition in the metabolism of drugs. *Proc. Roy. Soc. Med.* 58: 955-960, 1965.

1260. Adams, H.R. and B.N. Dixit. Prolongation of pentobarbital anesthesia by chloramphenical in dogs and cats. *J.A.V.M.A.* 156: 902-905, 1970.

1261. VanDyke, R.A. and M.B. Chenoweth. Metabolism of volatile anesthetics. *Anesthesiology* 26: 348-357, 1965.

1262. VanDyke, R.A. Metabolism of volatile anesthetics. III. Induction of microsomal dechlorinating and ether-cleaving enzymes. *J. Pharmacol. Exp. Ther.* 154: 364-369, 1966.

1263. Miller, E.V., *et al.* (Ed.) Comparative anesthesia in laboratory animals. *Fed. Proc.* 28: 1373-1586, 1969.

1264. Priano, L.L., *et al.* Barbiturate anesthesia: An abnormal physiologic situation. *J. Pharmacol. Exp. Ther.* 165: 126-135, 1969.

1265ò &amWissehr- HòXò- *et al.* Left ventricular dynamics in dogs during anesthesia with α-chloralose and sodium pentobarbital. *Am. J. Cardio.* 13: 349-354, 1964.

1266. Buss, B.G. and N.M. Buckley. Chloralose anesthesia in the dog: A study of drug actions and analytical methodology. *Am.J. Physiol.* 210: 854-862, 1966.

1267. Maynert, E.W. The usefulness of clinical signs for the comparison of intravenous anesthetics in dogs. *J. Pharmacol. Exp. Ther.* 128: 182-191, 1960.

1268. Maynert, E.W., *et al.* Acute tolerance to intravenous anesthetics in dogs. *J. Pharmacol. Exp. Ther.* 128: 192-200, 1960.

Bibliography

1269. Smith, T.C. and H. Wollman. History and principles of anesthesiology. In: *The Pharmacological Basis of Therapeutics,* ed. Goodman and Gilman. 7th edition, MacMillan Co., New York, 1985.

1270. Stevens, W.C., *et al.* The cardiovascular effects of a new inhalation anesthetic, Forane, in human volunteers at constant arterial carbon dioxide tension. *Anesthesiology* 35: 8-16, 1971.

1271. Merkel, G. and E. Eger, II. A comparative study of halothane and halopropane anesthesia. Including method for determining equipotency. *Anesthesiology* 24: 346-357, 1963.

1272. Waizer, P., *et al.* Microvascular reactions at known depth of anesthesia. *Fed. Proc.* 29: 354, 1970.

1273. Johnson, E.S., *et al.* The responses of cortical neurons to monoamines under differing anesthetic conditions. *J. Physiol.* 203: 261-280, 1969.

1274. Eger, E.I., II., *et al.* Temperature dependence of halothane and cyclopropane anesthesia in dogs: Correlation with some theories of anesthetic action. *Anesthesiology* 26: 764-770, 1965.

1275. Eger, E.I., II., *et al.* Equipotent alveolar concentrations of methoxyflurane, halothane, diethyl ether, fluroxene, cyclopropane, xeron and nitrous oxide in the dog. *Anesthesiology* 26: 771-777, 1965.

1276. Skorobogatov, V.I. The central action of curarizing drugs. In: *Progress in Brain Research* 20: 243-255, 1967.

1277. Severinghaus, J.W. and C.P. Larson, Jr. Respiration in anesthesia. In: Fenn, W. O. and H. Rahn. *Handbook of Physiology-Respiration II,* 1219-1264, American Physiology Soc., Washington, D.C., 1965.

1278. Venes, J.L., *et al.* Nitrous oxide: an anesthetic for experiments in cats. *Am. J. Physiol.* 220: 2028-2031, 1971.

1279. Carpenter, H.M. and G.H. Mudge. Acetaminophen nephrotoxicity: Studies on renal acetylation and deacetylation. *J. Pharmacol. Exp. Ther.* 218: 161-167, 1981.

1280. Corcoran, G.B. and B.K. Wong. Obesity as a risk factor in drug-induced organ injury: Increased liver and kidney damage by acetaminophen in the obese overfed rat. *J. Pharmacol. Exp. Ther.* 241: 921-927, 1987.

1281. Letteron, P., *et al.* Pre- or post-treatment with methoxsalen prevents the hepatotoxicity of acetaminophen in mice. *J. Pharmacol. Exp. Ther.* 239: 559-567, 1986.

1282. Speeg, K.V., *et al.* Additive protection of cimetidine and N-acetylcysteine treatment against acetaminophen-induced hepatic necrosis in the rat. *J. Pharmacol. Exp. Ther.* 234: 550-554, 1985.

Bibliography

1283.   Wong, S. and J.F. Gardocki. Anti-inflammatory and antiarthritic evaluation of acetaminophen and its potentiation of tolmetin. *J. Pharmacol. Exp. Ther.* 226: 625-632, 1983.

1284.   Winter, C.A., *et al.* Analgesic activity of diflunisal [MK-647; 5-(2,4-difluorophenyl) salicylic acid] in rats with hyperalgesia induced by Freund's adjuvant. *J. Pharmacol. Exp. Ther.* 211: 678-685, 1979.

1285.   Gray, J.A. and R.J. Kavlock. Pharmacologic probing of mercuric chloride-induced renal dysfunction in the neonatal rat. *J. Pharmacol. Exp. Ther.* 242: 212-216, 1987.

1286.   Langberg, H., *et al.* Inhibitory effect of acetazolamide on renal tubular reabsorption of $NaHCO_3$ and $NaCl$ in dogs varies inversely with plasma pH. *J. Pharmacol. Exp. Ther.* 234: 747-753, 1985.

1287.   Vogh, B.P. and D.R. Godman. Addition of the effects of norepinephrine and acetazolamide to decrease formation of cerebrospinal fluid. *J. Pharmacol. Exp. Ther.* 229: 207-209, 1984.

1288.   Johanson, C.E. Differential effects of acetazolamide, benzolamide and systemic acidosis on hydrogen and bicarbonate gradients across the apical and basolateral membranes of the choroid plexus. *J. Pharmacol. Exp. Ther.* 231: 502-511, 1984.

1289.   Vogh, B. The relation of choroid plexus carbonic anhydrase activity to cerebrospinal fluid formation: Study of three inhibitors in the cat with extrapolation to man. *J. Pharmacol. Exp. Ther.* 213: 321-331, 1980.

1290.   Lineberry, M.D. and L.C. Waite. Acidosis inhibits the hypocalcemic effect of acetazolamide. *J. Pharmacol. Exp. Ther.* 211: 452-455, 1979.

1291.   Vinegar, R., *et al.* Quantitative comparison of the analgesic and antiinflammatory activity of aspirin, phenacetin, and acetaminophen in rodents. *Eur. J. Pharmacol.* 37: 23-30, 1976.

1292.   Torchiana, M.L., *et al.* The anticonvulsant effect of carbonic anhydrase inhibitors in mice--A noradrenergic mechanism of action. *Eur. J. Pharmacol.* 21: 343-349, 1973.

1293.   Michael-Titus, A., *et al.* Role of endogenous enkephalins in locomotion evidenced by acetorphan, an "enkephalinase" inhibitor. *J. Pharmacol. Exp. Ther.* 243: 1062-1066, 1987.

1294.   Lecomte, J., *et al.* Pharmacological properties of acetorphan, a parenterally active "enkephalinase" inhibitor. *J. Pharmacol. Exp. Ther.* 237: 937-944, 1986.

1295.   Nayler, R.A. and H.W. Mitchell. Airways hyperreactivity and bronchoconstriction induced by vanadate in the guinea-pig. *Brit. J. Pharmacol.* 92: 173-180, 1987.

1296.   Hackett, D. and W.R. Buckett. Drug effects in a novel biphasic writhing syndrome induced by acetylcholine in mice. *Eur. J. Pharmacol.* 30: 280-287, 1975.

603

Bibliography

1297.   Carrier, G.O. and R.S. Aronstam. Altered muscarinic receptor properties and function in the heart in diabetes. *J. Pharmacol. Exp. Ther.* 242: 531-535, 1987.

1298.   Kalsner, S. and M. Quillan. Presynaptic interactions between acetylcholine and adrenergic antagonists on norepinephrine release. *J. Pharmacol. Exp. Ther.* 244: 879-891, 1988.

1299.   Ichihara, K., *et al.* Inhibition of ischemia-induced subcellular redistribution of lysosomal enzymes in the perfused rat heart by the calcium entry blocker, diltiazem. *J. Pharmacol. Exp. Ther.* 242: 1109-1113, 1987.

1300.   Hjelle, J.J., *et al.* Comparison of the effects of sodium sulfate and N-acetyl-cysteine on the hepatotoxicity of acetaminophen in mice. *J. Pharmacol. Exp. Ther.* 236: 526-534, 1986.

1301.   Corcoran, G.B., *et al.* Effects of N-acetylcysteine on the disposition and metabolism of acetaminophen in mice. *J. Pharmacol. Exp. Ther.* 232: 857-863, 1985.

1302.   Tariq, M., *et al.* Gastric and duodenal antiulcer and cytoprotective effects of proglumide in rats. *J. Pharmacol. Exp. Ther.* 241: 602-607, 1987.

1303.   Cavanagh, R.L., *et al.* Prevention of aspirin-induced gastric mucosal injury by Histamine H_2 receptor antagonists: A crossover endoscopic and intragastric pH study in the dog. *J. Pharmacol. Exp. Ther.* 243: 1179-1184, 1987.

1304.   Gerkens, J.F., *et al.* Effect of indomethacin and aspirin on gastric blood flow and acid secretion. *J. Pharmacol. Exp. Ther.* 203: 646-652, 1977.

1305.   DiMinno, G. and M.J. Silver. Mouse antithrombotic assay: A simple method for the evaluation of antithrombotic agents in vivo. Potentiation of antithrombotic activity by ethyl alcohol. *J. Pharmacol. Exp. Ther.* 225: 57-60, 1983.

1306.   Gambino, M.C., *et al.* Selectivity of oral aspirin as an inhibitor of platelet vs vascular cyclooxygenase activity is reduced by portacaval shunt in rats. *J. Pharmacol. Exp. Ther.* 245: 287-293, 1988.

1307.   Weselcouch, E.O., *et al.* Effects of low doses of aspirin and dipyridamole on platelet aggregation in the dog coronary artery. *J. Pharmacol. Exp. Ther.* 240: 37-43, 1987.

1308.   Tuttle, R.S., *et al.* Inhibition by metoprolol of the antihypertensive effect of aspirin in young rats. *J. Pharmacol. Exp. Ther.* 234: 166-171, 1985.

1309.   Halushka, P.V., *et al.* Protective effects of aspirin in endotoxic shock. *J. Pharmacol. Exp. Ther.* 218: 464-469, 1981.

1310.   Maggi, C.A., *et al.* Evidence for the involvement of arachidonic acid metabolites in spontaneous and drug-induced contractions of rat urinary bladder. *J. Pharmacol. Exp. Ther.* 230: 500-513, 1984.

Bibliography

1311. Sancilio, L.F. and S. Cheung. Analysis of the bradykinin response in dogs and its antagonism by analgesic drugs. *J. Pharmacol. Exp. Ther.* 207: 469-475, 1978.

1312. Kadokawa, T., *et al.* Effects of nonsteroidal anti-inflammatory drugs (NSAID) on renal excretion of sodium and water, and on body fluid volume in rats. *J. Pharmacol. Exp. Ther.* 209: 219-224, 1979.

1313. Karmazyn, M., *et al.* Effect of nonsteroidal antiinflammatory drugs on the hypoxic rat heart. *J. Pharmacol. Exp. Ther.* 218: 488-496, 1981.

1314. Satoh, H., *et al.* Development of histamine tachyphylaxis in the guinea-pig mesenteric artery. *J. Pharmacol. Exp. Ther.* 229: 527-531, 1984.

1315. Catravas, J.D., *et al.* Effects of acetylcholine in the pulmonary circulation of rabbits. *J. Pharmacol. Exp. Ther.* 231: 236-241, 1984.

1316. Chen, G., *et al.* Studies of drug effects on electrically induced extensor seizures and clinical implications. *Arch. Int. Pharmacodyn. Ther.* 172: 183-218, 1968.

1317. Dashputra, P.G., *et al.* Modification of metrazol induced convulsions in rats by antihistaminics. *Arch. Int. Pharmacodyn. Ther.* 160: 106-112, 1966.

1318. Roba, J., *et al.* Antiplatelet and antithrombogenic effects of suloctidil. *Eur. J. Pharmacol.* 37: 265-274, 1976.

1319. Evoniuk, G., *et al.* Antagonism of the cardiovascular effects of adenosine by caffeine or 8-(p-sulfophenyl) theophylline. *J. Pharmacol. Exp. Ther.* 240: 428-432, 1987.

1320. Perez, J.E., *et al.* Inotropic and chronotropic effects of vasodilators. *J. Pharmacol. Exp. Ther.* 221: 609-613, 1982.

1321. Rardon, D.P. and J.C. Bailey, Adenosine attenuation of the electrophysiological effects of isoproterenol on canine cardiac purkinje fibers. *J. Pharmacol. Exp. Ther.* 228: 792-798, 1984.

1322. Markley, K., *et al.* The role of histamine in burn, tourniquet and endotoxin shock in mice. *Eur. J. Pharmacol.* 33: 255-265, 1975.

1323. Gessner, P.K. and M.P. Shakarjian. Interactions of paraldehyde with ethanol and chloral hydrate. *J. Pharmacol. Exp. Ther.* 235: 32-36, 1985.

1324. Rees, D.C. and R.L. Balster. Attenuation of the discriminative stimulus properties of ethanol and oxazepam, but not of pentobarbital, by Ro 15-4513 in mice. *J. Pharmacol. Exp. Ther.* 244: 592-598, 1988.

1325. Barrett, J.E., *et al.* Behavioral studies with anxiolytic drugs. 1. Interactions of the benzodiazepine antagonist Ro15-1788 with chlordiazepoxide, pentobarbital and ethanol. *J. Pharmacol. Exp. Ther.* 233: 554-559, 1985.

Bibliography

1326. French, T.A., *et al.* Ethanol-induced changes in tyrosine hydroxylase activity in adrenal glands of mice selectively bred for differences in sensitivity to ethanol. *J. Pharmacol. Exp. Ther.* 232: 315-321, 1985.

1327. Chandrasekhar, R., *et al.* Alterations in rat brain polyphosphoinositide metabolism due to acute ethanol administration. *J. Pharmacol. Exp. Ther.* 245: 120-123, 1988.

1328. Lauterburg, B.H., *et al.* Ethanol suppresses hepatic glutathione synthesis in rats in vivo. *J. Pharmacol. Exp. Ther.* 230: 7-11, 1984.

1329. Impeduglia, G., *et al.* Influence of thiamine deficiency on the response to ethanol in two inbred rat strains. *J. Pharmacol. Exp. Ther.* 240: 755-763, 1987.

1330. Kosobud, A. and J.C. Crabbe. Ethanol withdrawal in mice bred to be genetically prone or resistant to ethanol withdrawal seizures. *J. Pharmacol. Exp. Ther.* 238: 170-177, 1986.

1331. Zgombick, J.M., *et al.* Ethanol-induced adrenomedullary catecholamine secretion in LS/lbg and SS/lbg mice. *J. Pharmacol. Exp. Ther.* 236: 634-640, 1986.

1332. Willis, B.R., *et al.* Ethanol-induced male reproductive tract pathology as a function of ethanol dose and duration of exposure. *J. Pharmacol. Exp. Ther.* 225: 470-478, 1983.

1333. Mello, N.K., *et al.* Alcohol effects on luteinizing hormone-releasing hormone-stimulated luteinizing hormone and follicle-stimulating hormone in female rhesus monkeys. *J. Pharmacol. Exp. Ther.* 237: 590-595, 1986.

1334. Breese, G.R., *et al.* Ethanol-induced locomotor stimulation in rats after thyrotropin-releasing hormone. *J. Pharmacol. Exp. Ther.* 229: 731-737, 1984.

1335. Frye, G.D., *et al.* Differential sensitivity of ethanol withdrawal signs in the rat to γ-aminobutyric acid (GABA) mimetics: Blockade of audiogenic seizure but not forelimb tremors. *J. Pharmacol. Exp. Ther.* 226: 720-725, 1983.

1336. Crabbe, J.C., *et al.* Rapid development of tolerance to the hypothermic effect of ethanol in mice. *J. Pharmacol. Exp. Ther.* 208: 128-133, 1979.

1337. Mullin, M.J. and A.P. Ferko. Ethanol and functional tolerance: Interactions with pimozide and clonidine. *J. Pharmacol. Exp. Ther.* 216: 459-464, 1981.

1338. Deimling, M.J. and R.C. Schnell. Circadian rhythms in the biological responses and disposition of ethanol in mouse. *J. Pharmacol. Exp. Ther.* 213: 1-8, 1980.

1339. Zysset, T., *et al.* Increased systemic availability of drugs during acute ethanol intoxication. Studies with mephenytoin in the dog. *J. Pharmacol. Exp. Ther.* 213: 173-178, 1980.

1340. Chapin, R.E., *et al.* Possible mechanisms of reduction of plasma luteinizing hormone by ethanol. *J. Pharmacol. Exp. Ther.* 212: 6-10, 1980.

Bibliography

1341. Abel, E.L. and H.B. Greizerstein. Ethanol-induced prenatal growth deficiency: Changes in fetal body composition. *J. Pharmacol. Exp. Ther.* 211: 668-671, 1979.

1342. Brown, F.C., *et al.* Interactions of pyrazole and ethanol on norepinephrine-metabolism in rat brain. *J. Pharmacol. Exp. Ther.* 206: 75-80, 1978.

1343. Ogiwara, Y., *et al.* Blocking effects of alinidine on negative chronotropic and inotropic responses to vagal stimulating and injected acetylcholine and carbachol in dogs. *J. Pharmacol. Exp. Ther.* 243: 1113-1120, 1987.

1344. Tibaldi, J., *et al.* Protection against alloxan-induced diabetes by various urea derivatives: Relationship between protective effects and reactivity with the hydroxyl radical. *J. Pharmacol. Exp. Ther.* 211: 415-418, 1979.

1345. Belanger, P.-M., *et al.* Depression of hepatic microsomal enzyme systems by amantatine hydrochloride in the rat. *J. Pharmacol. Exp. Ther.* 211: 485-490, 1979.

1346. Cox, B. and S.J. Tha. Amantadine tremor, a 5-hydroxytryptamine- mediated response? *Eur. J. Pharmacol.* 30: 344-351, 1975.

1347. Menon, M.K., *et al.* Blockade of the central effects of *d*-amphetamine sulfate by amantadine hydrochloride. *Eur. J. Pharmacol.* 21: 311-317, 1973.

1348. Way, E.L., *et al.* Precipitation of abstinence-like syndrome in morphine-dependent mice by pargyline. *J. Pharmacol. Exp. Ther.* 199: 400-407, 1976.

1349. Wesseling, H., *et al.* Effects of diazepam and pentobarbitone on convulsions induced by local anesthetics in mice. *Eur. J. Pharmacol.* 13: 150-154, 1971.

1350. de Jonge, A., *et al.* Inhibitory effect of alpha-1 adrenoceptor stimulation on cardiac sympathetic neurotransmission in pithed normotensive rats. *J. Pharmacol. Exp. Ther.* 236: 500-504, 1986.

1351. McGrath, J.C. and J.W. O'Brien. Blockade by nifedipine of responses to intravenous bolus injection or infusion of α_1- and α_2-adrenoceptor agonists in the pithed rat. *Br. J. Pharmacol.* 91: 355-365, 1987.

1352. Barrett, R.J. and S.T. Kau. Myocardial and vascular actions of amiloride in spontaneously hypertensive rats. *J. Pharmacol. Exp. Ther.* 239: 365-374, 1986.

1353. Marchese, A.C., *et al.* Electrophysiologic effects of amiloride in canine purkinje fibers: Evidence for a delayed effect on repolarization. *J. Pharmacol. Exp. Ther.* 232: 485-491. 1985.

1354. Horton, R.W. and B.S. Meldrum. Seizures induced by allylglycine, 3-mercaptopropionic acid and 4-deoxypyridoxine in mice and photosensitive baboons, and different modes of inhibition of cerebral glutamic acid decarboxylase. *Brit. J. Pharmacol.* 49: 52-63, 1973.

Bibliography

1355.   Lundberg, D.B., *et al.* Aminophylline may stimulate respiration in rats by activation of dopaminergic receptors. *J. Pharmacol. Exp. Ther.* 217: 215-221, 1981.

1356.   Romson, J.L., *et al.* Potentiation of the antithrombotic effect of prostacyclin by simultaneous administration of aminophylline in a canine model of coronary artery thrombosis. *J. Pharmacol. Exp. Ther.* 227: 288-294, 1983.

1357.   Gerkens, J.F., *et al.* Aminophylline inhibits renal vasoconstriction produced by intrarenal hypertonic saline. *J. Pharmacol. Exp. Ther.* 225: 611-615, 1983.

1358.   Rossing, T.H. and J.M. Drazen. Effects of milrinone on contractile responses of guinea pig trachea, lung parenchyma and pulmonary artery. *J. Pharmacol. Exp. Ther.* 238: 874-879, 1986.

1359.   Sirotnak, F.M. and R.C. Donsbach. A basis for the difference in toxicity of methotrexate, aminopterin, and methaguin in mice. *Biochem. Pharmacol.* 24: 156-158, 1975.

1360.   Ikushima, S., *et al.* Effects of 4-aminopyridine on the adrenergic nerve terminals of rabbit arteries. *J. Pharmacol. Exp. Ther.* 219: 792-797, 1981.

1361.   Lamarca, M.V. and B. Collier. Effects of 4-aminopyridine on the cat superior cervical ganglion. *J. Pharmacol. Exp. Ther.* 226: 249-257, 1983.

1362.   Lambert, C., *et al.* Lack of relation between the ventricular refractory period prolongation by amiodarone and the thyroid state in rats. *J. Pharmacol. Exp. Ther.* 242: 320-325, 1987.

1363.   Cambert, C., *et al.* Effect of the induction of amiodarone biotransformation on ventricular refractory periods in rats. *J. Pharmacol. Exp. Ther.* 238: 307-312, 1986.

1364.   Patterson, E., *et al.* Cardiac electrophysiologic effects of acute and chronic amiodarone administration in the isolated perfused rabbit heart: Altered thyroid hormone metabolism. *J. Pharmacol. Exp. Ther.* 239: 179-184, 1986.

1365.   Shank, R.P., *et al.* Preclinical evaluation of McN-5707 as a potential antidepressant. *J. Pharmacol. Exp. Ther.* 242: 74-84, 1987.

1366.   Lloyd, K.G., *et al.* Upregulation of γ aminobutyric acid (GABA) B binding sites in rat frontal cortex: A common action of repeated administration of different classes of antidepressants and electroshock. *J. Pharmacol. Exp. Ther.* 235: 191-199, 1985.

1367.   Follmer, C.H. and B.K.B. Lum. Protective action of diazepam and of sympathomimetic amines against amitriptyline-induced toxicity. *J. Pharmacol. Exp. Ther.* 222: 424-429, 1982.

1368.   Nattel, S. and M. Mittleman. Treatment of ventricular tachyarrhythmias resulting from amitryptyline in dogs. *J. Pharmacol. Exp. Ther.* 231: 430-435, 1984.

1369. Sasyniuk, B.I. and V. Jhamandas. Mechanisms of reversal of toxic effects of amitriptyline on cardiac purkinje fibers by sodium bicarbonate. *J. Pharmacol. Exp. Ther.* 231: 387-394, 1984.

1370. McKearney, J.W. Effects of tricyclic antidepressant and anticholinergic drugs on fixed-interval responding in the squirrel monkey. *J. Pharmacol. Exp. Ther.* 222: 215-219, 1982.

1371. Christensen, A.V., *et al.* Pharmacology of a new phthalane (LU-10-171), with specific 5-HT uptake inhibiting properties. *Eur. J. Pharmacol.* 41: 153-162, 1977.

1372. Shintomi, K. Effects of psychotropic drugs on methamphetamine-induced behavioral excitation in grouped mice. *Eur. J. Pharmacol.* 31: 195-206, 1975.

1373. Preskorn, S.H., *et al.* The effect of dibenzazepines (tricyclic antidepressants) on cerebral capillary permeability in the rat in vivo. *J. Pharmacol. Exp. Ther.* 213: 313-320, 1980.

1374. VonVoightlander, P.F., *et al.* Corneal lesions induced by antidepressants: A selective effect upon young Fischer 344 rats. *J. Pharmacol. Exp. Ther.* 222: 282-286, 1982.

1375. Catravas, J.D., *et al.* The effects of haloperidol, chlorpromazine and propranolol on acute amphetamine poisoning in the conscious dog. *J. Pharmacol. Exp. Ther.* 202: 230-243, 1977.

1376. Barnett, J.V., *et al.* Repeated amphetamine pretreatment alters the responsiveness of striatal dopamine-stimulated adenylate cyclase to amphetamine-induced desensitization. *J. Pharmacol. Exp. Ther.* 242: 40-47, 1987.

1377. Bergman, J. and R.D. Spealman. Some behavioral effects of histamine H_1 antagonists in squirrel monkeys. *J. Pharmacol. Exp. Ther.* 239: 104-110, 1986.

1378. Trulson, M.E. and B.L. Jacobs. Chronic amphetamine administration to cats: Behavioral and neurochemical evidence for decreased central serotonergic function. *J. Pharmacol. Exp. Ther.* 211: 375-384, 1979.

1379. Chou, D.T., *et al.* Unit activity in medial thalamus: Comparative effects of caffeine and amphetamines. *J. Pharmacol. Exp. Ther.* 213: 580-585, 1980.

1380. Piercey, M.F., *et al.* Electrophysiological evaluation of a partial agonist of dopamine receptors. *J. Pharmacol. Exp. Ther.* 243: 391-396, 1987.

1381. Kuhr, W.G., *et al.* Amphetamine attenuates the stimulated release of dopamine in vivo. *J. Pharmacol. Exp. Ther.* 232: 388-394, 1985.

1382. Segal, D.S. and R. Kuczenski. Individual differences in responsiveness to single and repeated amphetamine administration: Behavioral characteristics and neurochemical correlates. *J. Pharmacol. Exp. Ther.* 242: 917-926, 1987.

Bibliography

1383.   Bhakthavatsalam, P., *et al*. Dissociation of receptor sensitivity changes in rat perifornical hypothalamus: A role for dopaminergic receptors in amphetamine anorexic tolerance. *J. Pharmacol. Exp. Ther*. 240: 196-202, 1987.

1384.   Klemfuss, H. and M.W. Alder. Autonomic mechanisms for morphine and amphetamine mydriasis the rat. *J. Pharmacol. Exp. Ther*. 238: 788-793, 1986.

1385.   Koss, M.C. Studies on the mechanism of amphetamine mydriasis in the cat. *J. Pharmacol. Exp. Ther*. 213: 49-53, 1980.

1386.   Hernandez, L., *et al*. Amphetamine-induced hyperphagia and obesity caused by intraventricular or lateral hypothalamic injections in rats. *J. Pharmacol. Exp. Ther*. 227: 524-530, 1983.

1387.   van Ree, J.M., *et al*. Intravenous self-administration of drugs in rats. *J. Pharmacol. Exp. Ther*. 204: 547-557, 1978.

1388.   Woolverton, W.L., *et al*. Intravenous self-administration of dopamine receptor agonists by rhesus monkeys. *J. Pharmacol. Exp. Ther*. 230: 678-683, 1984.

1389.   Carroll, M.E. and D.C. Stotz. Oral d-amphetamine and ketamine self-administration by rhesus monkeys: Effects of food deprivation. *J. Pharmacol. Exp. Ther*. 227: 28-34, 1983.

1390.   Kamal, L.A., *et al*. Amphetamine inhibits the electrically evoked release of [^{3}H]dopamine from slices of the rabbit caudate. *J. Pharmacol. Exp. Ther*. 227: 446-458, 1983.

1391.   Abdallah, A.H., *et al*. Interaction of *d*-amphetamine with central nervous system depressants on food intake and spontaneous motor activity of mice. *Eur. J. Pharmacol*. 26: 119-121, 1974.

1392.   Abdallah, A.H., *et al*. Role of dopamine in the anorexigenic effect of DITA: Comparison with *d*-amphetamine. *Eur. J. Pharmacol*. 40: 39-44, 1976.

1393.   Kostrzewa, R. and D. Jacobowitz. Acute effect of 6-hydroxydopa on central monoaminergic neurons. *Eur. J. Pharmacol*. 21: 70-80, 1973.

1394.   Malecot, C.O., *et al*. Amrinone effects on electromechanical coupling and depolarization-induced automaticity in ventricular muscle of guinea pigs and ferrets. *J. Pharmacol. Exp. Ther*. 232: 10-19, 1985.

1395.   Lukas, A. and G.R. Ferrier. Electrophysiological effects of amrinone and milrinone in an isolated canine cardiac tissue model of ischemia and reperfusion. *J. Pharmacol. Exp. Ther*. 244: 348-354, 1988.

1396.   Hayes, J.S., *et al*. Molecular basis for the cardiovascular activities of amrinone and AR-L57. *J. Pharmacol. Exp. Ther*. 230: 124-132, 1984.

Bibliography

1397. Bayorh, M., *et al.* Leukotriene D$_4$ inhibits cardiovascular responses to sympathetic stimulation, angiotensin and vasopressin in the pithed spontaneously hypersensitive rats. *J. Pharmacol. Exp. Ther.* 231: 85-90, 1984.

1398. Kushiku, K., *et al.* Increment of calmodulin in proportion to enhancement of non-nicotinic responses after preganglionic stimulation of the dog cardiac sympathetic ganglia. *J. Pharmacol. Exp. Ther.* 245: 311-318, 1988.

1399. Susic, H., *et al.* Inhibition by bradykinin of the vascular action of angiotensin II in the dog kidney. *J. Pharmacol. Exp. Ther.* 218: 103-107, 1981.

1400. Campbell, W.B. and W.A. Pettinger. Organ specificity of angiotensin II and des-aspartyl angiotensin II in the conscious rat. *J. Pharmacol. Exp. Ther.* 198: 450-456, 1976.

1401. Costello, D.J. and H.L. Borison. Naloxone antagonizes narcotic self-blockade of emesis in the cat. *J. Pharmacol. Exp. Ther.* 203: 222-230, 1977.

1402. Imperato, A., *et al.* Pharmacological profile of dopamine receptor agonists as studies by brain dialysis in behaving rats. *J. Pharmacol. Exp. Ther.* 245: 257-264, 1988.

1403. Cunningham, K.A., *et al.* Discriminative stimulus properties of lergotrile. *J. Pharmacol. Exp. Ther.* 230: 47-52, 1984.

1404. Swerdlow, N.R., *et al.* Effects of chronic dietary lithium on behavioral indices of dopamine denervation supersensitivity in the rat. *J. Pharmacol. Exp. Ther.* 235: 324-329, 1985.

1405. Snow, A.E. and A. Horita. Interaction of apomorphine and stressors in the production of hyperthermia in the rabbit. *J. Pharmacol. Exp. Ther.* 220: 335-339, 1982.

1406. Woolverton, W.L., *et al.* Pharmacological analysis of the apomorphine discriminative stimulus in rhesus monkeys. *J. Pharmacol. Exp. Ther.* 241: 213-222, 1987.

1407. Winkler, J.D. and B. Weiss. Reversal of supersensitive apomorphine-induced rotational behavior in mice by continuous exposure to apomorphine. *J. Pharmacol. Exp. Ther.* 238: 242-247, 1986.

1408. Yamawaki, S., *et al.* Dopaminergic and serotonergic mechanisms of thermoregulation: Mediation of thermal effects of apomorphine and dopamine. *J. Pharmacol. Exp. Ther.* 227: 383-388, 1983.

1409. Helke, C.J. and R.A. Gillis. Centrally mediated protective effects of dopamine agonists on digitalis-induced ventricular arrhythmias. *J. Pharmacol. Exp. Ther.* 207: 263-270, 1978.

Bibliography

1410. Misu, Y., *et al.* Presynaptic inhibitory dopamine receptors on noradrenergic nerve terminals: Analysis of biphasic actions of dopamine and apomorphine on the release of endogenous norepinephrine in rat hypothalamic slices. *J. Pharmacol. Exp. Ther.* 235: 771-777, 1985.

1411. Nowak, J.Z., *et al.* Changes in sensitivity of release modulating dopamine autoreceptors after chronic treatment with haloperidol. *J. Pharmacol. Exp. Ther.* 226: 558-564, 1983.

1412. Buylaert, W.A., *et al.* Vasodilation produced by apomorphine in the hindleg of the dog. *J. Pharmacol. Exp. Ther.* 201: 738-746, 1977.

1413. Grabowska, M., *et al.* Possible involvement of brain serotonin in apomorphine-induced hypothermia. *Eur. J. Pharmacol.* 23: 82-89, 1973.

1414. Puech, A.J., *et al.* Antagonism by sulpiride of three apomorphine- induced effects in rodents. *Eur. J. Pharmacol.* 36: 439-441, 1976.

1415. Weissman, A. Penfluridol blockade of apomorphine dependence of duration on species and endpoint. *Eur. J. Pharmacol.* 33: 267-275, 1975.

1416. Hodge, G.K. and L.L. Butcher. Catecholamine correlates of isolation-induced aggression in mice. *Eur. J. Pharmacol.* 31: 81-93, 1975.

1417. Tulanay, F.C., *et al.* The effect of biogenic amine modifiers on morphine analgesia and its antagonism by naloxone. *Eur. J. Pharmacol.* 35: 285-292, 1976.

1418. Nakamura, M. and H. Fukushima. The effect of tricyclic antidepressants and neuroleptics on the peripheral and central action of norepinephrine in reserpine treated mice. *Eur. J. Pharmacol.* 38: 343-348, 1976.

1419. Maggi, C.A., *et al.* Four motor effects of capsaicin on guinea-pig distal colon. *Brit. J. Pharmacol.* 90: 651-660, 1987.

1420. Bass, A.S., *et al.* Mechanisms mediating the positive inotropic and chronotropic changes induced by dopexamine in the anesthetized dog. *J. Pharmacol. Exp. Ther.* 242: 940-944, 1987.

1421. Johnson, M.D., *et al.* Paradoxical elevation of sympathetic activity during catecholamine infusion in rats. *J. Pharmacol. Exp. Ther.* 227: 254-259, 1983.

1422. Kimura, T., *et al.* Predominance of postsynaptic mechanism in vagal suppression of sympathetic tachycardia in the dog. *J. Pharmacol. Exp. Ther.* 235: 793-797, 1985.

1423. Nishikawa, H., *et al.* Catecholamine receptors involved in the inhibitory effects of dopamine on vagally stimulated gastric acid secretion and mucosal blood flow in rats. *J. Pharmacol. Exp. Ther.* 240: 966-971, 1987.

1424. Durant, P.A.C., *et al.* Micturition in the unanesthetized rat: Spinal vs. peripheral pharmacology of the adrenergic system. *J. Pharmacol. Exp. Ther.* 245: 426-435, 1988.

Bibliography

1425. Kaniucki, M.D., *et al.* Sympathetic and parasympathetic nerves regulate postsynaptic alpha-2 adrenoceptor in salivary glands. *J. Pharmacol. Exp. Ther.* 239: 488-493, 1986.

1426. Edwards, R.M. and M. Gellai. Inhibition of vasopressin-stimulated cyclic AMP accumulation by alpha-2 adrenoceptor agonists in isolated papillary collecting ducts. *J. Pharmacol. Exp. Ther.* 244: 526-530, 1988.

1427. Goover, G.J., *et al.* Beta adrenoceptor control of the microvascular reserve in rabbit myocardium. *J. Pharmacol. Exp. Ther.* 238: 868-873, 1986.

1428. Sakai, K. and Y. Abiko. Attenuation by atenolol of myocardial acidosis during ischemia in dogs: Contribution of beta-1 adrenoceptors to myocardial acidosis. *J. Pharmacol. Exp. Ther.* 232: 810-816, 1985.

1429. Osborn, J.L., *et al.* Beta-1 receptor mediation of renin secretion elicited by low-frequency renal nerve stimulation. *J. Pharmacol. Exp. Ther.* 216: 265-269, 1981.

1430. Galligan, J.J. and T.F. Burks. Cholinergic neurons mediate intestinal propulsion in the rat. *J. Pharmacol. Exp. Ther.* 238: 594-598, 1986.

1431. Yokotani, K., *et al.* Effects of the sympathetic nervous system on bethanechol-induced elevation of gastric acid secretion and mucosal blood flow in rats. *J. Pharmacol. Exp. Ther.* 227: 478-483, 1983.

1432. Ruwart, M.J., *et al.* Evidence for noncholinergic mediation of small intestinal transit in the rat. *J. Pharmacol. Exp. Ther.* 209: 462-465, 1979.

1433. Pendleton, R.G., *et al.* Effects of atropine upon various components mediating postprandial gastric acid secretion in dogs. *J. Pharmacol. Exp. Ther.* 240: 396-399, 1987.

1434. Witkin, J.M., *et al.* Comparison of in vitro actions with behavioral effects of antimuscarinic agents. *J. Pharmacol. Exp. Ther.* 242: 796-803, 1987.

1435. Roszkowski, A.P., *et al.* Gastric antisecretory and antiulcer properties of enprostil, (±)-oxoprosta-4,5,13(t)-trienoic acid methyl ester. *J. Pharmacol. Exp. Ther.* 239: 382-389, 1986.

1436. Abraham, S., *et al.* Studies on the hypotensive response to atropine in hypertensive rats. *J. Pharmacol. Exp. Ther.* 218: 662-668, 1981.

1437. McArdle, S., *et al.* Cholinergic stimulation of phosphoinositide hydrolysis in rabbit kidney. *J. Pharmacol. Exp. Ther.* 244: 586-591, 1988.

1438. Woodman, O.L. and S.F. Vatner. Cardiovascular responses to the stimulation of alpha-1 and alpha-2 adrenoceptors in the conscious dog. *J. Pharmacol. Exp. Ther.* 237: 86-91, 1986.

Bibliography

1439.   Koe, B.K., *et al.* Sertraline, 1S,4S-N-methyl-4-(3,4-dichlorophenyl)-1,2,3,4-tetrahydro-1-napththylamine, a new uptake inhibitor with selectivity for serotonin. *J. Pharmacol. Exp. Ther.* 226: 686-700, 1983.

1440.   Delbarre, B. and H. Schmitt. Sedative effects of α-sympathomimetic drugs and their antagonism by adrenergic and cholinergic blocking drugs. *Eur. J. Pharmacol.* 13: 356-363, 1971.

1441.   Gerald, M.C., *et al.* Effects of various antihistamines on oxotremorine-induced hypothermia in mice. *Eur. J. Pharmacol.* 17: 189-193, 1972.

1442.   Leszkovsky, G.P. and L. Tardos. Antagonism of centrally mediated oxotremorine effects by a peripherally acting drug. *Eur. J. Pharmacol.* 15: 310-317, 1971.

1443.   Lundholm, B. and B. Sparf. The effect of atropine on the turnover of acetylcholine in the mouse brain. *Eur. J. Pharmacol.* 32: 287-292, 1975.

1444.   Tsubomura, T., *et al.* Gastric excitation by stimulation of the vagal trunk after chronic supranodose vagotomy in cats. *J. Pharmacol. Exp. Ther.* 241: 650-654, 1987.

1445.   Koranda, F.C., *et al.* Accelerated induction of skin cancers by ultraviolet radiation in hairless mice treated with immunosuppressive agents. *Surg. Forum* 26: 145-146, 1975.

1446.   Otterness, I.G. and Yi-Han Chang. Comparative study of cyclophosphamide, 6-mercaptopurine, azathiopurine and methotrexate. *Clin. Exp. Immunol.* 26: 346-354, 1976.

1447.   Tripod, J., *et al.* Experimental differentiation of inhibitors of the central nervous system. *Arch. Int. Pharmacodyn. Ther.* 112: 319-341, 1957.

1448.   Ault, B., *et al.* Efficacy of baclofen and phenobarbital against the kainic acid limbic seizure-brain damage syndrome. *J. Pharmacol. Exp. Ther.* 239: 612-617, 1986.

1449.   Levy, R.A. and H.K. Proudfit. The analgesic action of baclofen [ß-(4-chlorophenyl)-ɑ-aminobutyric acid]. *J. Pharmacol. Exp. Ther.* 202: 437-445, 1977.

1450.   Gianutsos, G. and K.E. Moore. Tolerance to the effects of baclofen and γ-butyrolactone on locomotor activity and dopaminergic neurons in the mouse. *J. Pharmacol. Exp. Ther.* 207: 859-869, 1978.

1451.   Lalley, P.M. Biphasic effects of baclofen on phrenic motorneurons: Possible involvement of two types of γ-aminobutyric acid (GABA) receptors. *J. Pharmacol. Exp. Ther.* 226: 616-624, 1983.

1452.   Ulloque, R.A., *et al.* Effects γ-aminobutyric acid (GABA) receptor agonists on the neurotoxicity and anticonvulsant activity of barbiturates in mice. *J. Pharmacol. Exp. Ther.* 237: 468-472, 1986.

1453.   Bartolini, A., *et al.* Antinociception induced by systemic administration of local anaesthetics depends on a central cholinergic mechanism. *Brit. J. Pharmacol.* 92: 711-721, 1987.

1454.   Gray, J.A., *et al.* Hypothermia induced by baclofen, a possible index of GABA$_B$ receptor function in mice, is enhanced by antidepressant drugs and ECS. *Brit. J. Pharmacol.* 92: 863-870, 1987.

1455.   Levy, R.A. and H.K. Proudfit. The analgesic action of baclofen [ß-(4-chlorophenyl-γ-aminobutyric acid]. *J. Pharmacol. Exp. Ther.* 202: 437-445, 1977.

1456.   Darwish, S.A.E. and B.L. Furman. Effects of levodopa and dopamine on plasma glucose concentration in mice. *Eur. J. Pharmacol.* 41: 351-360, 1977.

1457.   Brase, D.A., *et al.* Cholinergic modification of naloxone-induced jumping in morphine dependent mice. *Eur. J. Pharmacol.* 26: 1-8, 1974.

1458.   Menon, M.K., *et al.* The central stimulant and potential antiparkinsonism effects of 2(*p*-nitrobenzylthio)-imidazoline (^{3}H)-HCl. *Eur. J. Pharmacol.* 19: 43-51, 1972.

1459.   Lynch, J.J., *et al.* The effects of calcium entry blockade on the vulnerability of infarcted canine myocardium toward ventricular fibrillation. *J. Pharmacol. Exp. Ther.* 239: 340-345, 1986.

1460.   Suzuki, H., *et al.* Mechanisms of the bepridil-induced vasodilation of the rabbit mesenteric artery. *J. Pharmacol. Exp. Ther.* 235: 749-756, 1985.

1461.   Cruz, C., *et al.* Protective effects of bepridil on calcium injury of anoxic myocytes isolated from adult rat heart ventricular muscle. *J. Pharmacol. Exp. Ther.* 242: 1126-1132, 1987.

1462.   Hirschowitz, B.I. Somatostatin effects on gastric electrolytes and pepsin in dogs with various secretory stimuli. *J. Pharmacol. Exp. Ther.* 243: 501-506, 1987.

1463.   Gonsalves, S.F. and H.L. Borison. Atropine-resistant central respiratory stimulation by bethanechol in cats. *J. Pharmacol. Exp. Ther.* 214: 279-305, 1980.

1464.   Neumaier, J.F., *et al.* Opioid receptor-mediated responses in the dentate gyrus and CA1 region of the rat hippocampus. *J. Pharmacol. Exp. Ther.* 244: 564-570, 1988.

1465.   Fujimoto, M., *et al.* Effect of γ-aminobutyric acid$_A$ receptor antagonists on the release of enkephalin-containing peptides from dog adrenal gland. *J. Pharmacol. Exp. Ther.* 243: 195-199, 1987.

1466.   LLoyd, K.G., *et al.* Fengabine, a novel antidepressant GABAergic agent. 1. Activity in models for antidepressant drugs and psychopharmacological profile. *J. Pharmacol. Exp. Ther.* 241: 245-257, 1987.

Bibliography

1467.   Maggi, C.A., *et al*. Spinal and supraspinal components of GABAergic inhibition of the micturition reflex in rats. *J. Pharmacol. Exp. Ther.* 240: 998-1005, 1987.

1468.   Lima, L. and T.L. Sourkes. Cholinergic and GABAergic regulation of dopamine beta-hydroxylase activity in the adrenal gland of the rat. *J. Pharmacol. Exp. Ther.* 237: 265-270, 1986.

1469.   Humphrey, S.J. and R.B. McCall. Evidence for γ-aminobutyric acid mediation of the sympathetic nerve inhibitory response to vagal afferent stimulation. *J. Pharmacol. Exp. Ther.* 234: 288-297, 1985.

1470.   Piredda, S.G., *et al*. Effect of stimulus intensity on the profile of anticonvulsant activity of phenytoin, ethosuximide and valproate. *J. Pharmacol. Exp. Ther.* 232: 741-745, 1985.

1471.   Yamada, K.A., *et al*. Pentobarbital causes cardiorespiratory depression by interacting with a GABAergic system at the ventral surface of the medulla. *J. Pharmacol. Exp. Ther.* 226: 349-355, 1983.

1472.   DiMicco, J.A. and R.A. Gillis. Neuro-cardiovascular effects produced by bicuculline in the cat. *J. Pharmacol. Exp. Ther.* 210: 1-6, 1979.

1473.   Harrison, J.H., Jr. and J.S. Lazo. High dose continuous infusion of bleomycin in mice: A new model for drug-induced pulmonary fibrosis. *J. Pharmacol. Exp. Ther.* 243: 1185-1194, 1987.

1474.   Counts, D.F., *et al*. Collagen lysloxidase activity in the lung increases during bleomycin-induced lung fibrosis. *J. Pharmacol. Exp. Ther.* 219: 675-678, 1981.

1475.   Koslo, R.J., *et al*. Centrally administered bombesin affects gastrointestinal transit and colonic bead expulsion through supraspinal mechanisms. *J. Pharmacol. Exp. Ther.* 238: 62-67, 1986.

1476.   Kachur, J.F., *et al*. Neurohumoral control of ileal electrolyte transport. 1. Bombesin and related peptides. *J. Pharmacol. Exp. Ther.* 220: 449-455, 1982.

1477.   Moerschbaecher, J.M., *et al*. Effects of kappa agonists and dexoxadrol on the acquisition of conditional discriminations in monkeys. *J. Pharmacol. Exp. Ther.* 243: 737-744, 1987.

1478.   Leander, J.D., *et al*. Kappa agonist-induced diuresis: Evidence for stereo selectivity, strain differences, independence of hydration variables and a result of decreased plasma vasopressin levels. *J. Pharmacol. Exp. Ther.* 242: 33-39, 1987.

1479.   Dykstra, L.A., *et al*. Kappa opioids in rhesus monkeys. I. Diuresis, sedation, analgesia and discriminative stimulus effects. *J. Pharmacol. Exp. Ther.* 242: 413-420, 1987.

Bibliography

1480. DiChiara, G. and A. Imperato. Opposite effects of mu and kappa opiate agonists on dopamine release in the nucleus accumbens and in the dorsal caudate of freely moving rats. *J. Pharmacol. Exp. Ther.* 244: 1067-1080, 1988.

1481. Clark, R.W. and T.W. Ford. The contributions of μ-, δ- k-opioid receptors to the actions of endogenous opioids on spinal reflexes in the rabbit. *Brit. J. Pharmacol.* 91: 579-589, 1987.

1482. Hayes, A.G., *et al.* Differential sensitivity of models of antinociception in the rat, mouse and guinea-pig to μ- and k-opioid receptor agonists. *Brit. J. Pharmacol.* 91: 823-832, 1987.

1483. Marcais-Collado, H., *et al.* Inhibition of the spontaneous climbing behavior elicited in mice by opiates. *J. Pharmacol. Exp. Ther.* 227: 466-471, 1983.

1484. VonVoightlander, P.F., *et al.* U-50,488: A selective and structurally novel non-mu (kappa) opioid agonist. *J. Pharmacol. Exp. Ther.* 224: 7-12, 1983.

1485. Ensinger, H., *et al.* Neuronal and postjunctional components in the blood pressure effects of dopamine and bromocriptine in rabbits. *J. Pharmacol. Exp. Ther.* 234: 681-690, 1985.

1486. Nagahama, S., *et al.* Mechanisms of the depressor effect of bromocriptine in the spontaneously hypertensive rat. *J. Pharmacol. Exp. Ther.* 228: 370-375, 1984.

1487. Stier, C.T., *et al.* Effects of bromocriptine on single nephron and whole-kidney function in rats. *J. Pharmacol. Exp. Ther.* 220: 366-370, 1982.

1488. Anlezark, G., *et al.* Ergot alkaloids as dopamine agonists: Comparison in two rodent models. *Eur. J. Pharmacol.* 37: 295-302, 1976.

1489. Zimmerman, D.M., *et al.* Use of ß-funaltrexamine to determine mu opioid receptor involvement in the analgesic activity of various opioid ligands. *J. Pharmacol. Exp. Ther.* 241: 374-378, 1987.

1490. Sadee, W., *et al.* Buprenorphine: Differential interaction with opiate receptor subtypes in vivo. *J. Pharmacol. Exp. Ther.* 223: 157-162, 1982.

1491. Dykstra, L.A. Effects of buprenorphine on shock titration in squirrel monkeys. *J. Pharmacol. Exp. Ther.* 235: 20-25, 1985.

1492. Hayes, A.G., *et al.* Evaluation of the receptor selectivities of opioid drugs by investigating the block of their effect on urine output by ß-funaltrexamine. *J. Pharmacol. Exp. Ther.* 240: 984-988, 1987.

1493. Shannon, H.E., *et al.* Morphine-like discriminative stimulus effects of buprenorphine and demethoxybuprenorphine in rats: Quantitative antagonism by naloxone. *J. Pharmacol. Exp. Ther.* 229: 768-774, 1984.

Bibliography

1494. DeRossett, S.E. and S.G. Holtzman. Discriminative stimulus effects of the opioid antagonist diprenorphine in the squirrel monkey. *J. Pharmacol. Exp. Ther.* 237: 437-444, 1986.

1495. Rosow, C.E., *et al.* Opiates and thermoregulation in mice. III. Agonist-antagonists. *J. Pharmacol. Exp. Ther.* 220: 468-475, 1982.

1496. Geller, E.B., *et al.* Subclasses of opioids based on body temperature changes in rats: Acute subcutaneous administration. *J. Pharmacol. Exp. Ther.* 225: 391-398, 1983.

1497. Lukas, S.E., *et al.* Comparison of opioid self-injection and disruption of schedule-controlled performance in the baboon. *J. Pharmacol. Exp. Ther.* 238: 924-931, 1986.

1498. Jacob, J.J.C. and K. Ramabadran. Opioid antagonists, endogenous ligands and nociception. *Eur. J. Pharmacol.* 46: 393-394, 1977.

1499. Leander, J.D., *et al.* Kappa agonist-induced diuresis: Evidence for stereoselectivity, strain differences independence of hydration variables and a result of decreased plasma vasopressin levels. *J. Pharmacol. Exp. Ther.* 242: 33-39, 1987.

1500. Steinfels, G.F. and L. Cook. Antinociceptive profiles of mu and kappa opioid agonists in a rat tooth pulp stimulation procedure. *J. Pharmacol. Exp. Ther.* 236: 111-117, 1986.

1501. Holtzman, S.G. Discriminative stimulus properties of caffeine in the rat: Noradrenergic mediation. *J. Pharmacol. Exp. Ther.* 239: 706-714, 1986.

1502. Katz, J.L. and S.R. Goldberg. Psychomotor stimulant effects of caffeine alone and in combination with an adenosine analog in the squirrel monkey. *J. Pharmacol. Exp. Ther.* 242: 179-187, 1987.

1503. Winsky, L. and J.A. Harvey. Effects of N^6-(L-phenylisopropyl) adenosine, caffeine, theophylline and rolipram on the acquisition of conditioned responses in the rabbit. *J. Pharmacol. Exp. Ther.* 241: 223-229, 1987.

1504. Finn, I.B. and S.G. Holtzman. Tolerance to caffeine-induced stimulation of locomotor activity in rats. *J. Pharmacol. Exp. Ther.* 238: 542-546, 1986.

1505. Satch, H. and M. Vassalle. Reversal of caffeine-induced calcium overload in cardiac purkinje fibers. *J. Pharmacol. Exp. Ther.* 234: 172-179, 1985.

1506. Concannon, J.T., *et al.* Pre- and postnatal effects of caffeine on brain biogenic amines, cyclic nucleotides and behavior in developing rats. *J. Pharmacol. Exp. Ther.* 226: 673-679, 1983.

1507. Spindel, E., *et al.* Neuroendocrine effects of caffeine. II. Effects on thyrotropin and corticosterone secretion. *J. Pharmacol. Exp. Ther.* 225: 346-350, 1983.

Bibliography

1508.	Chernow, B., *et al*. Glucagon's chronotropic action is calcium dependent. *J. Pharmacol. Exp. Ther.* 241: 833-837, 1987.

1509.	Cory-Slechta, D.A., *et al*. Mobilization and redistribution of lead over the course of calcium disodium ethylenediamine tetraacetate chelation. *J. Pharmacol. Exp. Ther.* 243: 804-813, 1987.

1510.	Quest, J.A., *et al*. Central nervous system site of action of capsaicin-induced cardiovascular changes in the cat. *J. Pharmacol. Exp. Ther.* 228: 719-724, 1984.

1511.	Amann, R. and F. Lembeck. Stress induced ACTH release in capsaicin treated rats. *Brit. J. Pharmacol.* 90: 727-731, 1987.

1512.	Shimizu, T., *et al*. Capsaicin-induced corneal lesions in mice and the effects of chemical sympathectomy. *J. Pharmacol. Exp. Ther.* 243: 690-695, 1987.

1513.	Kaufman, L.J. and R.R. Vollmer. Endogenous angiotensin II facilitates sympathetically mediated hemodynamic responses in pithed rats. *J. Pharmacol. Exp. Ther.* 235: 128-134, 1985.

1514.	Chen, X., *et al*. Correlation between lung and plasma angiotensin converting enzyme and the hypotensive effect of captopril in conscious rabbits. *J. Pharmacol. Exp. Ther.* 229: 649-653, 1984.

1515.	Panzenbeck, M.J., *et al*. Prostaglandins mediate the increased sensitivity of left ventricular reflexes after captopril treatment in conscious dogs. *J. Pharmacol. Exp. Ther.* 244: 384-390, 1988.

1516.	Cohen, M.L. and K.D. Kurz. Angiotensin converting enzyme inhibition in tissues from spontaneously hypertensive rats after treatment with captopril on MK-421. *J. Pharmacol. Exp. Ther.* 220: 63-69, 1982.

1517.	Vollmer, R.R., *et al*. Antihypertensive activity of captopril (SQ 14,225), an orally active inhibitor of angiotensin converting enzyme in conscious two-kidney perinephritic hypertensive drugs. *J. Pharmacol. Exp. Ther.* 216: 225-231, 1981.

1518.	Evered, M.D. and M.M. Robinson. Effects of captopril on salt appetite in sodium-replete rats and rats treated with desoxycorticosterone acetate (DOCA). *J. Pharmacol. Exp. Ther.* 225: 416-421, 1983.

1519.	Wong, P.C., *et al*. Pharmacological evaluation in conscious dogs of factors involved in the renal vasodilator effect of captopril. *J. Pharmacol. Exp. Ther.* 219: 646-650, 1981.

1520.	Wu, Y.Y. and E.T. Wei. Mechanisms underlying the pressor responses to acute and chronic intraventricular administration of carbachol in the rat. *J. Pharmacol. Exp. Ther.* 228: 354-363, 1984.

1521.	Maggi, C.A., *et al*. Motor effect of neurokinins on the rat duodenum: Evidence for the involvement of substance K and substance P receptors. *J. Pharmacol. Exp. Ther.* 238: 341-351, 1986.

Bibliography

1522. Vadlamudi, R.V.S.V. and J.H. McNeill. Effect of alloxan- and streptozotocin-induced diabetes on isolated rat heart. *J. Pharmacol. Exp. Ther.* 225: 410-415, 1983.

1523. Waldmeier, P.C., *et al.* Carbamazepine decreases catecholamine turnover in the rat brain. *J. Pharmacol. Exp. Ther.* 231: 166-172, 1984.

1524. Hershkowitz, N., *et al.* Effects of carbamazepine on muscle tone in the decerebrate cat. *J. Pharmacol. Exp. Ther.* 224: 473-481, 1983.

1525. O'Dell, T.B. Experimental parameters in the evaluation of analgesics. *Arch. Int. Pharmacodyn. Ther.* 134: 154-174, 1961.

1526. Dhawan, B.N. and R.C. Srimal. Anti-inflammatory and some other pharmacological effects of 3,4-trans-2,2-dimethyl-3-phenyl-4 [p-(ß-pyrrolidinoethoxy)-phenyl]-7-methoxy-chroman (centchroman). *Brit. J. Pharmacol.* 49: 64-73, 1973.

1527. Coffin, V.L. and R.D. Spealman. Modulation of the behavioral effects of chlordiazepoxide by methylxanthines and analogs of adenosine in squirrel monkeys. *J. Pharmacol. Exp. Ther.* 235: 724-728, 1985.

1528. Ervin, G.N. and B.R. Cooper. Use of conditioned taste aversion as a conflict model: Effects of anxiolytic drugs. *J. Pharmacol. Exp. Ther.* 245: 137-146, 1988.

1529. Boisse, N.R., *et al.* Pharmacologic characterization of acute chlordiazepoxide dependence in the rat. *J. Pharmacol. Exp. Ther.* 239: 775-783, 1986.

1530. Soubrie, P., *et al.* Chlordiazepoxide reduces in vivo serotonin release in the basal ganglia of encephale isole but not anesthetized cats: Evidence for a dorsal raphe site of action. *J. Pharmacol. Exp. Ther.* 226: 526-532, 1983.

1531. Goldberg, S.R. Histamine as a punisher in squirrel monkeys: Effects of pentobarbital, chlordiazepoxide and H_1- and H_2-receptor antagonists on behavior and cardiovascular responses. *J. Pharmacol. Exp. Ther.* 214: 726-736, 1980.

1532. McMillan, D.E. and J.D. Leander. Chronic chlordiazepoxide and pentobarbital interactions on punished and unpunished behavior. *J. Pharmacol. Exp. Ther.* 207: 515-520, 1978.

1533. Silvestrini, B. and E. Quadri. Investigations of the specificity of the so-called analgesic activity of non-narcotic drugs. *Eur. J. Pharmacol.* 12: 231-235, 1970.

1534. Crews, F.T. and C.B. Smith. Potentiation of responses to adrenergic nerve stimulation in isolated rat atria during chronic tricyclic antidepressant administration. *J. Pharmacol. Exp. Ther.* 215: 143-149, 1980.

1535. Wilkerson, R.D. Antiarrhythmic effects of tricyclic antidepressant drugs in ouabain-induced arrhythmias in the dog. *J. Pharmacol. Exp. Ther.* 205: 666-674, 1978.

1536. Lassen, J.B., *et al.* Comparative studies of a new 5-HT uptake inhibitor and some tricyclic thymoleptics. *Eur. J. Pharmacol.* 32: 108-115, 1975.

1537. Chelly, J.E., *et al.* Role of isoflurane on hemodynamic properties and disposition of nicardipine. *J. Pharmacol. Exp. Ther.* 241: 899-906, 1987.

1538. Gardier, R.W., *et al.* The effect of pancuronium and gallamine on muscarinic transmission in the superior cervical ganglion. *J. Pharmacol. Exp. Ther.* 204: 46-53, 1978.

1539. Nabeshima, T., *et al.* Potentiation in phencyclidine-induced serotonin-mediated behaviors after intracerebroventricular administration of 5,7 dihydroxytryptamine in rats. *J. Pharmacol. Exp. Ther.* 243: 1139-1146, 1987.

1540. Alper, R.H., *et al.* Hemodynamic pharmacology of p-chloroamphetamine, a serotonin agonist, in conscious rats. *J. Pharmacol. Exp. Ther.* 243: 446-454, 1987.

1541. Oishi, R., *et al.* Δ^9-Tetrahydrocannabinol decreases turnover of brain histamine. *J. Pharmacol. Exp. Ther.* 232: 513-518, 1985.

1542. Ormsbee, H.S., *et al.* Serotonin regulation of the canine migrating motor complex. *J. Pharmacol. Exp. Ther.* 231: 436-440, 1984.

1543. Hoskins, B. and C.W. Jackson III. The mechanism of chlorothiazide- induced carbohydrate intolerance. *J. Pharmacol. Exp. Ther.* 206: 423-430, 1978.

1544. Nishibori, M., *et al.* Mechanism of the central hyperglycemic action of histamine in mice. *J. Pharmacol. Exp. Ther.* 241: 582-586, 1987.

1545. Rigel, D.F. and P.G. Katona. Effects of antihistamines and local anesthetics on excess tachycardia in conscious dogs. *J. Pharmacol. Exp. Ther.* 238: 367-371, 1986.

1546. Catravas, J.D. and I.W. Waters. Acute cocaine intoxication in the conscious dog: Studies on the mechanism of lethality. *J. Pharmacol. Exp. Ther.* 217: 350-356, 1981.

1547. Nose, T. and H. Takemoto. The effect of penfluridol and some psychotropic drugs on monoamine metabolism in central nervous system. *Eur. J. Pharmacol.* 31: 351-359, 1975.

1548. Katz, L.B., *et al.* Pharmacological comparison of ORF 17910, a potent, long-acting histamine H_2-receptor antagonist, to cimetidine and ranitidine. *J. Pharmacol. Exp. Ther.* 238: 587-593, 1986.

1549. Katz, L.B., *et al.* Selective gastric antilesion properties of rioprostil, a prostaglandin E_1 analog, in rats and dogs. *J. Pharmacol. Exp. Ther.* 242: 927-933, 1987.

1550. Lin, T., *et al.* Actions of nizatidine on the rat uterus, dog stomach and experimentally induced gastric lesions. *J. Pharmacol. Exp. Ther.* 239: 400-405, 1986.

Bibliography

1551. Lin, T., *et al.* Actions of nizatidine, a selective histamine H_2-receptor antagonist, on gastric acid secretion in dog, rats and frogs. *J. Pharmacol. Exp. Ther.* 239: 406-410, 1986.

1552. Sawamura, A., *et al.* Stimulation of cardiac slow Ca^{++} current by high concentration of cimetidine. *J. Pharmacol. Exp. Ther.* 236: 192-196, 1986.

1553. Mokler, D.J., *et al.* Blockade of the behavioral effects of lysergic acid diethylamide, 2,5-dimethoxy-4-methylamphetamin, quipazine and lisuride by 5-hydroxytryptamine antagonists. *J. Pharmacol. Exp. Ther.* 227: 557-562, 1983.

1554. Brady, L.S. and J.E. Barrett. Effects of serotonin receptor agonists and antagonists on schedule-controlled behavior of squirrel monkeys. *J. Pharmacol. Exp. Ther.* 235: 436-441, 1985.

1555. McCall, R.B. and S.J. Humphrey. Involvement of serotonin in the central regulation of blood pressure: Evidence for a facilitating effect on sympathetic nerve activity. *J. Pharmacol. Exp. Ther.* 222: 94-102, 1982.

1556. Gellai, M. and R.R. Ruffolo, Jr. Renal effects of selective alpha-1 and alpha-2 adrenoceptor agonists in conscious, normotensive rats. *J. Pharmacol. Exp. Ther.* 240: 723-728, 1987.

1557. Daugaard, G., *et al.* Effect of cisplatin on proximal convoluted and straight segments of the rat kidney. *J. Pharmacol. Exp. Ther.* 244: 1081-1085, 1988.

1558. O'Donnell, J.M. Effects of clenbuterol and prenalterol on behavior maintained under a multiple fixed-interval, fixed-ratio schedule. *J. Pharmacol. Exp. Ther.* 242: 588-594, 1987.

1559. Vos, P., *et al.* Selective regulation of beta-2 adrenergic receptors by the chronic administration of the lipophilic beta adrenergic receptor agonist clenbuterol: An autoradiographic study. *J. Pharmacol. Exp. Ther.* 242: 707-712, 1987.

1560. Lassen, J.B. Piperoxane reduces the effects of clonidine on aggression in mice and on noradrenaline dependent hypermotility in rats. *Eur. J. Pharmacol.* 47: 45-49, 1978.

1561. Ross, S.B. Anti-aggressive action of dopamine-ß-hydroxylase inhibitors in mice. *J. Pharm. Pharmacol.* 28: 590, 1976.

1562. Razzak, A., *et al.* Automutilation induced by clonidine in mice. *Eur. J. Pharmacol.* 30: 356-359, 1975.

1563. Yoshioka, M., *et al.* Central Sympatho-inhibitory action of ketanserin in rats. *J. Pharmacol. Exp. Ther.* 243: 1174-1178, 1987.

1564. Tangri, K.K., *et al.* Mechanism of cardiovascular effects of clonidine in conscious and anesthetized rabbits. *J. Pharmacol. Exp. Ther.* 202: 69-75, 1977.

Bibliography

1565. Cavero, I., *et al.* Pharmacological, hemodynamic and biochemical mechanisms involved in the blood pressure lowering effects of pergolide, in normotensive and hypertensive dogs. *J. Pharmacol. Exp. Ther.* 235: 798-809, 1985.

1566. Oates, H.F., *et al.* Withdrawal of clonidine: Effects of varying dosage or duration of treatment on subsequent blood pressure and heart rate responses. *J. Pharmacol. Exp. Ther.* 206: 268-273, 1978.

1567. Primm, R.K., *et al.* Selective effects of clonidine on the canine sinus node. *J. Pharmacol. Exp. Ther.* 214: 223-228, 1980.

1568. Hom, G.J. and B.S. Jandhyala. Effects of cerebroventricular administration of ouabain on renal hemodynamics in anesthetized dogs: Evidence for the participation of renal dopaminergic vasodilator fibers. *J. Pharmacol. Exp. Ther.* 230: 275-283, 1984.

1569. Hayashi, S., *et al.* Postsynaptic alpha adrenoceptors in baboon cerebral and mesenteric arteries. *J. Pharmacol. Exp. Ther.* 235: 113-121, 1985.

1570. Tibirica, E., *et al.* Differences in the ability of yohimbine to antagonize the hypotensive effect of clonidine in normotensive and spontaneously hypertensive rats. *J. Pharmacol. Exp. Ther.* 244: 1062-1066, 1988.

1571. Shropshire, A.T. and R.L. Wendt. Failure of naloxone to reduce clonidine-induced changes in blood pressure, heart rate and sympathetic nerve firing in cats. *J. Pharmacol. Exp. Ther.* 224: 494-500, 1983.

1572. Armstrong, J.M., *et al.* Urethane inhibits cardiovascular responses mediated by the stimulation of alpha-2 adrenoceptors in the rat. *J. Pharmacol. Exp. Ther.* 223: 524-535, 1982.

1573. Sybertz, E.J. and B.G. Zimmerman. Influence of hypoxic stimulation of carotid body chemoreceptors on clonidine and l-dopa-induced hypotension. *J. Pharmacol. Exp. Ther.* 207: 950-957, 1978.

1574. Kubo, T., *et al.* Pharmacological characterization of spinal alpha adrenoceptors related to blood pressure control in rats. *J. Pharmacol. Exp. Ther.* 240: 298-302, 1987.

1575. Colpaert, F.C. and P.A.J. Janssen. Discriminative stimulus properties of xylazine in rat: Discriminability and effects of putative alpha-2 adrenoceptor agonists and antagonists. *J. Pharmacol. Exp. Ther.* 235: 521-527, 1985.

1576. Smith, J.B. Effects of single and repeated daily injections of morphine, clonidine and l-nantradol on responding of squirrel monkeys under escape titration. *J. Pharmacol. Exp. Ther.* 234: 94-99, 1985.

1577. Curtis, A.L. and J. Marwah. Evidence for alpha adrenoceptor modulation of the nociceptive jaw-opening reflex in rats and rabbits. *J. Pharmacol. Exp. Ther.* 238: 576-580, 1986.

Bibliography

1578. Doherty, N.S., *et al.* The role of prostaglandins in the nociceptive response induced by intraperitoneal injection of zymosan in mice. *Brit. J. Pharmacol.* 91: 39-47, 1987.

1579. Thomas, G.P. and R.M. Tripathi. Effects of α-adrenoceptor agonists and antagonists on ouabain-induced arrhythmias and cardiac arrest in guinea-pig. *Brit. J. Pharmacol.* 89: 385-388, 1986.

1580. Gellman, R.L., *et al.* Alpha-2 receptors mediate an endogenous noradrenergic suppression of kindling development. *J. Pharmacol. Exp. Ther.* 241: 891-898, 1987.

1581. Moroni, F., *et al.* Modulation of cortical acetylcholine and γ-aminobutyric acid release in freely moving guinea pigs: Effects of clonidine and other adrenergic drugs. *J. Pharmacol. Exp. Ther.* 227: 435-440, 1983.

1582. Cheng, H.C., *et al.* Effects of clonidine on gastric acid secretion in the rat. *J. Pharmacol. Exp. Ther.* 217: 121-126, 1981.

1583. Fox, D.A. and P. Bass. Ablation of the myenteric plexus impairs alpha but not beta jejunal longitudinal muscle. *J. Pharmacol. Exp. Ther.* 239: 9-14, 1986.

1584. Buccafusco, J.J. and R.S. Aronstam. Clonidine protection from the toxicity of Soman, an organophosphate acetylcholinesterase inhibitor, in the mouse. *J. Pharmacol. Exp. Ther.* 239: 43-47, 1986.

1585. Di Tullio, N.W., *et al.* Mechanisms involved in the hyperglycemic response induced by clonidine and other alpha-2 adrenoceptor agonists. *J. Pharmacol. Exp. Ther.* 228: 168-173, 1984.

1586. Humphreys, M.H. and I.A. Reid. Effects of clonidine on glucose and phosphate metabolism in the anesthetized dog. *J. Pharmacol. Exp. Ther.* 208: 243-247, 1979.

1587. Roman, R.J., *et al.* Water diuretic and natriuretic effect of clonidine in the rat. *J. Pharmacol. Exp. Ther.* 211: 385-393, 1979.

1588. Miller, M. Clonidine-induced diuresis in the rat: Evidence for a renal site of action. *J. Pharmacol. Exp. Ther.* 214: 608-613, 1980.

1589. Buccafusco, J.J. Mechanism of the antihypertensive action of clonidine on the pressor response to physostigmine. *J. Pharmacol. Exp. Ther.* 212: 58-63, 1980.

1590. Ruwart, M.J., *et al.* Clonidine delays small intestinal transit in the rat. *J. Pharmacol. Exp. Ther.* 212: 487-490, 1980.

1591. Braestrup, C. and M. Nielsen. Regulation in the central norepinephrine neurotransmission induced in vivo by alpha adrenoceptor active drugs. *J. Pharmacol. Exp. Ther.* 198: 596-608, 1976.

1592. DiStefano, P., *et al.* Characterization of the clonidine withdrawal syndrome in the normotensive rat. *J. Pharmacol. Exp. Ther.* 214: 263-268, 1980.

Bibliography

1593. Togashi, H. Central and peripheral effects of clonidine on the adrenal medullary function in spontaneously hypertensive rats. *J. Pharmacol. Exp. Ther.* 225: 191-197, 1983.

1594. Ishii, K. and R. Kato. Development of tolerance to alpha-2 adrenergic agonists in the vascular system of the rat after chronic treatment with clonidine. *J. Pharmacol. Exp. Ther.* 231: 685-691, 1984.

1595. Kaempf, G.L. and J.H. Porter. Differential effects of pimozide and clozapine on schedule-controlled and schedule-induced behaviors after acute and chronic administration. *J. Pharmacol. Exp. Ther.* 243: 437-445, 1987.

1596. Fromherz, K. Larocain, a new local anesthetic. *Naunyn-Schmiedebergs Arch. Exp. Pathol. Pharmakol.* 158: 368-380, 1930.

1597. Fekete, M. and J. Borsy. Chlorpromazine, cocaine antagonism: Its relation to changes of dopamine metabolism in the brain. *Eur. J. Pharmacol.* 16: 171-175, 1971.

1598. Blumberg, H. and C. Ikeda. Naltrexone, morphine and cocaine interactions in mice and rat. *J. Pharmacol. Exp. Ther.* 206: 303-310, 1978.

1599. Risner, M.E., *et al.* Effects of nicotine, cocaine and some of their metabolites on schedule-controlled responding by beagle dogs and squirrel monkeys. *J. Pharmacol. Exp. Ther.* 234: 113-119, 1985.

1600. Spealman, R.D., *et al.* Stereoselective behavioral effects of cocaine and a phenylpropane analog. *J. Pharmacol. Exp. Ther.* 225: 509-514, 1983.

1601. Reith, M.E.A., *et al.* Cocaine disposition in the brain after continuous or intermittent treatment and locomotor stimulation in mice. *J. Pharmacol. Exp. Ther.* 243: 281-287, 1987.

1602. Wood, D.M. and M.W. Emmett-Oglesby. Characteristics of tolerance, recovery of tolerance and cross-tolerance for cocaine used as a discriminative stimulus. *J. Pharmacol. Exp. Ther.* 237: 120-125, 1986.

1603. James, R.C., *et al.* Antagonism of cocaine-induced hepatotoxicity by the alpha adrenergic antagonists phentolamine and yohimbine. *J. Pharmacol. Exp. Ther.* 242: 726-732, 1987.

1604. Pitts, D.K. and J. Marwah. Electrophysiological actions of cocaine on noradrenergic neurons in rat locus ceruleus. *J. Pharmacol. Exp. Ther.* 240: 345-351, 1987.

1605. Carroll, M.E., *et al.* Effects of naltrexone on intravenous cocaine self administration in rats during food satiation and deprivation. *J. Pharmacol. Exp. Ther.* 238: 1-7, 1986.

1606. Risner, M.E. and S.R. Goldberg. A comparison of nicotine and cocaine self-administration in the dog: Fixed-ratio and progressive ratio schedules of intravenous drug infusion. *J. Pharmacol. Exp. Ther.* 224: 319-326, 1983.

Bibliography

1607.   Spealman, R.D. and R.T. Kelleher. Behavioral effects of self-administered cocaine: Responding maintained alternately by cocaine and electric shock in squirrel monkeys. *J. Pharmacol. Exp. Ther.* 210: 206-214, 1979.

1608.   Blumberg, H. and C. Ikeda. Naltrexone, morphine and cocaine interactions in mice and rats. *J. Pharmacol. Exp. Ther.* 206: 303-310, 1978.

1609.   Chaudhry, A. and M.M. Vohra. Mechanism and metabolic disposition of verapamil-evoked overflow of radioactivity from isolated atria preloaded with [^{3}H]norepinephrine. *J. Pharmacol. Exp. Ther.* 232: 850-856, 1985.

1610.   Kachur, J.F., *et al*. Effect of dextromethorphan on guinea pig ileal contractility in vitro: Comparison with levomethorphan, loperamide and codeine. *J. Pharmacol. Exp. Ther.* 239: 661-667, 1986.

1611.   Hoffmeister, F., *et al*. Intragastric self-administration in the Rhesus monkey: A comparison of the reinforcing effects of codeine, phenacetin and paracetamol. *J. Pharmacol. Exp. Ther.* 214: 213-218, 1980.

1612.   Bloss, J.L. and D.L. Hammond. Shock titration in the rhesus monkey: Effects of opiate and nonopiate analgesics. *J. Pharmacol. Exp. Ther.* 235: 423-430, 1985.

1613.   Rosow, C.E. Opiates and thermoregulation in mice. I. Agonists. *J. Pharmacol. Exp. Ther.* 213: 273-283, 1980.

1614.   Niemegeers, C.J.E., *et al*. Dissociation between opiate-like and antidiarrheal activities of antidiarrheal drugs. *J. Pharmacol. Exp. Ther.* 210: 327-333, 1979.

1615.   Foulkes, R., *et al*. Exogenous corticosterone acetate attenuates the hypotension induced by ganglionic blockade in conscious Long Evans and Brattleboro rats. *J. Pharmacol. Exp. Ther.* 243: 1048-1054, 1987.

1616.   Walzer, P.D., *et al*. Experimental *Pneumocystis carinii* pneumonia in different strains of cortisonized mice. *Infect. Immun.* 24: 939-947, 1979.

1617.   Müller, E. and M. Müntener. Short time observations of morphological changes and cholinesterase distribution in lymphatic organs and the mouse after corticosteroid and x-ray treatment. *Histochemistry* 60: 169-180, 1979.

1618.   Bedrick, A.D. and R.L. Ladda. Epidermal growth factor potentiates cortisone-induced cleft palate in the mouse. *Teratology* 17: 13-18, 1978.

1619.   Dolphin, A., *et al*. Modification of the L-dopa reversal of reserpine akinesia by inhibition of dopamine ß-hydroxylase. *Eur. J. Pharmacol.* 35: 135-144, 1976.

1620.   Harris, R.A., *et al*. Alterations in the efficacy of naloxone induced by stress, cyclic adenosine monophosphate, and morphine tolerance. *Eur. J. Pharmacol.* 39: 1-10, 1976.

Bibliography

1621.	Slifer, B.L. and R.L. Balster. Phencyclidine-like discriminative stimulus effects of the stereoisomers of alpha- and beta-cyclazocine in rats. *J. Pharmacol. Exp. Ther.* 244: 606-612, 1988.

1622.	White, J.M. and S.G. Holtzman. Three choice drug discrimination in the rat: Morphine, cyclazocine and saline. *J. Pharmacol. Exp. Ther.* 217: 254-262, 1981.

1623.	Teal, J.J. and S.G. Holtzman. Discriminative stimulus effects of cyclazocine in the rat. *J. Pharmacol. Exp. Ther.* 212: 368-376, 1980.

1624.	Bergman, J., *et al.* Behavioral effects of selected opiates and phencyclidine in the non-dependent and cyclazocine-dependent rhesus monkey. *J. Pharmacol. Exp. Ther.* 235: 463-469, 1985.

1625.	Dykstra, L.A. Discrimination of electric shock: Effects of some opioid and nonopioid drugs. *J. Pharmacol. Exp. Ther.* 213: 234-240, 1980.

1626.	Chau, T.T., *et al.* Antitussive effect of the optical isomers of mu, kappa and sigma opiate agonists/antagonists in the cat. *J. Pharmacol. Exp. Ther.* 226: 108-113, 1983.

1627.	Gilliam, J.N. and E.R. Hurd. The differential effects of 6-MP and cyclophosphamide on immunoglobulin deposition in the skin and kidney of NZB/NZW F_1 mice. *J. Immunol.* 119: 1285-1288, 1977.

1628.	Merletti, P.R., *et al.* Growth and inhibition of mouse or human tumors in "nude" (athymic) mice monitored by the extent of ^{125}I-5-iodo-2'-deoxyuridine (^{125}IUdR) uptake. *Eur. J. Cancer* 14: 1057-1064, 1978.

1629.	Levy, L., *et al.* Effect of pulse dose cyclophosphamide on the anamnestic immune response in NZB1W mice. *Agents Actions* 816: 644-651, 1978.

1630.	Stockman, G.D., *et al.* Differential effects of cyclophosphamide on the B and T cell compartments of adult mice. *J. Immunol.* 110: 277-282, 1973.

1631.	Jackson, N.M., *et al.* Alterations in renal structure and function in a rat model of cyclosporine nephrotoxicity. *J. Pharmacol. Exp. Ther.* 242: 749-756, 1987.

1632.	Babany, G., *et al.* Evaluation of the in vivo dose-response relationship of immunosuppressive drugs using a mouse heart transplant model: Application to cyclosporine. *J. Pharmacol. Exp. Ther.* 244: 259-262, 1988.

1633.	Perico, N., *et al.* Effect of short-term cyclosporine administration in rats on renin-angiotensin and thromboxane A_2: Possible relevance to the reduction in glomerular filtration rate. *J. Pharmacol. Exp. Ther.* 239: 229-235, 1986.

1634.	Winquist, R.J., *et al.* Calcium entry blocker activity of cyproheptadine in isolated cardiovascular preparations. *J. Pharmacol. Exp. Ther.* 230: 103-109, 1984.

Bibliography

1635.   Bush, L.R. Effects of the serotonin antagonists, cyproheptadine, ketanserin and mianserin, on cyclic flow reductions in stenosed canine coronary arteries. *J. Pharmacol. Exp. Ther.* 240: 674-682, 1987.

1636.   Clineschmidt, B.V., *et al.* Central serotonin-like activity of 6-chloro-2-[-1-piperazinyl]pyrazine (CPP; MK-212). *Eur. J. Pharmacol.* 44: 65-74, 1977.

1637.   Scarpignato, C., *et al.* Antisecretory and antiulcer effect of the H_2-receptor antagonist famotidine in the rat: Comparison with ranitidine. *Brit. J. Pharmacol.* 92: 153-159, 1987.

1638.   Oishi, T. and S. Szabo. Effect of tyrosine administration on duodenal ulcer induced by cysteamine in the rat. *J. Pharmacol. Exp. Ther.* 240: 879-882, 1987.

1639.   Cooper, C.L. and K.U. Malik. Mechanism of action of vasopressin on prostaglandin synthesis and vascular function in the isolated rat kidney: Effect of calcium antagonists and calmodulin inhibitors. *J. Pharmacol. Exp. Ther.* 229: 139-147, 1984.

1640.   Szikszay, M., *et al.* Interactions between verapamil and morphine on physiological parameters in rats. *J. Pharmacol. Exp. Ther.* 238: 192-197, 1986.

1641.   Salata, J.J. and J. Jalife. Effects of dantrolene sodium on the electrophysiological properties of canine cardiac purkinje fibers. *J. Pharmacol. Exp. Ther.* 220: 157-166, 1982.

1642.   Dennis, T., *et al.* Presynaptic alpha-2 adrenoceptors play a major role in the effects of idazoxan on cortical noradrenaline release (as measured by in vivo dialysis in the rat). *J. Pharmacol. Exp. Ther.* 241: 642-649, 1987.

1643.   O'Donnell, J.M and L.S. Seiden. Altered effects of desipramine on operant performance after 6-hydroxydopamine-induced depletion of brain dopamine or norepinephrine. *J. Pharmacol. Exp. Ther.* 229: 629-635, 1984.

1644.   Nomura, Y., *et al.* Influence of repeated administration of desmethylimipramine on beta adrenergic and muscarinic cholinergic receptors and $^{45}Ca^{++}$ binding to sarcoplasmic reticulum in the rat heart. *J. Pharmacol. Exp. Ther.* 223: 834-840, 1982.

1645.   Penten, P. and N. Benowitz. Efficacy and mechanisms of action of sodium bicarbonate in the treatment of desipramine toxicity in rats. *J. Pharmacol. Exp. Ther.* 230: 12-19, 1984.

1646.   Pals, D.T. and G.L. DeGraff. Cardiovascular effects of losulazine hydrochloride, a peripheral norepinephrine-depleting agent, in nonhuman primates. *J. Pharmacol. Exp. Ther.* 232: 407-412, 1985.

1647.   Szekely, A.M., *et al.* Effect of a protracted antidepressant treatment on signal transduction and [^{3}H] (-)-baclofen binding at $GABA_B$ receptors. *J. Pharmacol. Exp. Ther.* 243: 155-159, 1987.

Bibliography

1648. Nies, A.S., *et al.* Indomethacin-furosemide interaction: The importance of renal blood flow. *J. Pharmacol. Exp. Ther.* 226: 27-32, 1983.

1649. Honma, Y., *et al.* Prolongation of survival time of mice inoculated with myeloid leukemia cells by normal differentiation. *Cancer. Res.* 39: 3167-3171, 1979.

1650. Gillette, R.W. and D.A. Wunderlich. Accelerated growth of mammary tumor cells in normal and athymic mice after treatment *in vitro* with dexamethasone. *Cancer Res.* 38: 3146-3149, 1978.

1651. Gidari, A.S. and R.D. Levere. Glucocorticoid-mediated inhibition of erythroid colony formation by mouse bone marrow cells. *J. Lab. Clin. Med.* 93: 872-878, 1979.

1652. Wallace, J.L. and B.J.R. Whittle. Effects of inhibitors of arachidonic acid metabolism on Paf-induced gastric mucosal necrosis and haemoconcentration. *Brit. J. Pharmacol.* 89: 415-422, 1986.

1653. Terashita, Z., *et al.* A lethal role of platelet-activating factor in anaphylactic shock in mice. *J. Pharmacol. Exp. Ther.* 243: 378-383, 1987.

1654. Young, A.M. and J.H. Woods. Maintenance of behavior by ketamine and related compounds in Rhesus monkeys with different self-administration histories. *J. Pharmacol. Exp. Ther.* 218: 720-727, 1981.

1655. Jacobson, A.E., *et al.* Enantiomeric and diastereomeric dioxadrols: Behavioral, biochemical and chemical determination of the configuration necessary for phencyclidine-like properties. *J. Pharmacol. Exp. Ther.* 243: 110-117, 1987.

1656. Gaginella, T.S., *et al.* Effect of dextromethorphan and levomethorphan on gastric emptying and intestinal transit in the rat. *J. Pharmacol. Exp. Ther.* 240: 388-391, 1987.

1657. Domino, E.F., *et al.* Evidence for a central site of action for the antitussive effects of caramiphen. *J. Pharmacol. Exp. Ther.* 233: 249-253, 1985.

1658. Choi, D.W., *et al.* Dextrorphan and levorphanol selectively block N-methyl-D-aspartate receptor-mediated neurotoxicity on cortical neurons. *J. Pharmacol. Exp. Ther.* 242: 713-720, 1987.

1659. Marcucci, F., *et al.* Anticonvulsant activity and brain levels of diazepam and its metabolites in mice. *Eur. J. Pharmacol.* 16: 311-314, 1971.

1660. Wettstein, J.G. and R.D. Spealman. Behavioral effects of zopiclone, CL 218, 872 and diazepam in squirrel monkeys: Antagonism by RO 15-1788 and CGS 8216. *J. Pharmacol. Exp. Ther.* 238: 522-528, 1986.

1661. McCormick, G.Y., *et al.* Effects of diazepam on arterial blood gas concentrations and pH of adult rats acutely and chronically exposed to methadone. *J. Pharmacol. Exp. Ther.* 230: 353-359, 1984.

1662. Okamoto, M., *et al.* Comparison of effects of diazepam on barbiturate and on ethanol withdrawal. *J. Pharmacol. Exp. Ther.* 225: 589-594, 1983.

1663. Liu, S.-S., *et al.* Correlation of urinary excretion of methadone metabolites with methadone metabolism and analgesia in the rat. *J. Pharmacol. Exp. Ther.* 204: 67-76, 1978.

1664. Waszczak, B.L., *et al.* Effects of anticonvulsant drugs on substantia nigra pars reticulata neurons. *J. Pharmacol. Exp. Ther.* 239: 606-611, 1986.

1665. Gallaher, E.J., *et al.* Benzodiazepine dependence in mice after ingestion of drug-containing pellets. *J. Pharmacol. Exp. Ther.* 237: 462-467, 1986.

1666. McNicholas, L.F., *et al.* Precipitation of abstinence in nordiazepam and diazepam-dependent dogs. *J. Pharmacol. Exp. Ther.* 245: 221-224, 1988.

1667. Bennett, D.A. and C.L. Amrick. Home cage pretreatment with diazepam: Effects on subsequent conflict testing and rotorod assessment. *J. Pharmacol. Exp. Ther.* 242: 595-599, 1987.

1668. Emmett-Oglesby, M.W., *et al.* Withdrawal from diazepam substitutes for the discriminative stimulus properties of pentylenetetrazol. *J. Pharmacol. Exp. Ther.* 244: 892-897, 1988.

1669. Navarro, H.A., *et al.* Prenatal exposure to nicotine via maternal infusions: Effects on development of catecholamine systems. *J. Pharmacol. Exp. Ther.* 244: 940-944, 1988.

1670. Gray, W.D. and C.E. Rawh. The anticonvulsant action of the carbonic anhydrase inhibitor methazolamide: Possible involvement of a noradrenergic mechanism. *Eur. J. Pharmacol.* 28: 42-54, 1974.

1671. Ayachi, S. and A.M. Brown. Hypotensive effects of cardiac glycosides in spontaneously hypertensive rats. *J. Pharmacol. Exp. Ther.* 213: 520-524, 1980.

1672. Karagueuzian, H.S. and B.G. Katzung. Relative inotropic and arrhythmogenic effects of five cardiac steroids in ventricular myocardium: Oscillatory afterpotentials and the role of endogenous catecholamines. *J. Pharmacol. Exp. Ther.* 218: 348-356, 1981.

1673. Kim, D.-H., *et al.* Ischemia-induced enhancement of digitalis sensitivity in isolated guinea-pig heart. *J. Pharmacol. Exp. Ther.* 226: 335-342, 1983.

1674. Lechat, P., *et al.* Reversal of lethal digoxin toxicity in guinea pigs using monoclonal antibodies and Fab fragments. *J. Pharmacol. Exp. Ther.* 229: 210-213, 1984.

1675. Kim, D., *et al.* Role of sympathetic nervous system in ischemia-induced reduction of digoxin tolerance in anesthetized cats. *J. Pharmacol. Exp. Ther.* 228: 537-544, 1984.

Bibliography

1676. Pace, D.G. and R.A. Gillis. Neuroexcitatory effects of digoxin in the cat. *J. Pharmacol. Exp. Ther.* 199: 583-600, 1976.

1677. Mello, N.K., *et al.* Comparison of buprenorphine and methadone effects on opiate self-administration in primates. *J. Pharmacol. Exp. Ther.* 225: 378-386, 1983.

1678. Ruffolo, R.R., *et al.* Possible relationship between receptor reserve and the differential antagonism of alpha-1 and alpha-2 adrenoceptor-mediated pressor responses by calcium channel antagonists in the pithed rat. *J. Pharmacol. Exp. Ther.* 230: 587-594, 1984.

1679. Pearce, W.J. and J.A. Bevan. Diltiazem and autoregulation of canine cerebral blood flow. *J. Pharmacol. Exp. Ther.* 242: 812-817, 1987.

1680. Ritchie, D.M., *et al.* Evaluation of calcium entry blockers in several models of immediate hypersensitivity. *J. Pharmacol. Exp. Ther.* 229: 690-695, 1984.

1681. Cavero, I., *et al.* Diltiazem protects the isolated rabbit heart from the mechanical and ultrastructural damage produced by transient hypoxia, low-flow ischemia and exposure to Ca^{++}-free medium. *J. Pharmacol. Exp. Ther.* 226: 258-268, 1983.

1682. Hondeghen, L.N., *et al.* Verapamil, diltiazem and nifedipine block the depolarization-induced potentiation of norepinephrine contractions in rabbit aorta and porcine coronary arteries. *J. Pharmacol. Exp. Ther.* 239: 808-813, 1986.

1683. Narita, H., *et al.* Hypotensive and diuretic actions of diltiazem in spontaneously hypertensive and Wistar Kyoto rats. *J. Pharmacol. Exp. Ther.* 227: 472-477, 1983.

1684. Walsh, K.B., *et al.* Effect of calcium antagonist drugs on calcium currents in mammalian skeletal muscle fibers. *J. Pharmacol. Exp. Ther.* 236: 403-407, 1986.

1685. Downing, S.J., *et al.* Diltiazem pharmacokinetics in the rat and relationship between its serum concentration and uterine and cardiovascular effects. *Brit. J. Pharmacol.* 91: 735-745, 1987.

1686. Kadowitz, P.J., *et al.* Inhibitory effects of diltiazem on vasoconstrictor responses in the cat. *J. Pharmacol. Exp. Ther.* 244: 84-90, 1988.

1687. Weis, M.T. and K.U. Malik. Beta adrenergic receptor-stimulated prostaglandin syntheses in the isolated rabbit heart: Relationship to extra- and intracellular calcium. *J. Pharmacol. Exp. Ther.* 235: 178-185, 1985.

1688. Rubin, L.F. Toxicity of dimethyl sulfoxide alone and in combination. *Ann. N.Y. Acad. Sci.* 243: 98-103, 1975.

1689. Heikkila, R.E. The prevention of alloxan-induced diabetes in mice by dimethyl sulfoxide. *Eur. J. Pharmacol.* 44: 191-193, 1977.

1690. Debons, A.F., *et al.* Inhibition of cholesterol-induced atherosclerosis in rabbits by dimethylsulfoxide. *J. Pharmacol. Exp. Ther.* 243: 745-757, 1987.

Bibliography

1691. Dajani, E.Z., *et al.* Effects of E prostaglandins, diphenoxylate and morphine on intestinal motility *in vivo*. *Eur. J. Pharmacol.* 34: 105-113, 1975.

1692. Reynolds, I.J., *et al.* Loperamide: Blockade of calcium channels as a mechanism for antidiarrheal effects. *J. Pharmacol. Exp. Ther.* 231: 628-632, 1984.

1693. J.G. Gerber and N.A. Payne. Endogenous adenosine modulates gastric acid secretion to histamine in canine parietal cells. *J. Pharmacol. Exp. Ther.* 244: 190-194, 1988.

1694. Rardon, D.P., *et al.* Adenosine and prostacyclin independent electrophysiological effects of dipyridamole in guinea-pig papillary muscles and canine cardiac purkinje fibers. *J. Pharmacol. Exp. Ther.* 231: 206-213, 1984.

1695. Deneke, S.M., *et al.* Enhancement by disulfiram (antabuse) of toxic effects of 95 to 97% O_2 on the rat lung. *J. Pharmacol. Exp. Ther.* 208: 377-389, 1979.

1696. Hayes, J.S. and N. Bowling. Role of the alpha agonist activity of dobutamine in mediating cardiac output: Effects of prolonged isoproterenol infusion. *J. Pharmacol. Exp. Ther.* 241: 861-869, 1987.

1697. Wanless, R.B., *et al.* Regional blood flow and hemodynamics in the rabbit with adriamycin cardiomyopathy: Effects of isosorbide dinitrate, dobutamine and captopril. *J. Pharmacol. Exp. Ther.* 243: 1101-1106, 1987.

1698. Petein, M., *et al.* Hemodynamic and regional blood flow response to piroximone (MDL 19,205) in dogs with congestive heart failure: A comparison with dobutamine. *J. Pharmacol. Exp. Ther.* 241: 956-960, 1987.

1699. Hagahama, S., *et al.* Role of vasopressin in the cardiovascular effects of LY 171555, a selective dopamine D_2 receptor agonist: Studies in conscious Brattleboro and Long-Evans rats. *J. Pharmacol. Exp. Ther.* 242: 143-151, 1987.

1700. Szabo, B., *et al.* Dopamine receptor agonist and alpha-2 adrenoceptor antagonist effects of fenoldopam in rabbits. *J. Pharmacol. Exp. Ther.* 239: 881-886, 1986.

1701. Lokhandwala, M.F. and J.P. Buckley. The effect of L-dopa on peripheral sympathetic nerve function: Role of presynaptic dopamine receptors. *J. Pharmacol. Exp. Ther.* 204: 362-371, 1978.

1702. Dhasmana, K.M. and B.A. Spilker. On the mechanism of L-DOPA-induced postural hypotension in the cat. *Brit. J. Pharmacol.* 47: 437-451, 1973.

1703. Schriefer, J.A., *et al.* Effect of dopamine on length of gestation and on the release of fetal oxytocin in rats. *J. Pharmacol. Exp. Ther.* 212: 431-434, 1980.

1704. Cox, B., *et al.* A comparison between a melanocyte-stimulating hormone inhibitory factor (MIF-I) and substances known to activate central dopamine receptors. *Eur. J. Pharmacol.* 36: 141-147, 1976.

Bibliography

1705. Svensson, T.H. Dopamine release and direct dopamine receptor activation in the central nervous system by D-145, an amantadine derivative. *Eur. J. Pharmacol.* 23: 232-238, 1973.

1706. Yonehara, N. and D.H. Clouet. Effects of delta and mu opiopeptides on the turnover and release of dopamine in rat striatum. *J. Pharmacol. Exp. Ther.* 231: 38-42, 1984.

1707. Horst, W.D., *et al.* Correlation between brain dopamine levels and L-dopa activity in antiparkinson tests. *Eur. J. Pharmacol.* 21: 337-342, 1973.

1708. Pleuvry, B.J. Mouse brain catecholamines 5-hydroxytryptamine and the antinociceptive activity of pethidine. *Eur. J. Pharmacol.* 34: 351-361, 1975.

1709. Nichols, A.J. and R.R. Ruffolo. Evaluation of the alpha and beta adrenoceptor-mediated activitites of the novel, orally active inotropic agent, ibopamine in the cardiovascular system of the pithed rat: Comparison with epinine and dopamine. *J. Pharmacol. Exp. Ther.* 242: 455-463, 1987.

1710. Kusunoki, M., *et al.* Dopamine regulation of [^{3}H]acetylcholine release from guinea-pig stomach. *J. Pharmacol. Exp. Ther.* 234: 713-719, 1985.

1711. Grega, G.J., *et al.* Effects of dopamine (DA) and SKF 82526, a selective DA_1-receptor agonist, on vascular resistances in the canine forelimb. *J. Pharmacol. Exp. Ther.* 229: 756-762, 1984.

1712. Stoychkov, J.N., *et al.* Effects of adriamycin and cyclophosphamide treatment on induction of macrophage cytotoxic function in mice. *Cancer Res.* 39: 3014-3017, 1979.

1713. de Wildt, D.J., *et al.* Cardiovascular effects of doxorubicin-induced toxicity in the intact Lou/M rat and in isolated heart preparations. *J. Pharmacol. Exp. Ther.* 235: 234-240, 1985.

1714. Gilbeau, P.M., *et al.* Dynorphin effects on plasma concentrations of anterior pituitary hormones in the non-human primate. *J. Pharmacol. Exp. Ther.* 238: 974-977, 1986.

1715. Kiang, J.G. and E.T. Wei. Sensitivity to morphine-evoked bradycardia in rats in modified by dynorphin (1-13), leu- and met-enkephalin. *J. Pharmacol. Exp. Ther.* 229: 469-473, 1984.

1716. Garant, D.S. and K. Gale. Infusion of opiates into substantia nigra protects against maximal electroshock seizures in rats. *J. Pharmacol. Exp. Ther.* 234: 45-48, 1985.

1717. Grider, J.R. and G.M. Makhlouf. Suppression of inhibitory neural input to colonic circular muscle by opioid peptides. *J. Pharmacol. Exp. Ther.* 243: 205-210, 1987.

1718. Ueda, N., *et al.* Dual effects of dynorphin-(1-13) on cholinergic and substance P-ergic transmissions in the rabbit iris sphincter muscle. *J. Pharmacol. Exp. Ther.* 232: 545-550, 1985.

Bibliography

1719. Tseng, L.-F., *et al.* Inhibition of tail flick and shaking responses by intrathecal and intraventricular D-ala-D-Leu-enkephalin and ß-endorphin in anesthetized rats. *J. Pharmacol. Exp. Ther.* 224: 51-54, 1983.

1720. Davis, T.P., *et al.* ß-endorphin and its metabolites stimulate motility of the dog small intestine. *J. Pharmacol. Exp. Ther.* 227: 499-507, 1983.

1721. Wightman, J.M., *et al.* Decreased vascular resistance after intra-arterial injections of [met]enkephalin in the hindquarters of conscious rabbits. *J. Pharmacol. Exp. Ther.* 241: 314-320, 1987.

1722. Vaught, J.L. and A.E. Takemori. Differential effects of leucine and methionine enkephalin on morphine-induced analgesia, acute tolerance and dependence. *J. Pharmacol. Exp. Ther.* 208: 86-90, 1979.

1723. Evanich, M.J., *et al.* Ventilatory response to intravenous methionine enkephalin in awake dogs. *J. Pharmacol. Exp. Ther.* 234: 677-680, 1985.

1724. Kimura, T., *et al.* Inhibition by opioid agonists and enhancement by antagonists of the release of catecholamines from the dog adrenal gland in response to splanchnic nerve stimulation: Evidence for the functional role of opioid receptors. *J. Pharmacol. Exp. Ther.* 244: 1098-1102, 1988.

1725. Itoh, Y., *et al.* Involvement of Mu receptors in the opioid-induced increase in the turnover of mouse brain histamine. *J. Pharmacol. Exp. Ther.* 244: 1021-1026, 1988.

1726. Lurie, K.G., *et al.* Desensitization of alpha-1 adrenergic receptor-mediated vascular smooth muscle contraction. *J. Pharmacol. Exp. Ther.* 234: 147-152, 1985.

1727. DeRick, A.F., *et al.* Influence of enhanced alpha-1 acid glycoprotein concentration on protein binding, pharmacokinetics and antiarrhythmic effect of lidocaine in the dog. *J. Pharmacol. Exp. Ther.* 241: 289-293, 1987.

1728. Yorikane, R., *et al.* Effects of epinephrine, isoproterenol and IPS-339 on sympathetic transmission to the dog heart: Evidence against the facilitory role of presynaptic beta adrenoceptors. *J. Pharmacol. Exp. Ther.* 238: 334-340, 1986.

1729. Williams, P.B. Response to adrenergic agonists and antagonists by collateral arteries from the hind limb of the dog. *J. Pharmacol. Exp. Ther.* 214: 239-245, 1980.

1730. Pettibone, D.J. and G.P. Mueller. Adrenergic control of immunoreactive ß-endorphin release from the pituitary of the rat: In vitro and in vivo studies. *J. Pharmacol. Exp. Ther.* 222: 103-108, 1982.

1731. Itoh, H., *et al.* Comparison of the cardiovascular actions of dopamine and epinine in the dog. *J. Pharmacol. Exp. Ther.* 233: 87-93, 1985.

1732. Shebuski, R.J., *et al.* Comparison of the alpha adrenoceptor activity of dopamine, ibopamine and epinine in the pulmonary circulation of the dog. *J. Pharmacol. Exp. Ther.* 241: 6-12, 1987.

Bibliography

1733. Gisclard, V., *et al.* Effect of 17ß-estradiol on endothelium-dependent responses in the rabbit. *J. Pharmacol. Exp. Ther.* 244: 19-22, 1988.

1734. Perez, J., *et al.* Estrogen modulation of the γ-aminobutyric acid receptor complex in the central nervous system of rat. *J. Pharmacol. Exp. Ther.* 244: 1005-1010, 1988.

1735. Steen, P.A., *et al.* Ethacrynic acid inhibits transcellular NaCl reabsorption in dog kidneys in doses of 1 to 10 mg.kg^{-1} and proximal bicarbonate-dependent reabsorption at higher doses. *J. Pharmacol. Exp. Ther.* 219: 505-509, 1981.

1736. Foy, J.M. and B.L. Furman. Effect of single dose administration of diuretics on the blood sugar of alloxan-diabetic mice or mice made hyperglycaemic by acute administration of diazoxide. *Brit. J. Pharmacol.* 47: 124-132, 1973.

1737. Lin-Michell, E., *et al.* Effect of ethosuximide alone and in combination with γ-aminobutyric acid receptor agonists on brain γ-aminobutyric acid concentration, anticonvulsant activity and neurotoxicity in mice. *J. Pharmacol. Exp. Ther.* 237: 486-489, 1986.

1738. Paule, M.G. and E.K. Killam. Behavioral toxicity of chronic ethosuximide and sodium valproate treatment in the epileptic baboon, *Papio papio*. *J. Pharmacol. Exp. Ther.* 238: 32-38, 1986.

1739. Capek, R. and B. Esplin. Effects of ethosuximide on transmission of repetitive impulses and apparent rates of transmitter turnover in the spinal monosynaptic pathway. *J. Pharmacol. Exp. Ther.* 201: 320-325, 1977.

1740. Gwynn, G.J. and E.F. Domino. Genotype-dependent behavioral sensitivity to Mu vs. Kappa opiate agonists. I. Acute and chronic effects on mouse locomotor activity. *J. Pharmacol. Exp. Ther.* 231: 306-311, 1984.

1741. Katz J.L. and S.R. Goldberg. Effects of ethylketazocine and morphine on schedule-controlled behavior in pigeons and squirrel monkeys. *J. Pharmacol. Exp. Ther.* 239: 433-441, 1986.

1742. Wu, K.M. and W.R. Martin. An analysis of nicotinic and opioid processes in the medulla oblongata and nucleus ambiguus of the dog. *J. Pharmacol. Exp. Ther.* 229: 302-307, 1983.

1743. Sheldon, R.J., *et al.* Mu antagonist properties of kappa agonists in a model of rat urinary bladder motility in vivo. *J. Pharmacol. Exp. Ther.* 243: 234-240, 1987.

1744. Takemori, A.E., *et al.* Studies on the quantitative antagonism of analgesics by naloxone and diprenorphine. *Eur. J. Pharmacol.* 20: 85-92, 1972.

1745. Iyengar, S., *et al.* Kappa opiate agonists modulate the hypothalamic-pituitary-adrenocortical axis in the rat. *J. Pharmacol. Exp. Ther.* 238: 429-436, 1986.

Bibliography

1746. Clark, E.S. and D.N. Granger. Effects of fenoldopam on feline intestinal microcirculation. *J. Pharmacol. Exp. Ther.* 244: 983-986, 1988.

1747. Lappe, R.W., *et al.* Effects of fenoldopam on regional vascular resistance in conscious spontaneously hypertensive rats. *J. Pharmacol. Exp. Ther.* 236: 187-191, 1986.

1748. Sabouni, M.H., *et al.* Pharmacological characterization of dopamine receptors in the stellate ganglia with selective DA_1 and DA_2 receptor agonists and antagonists. *J. Pharmacol. Exp. Ther.* 236: 65-70, 1986.

1749. Fone, K.C.F. and H. Wilson. The effects of alfentanil and selected narcotic analgesics on the rate of action potential discharge of medullary respiratory neurones in anaesthetized rats. *Brit. J. Pharmacol.* 89: 67-76, 1986.

1750. Willette, R.M., *et al.* Stimulation of opiate receptors in the dorsal pontine tegmentum inhibits reflex contraction of the urinary bladder. *J. Pharmacol. Exp. Ther.* 244: 403-409, 1988.

1751. Emmett-Oglesby, M.W., *et al.* Tolerance and cross-tolerance to the discriminative stimulus properties of fentanyl and morphine. *J. Pharmacol. Exp. Ther.* 245: 17-23, 1988.

1752. Yaksh, T.L. and T.A. Rudy. Studies on the direct spinal action of narcotics in the production of analgesia in the rat. *J. Pharmacol. Exp. Ther.* 202: 411-428, 1977.

1753. Willette, R.N., *et al.* Activation of cholinergic mechanisms in the medulla oblongata reverse intravenous opioid-induced respiratory depression. *J. Pharmacol. Exp. Ther.* 240: 352-358, 1987.

1754. Rendig, S.V., *et al.* Comparative cardiac contractile actions of six narcotic analgesics: Morphine, meperidine, pentazocine, fentanyl, methadone and l-α-acetylmethadol (LAAM). *J. Pharmacol. Exp. Ther.* 215: 259-265, 1980.

1755. Vicini, S., *et al.* Actions of benzodiazepine and ß-carboline derivatives on GABA-activated Cl^- channels recorded from membrane patches of neonatal rat cortical neurons in culture. *J. Pharmacol. Exp. Ther.* 243: 1195-1201, 1987.

1756. Skinner, S.M. and R.W. Lewis. Antileukemia activity (L1210) of 6-mercaptopurine and its metallo complexes in mice. *Res. Commun. Chem. Pathol. Pharmacol.* 16: 183-186, 1977.

1757. Houghton, J.A., *et al.* Mechanism of induction of gastrointestinal toxicity in the mouse by 5-fluorouracil, 5-fluorouridine, and 5-fluoro-2'-deoxyuridine. *Cancer Res.* 39: 2406-2413, 1979.

1758. Heppner, G.H. and P. Calabresi. Effect of sequence of administration of methotrexate, leucovorin, and 5-fluorouracil on mammary tumor growth and survival in syngeneic C_3H mice. *Cancer Res.* 37: 4580-4583, 1977.

Bibliography

1759. Drago, J.R., *et al.* Chemotherapy of Nb rat adenocarcinoma of the prostate heterotransplanted into congenitally athymic (nude) mice: Report of 5-fluorouracil and cyclophosphamide. *J. Surg. Res.* 26: 400-403, 1979.

1760. Lassen, J.B. Potent and long-lasting potentiation of two 5-hydroxytryptophan-induced effects in mice by three selective 5-HT uptake inhibitors. *Eur. J. Pharmacol.* 47: 351-358, 1978.

1761. Takemori, A.E. and P.S. Portoghese. Evidence for the interaction of morphine with kappa and delta opioid receptors to induce analgesia in ß-funaltrexamine-treated mice. *J. Pharmacol. Exp. Ther.* 243: 91-94, 1987.

1762. Dykstra, L.A., *et al.* Kappa opioids in rhesus monkeys. II. Analysis of the antagonistic actions of quadazocine and ß-funaltrexamine. *J. Pharmacol. Exp. Ther.* 242: 421-427, 1987.

1763. Gmerek, D.E. and J.H. Woods. Effects of ß-funaltrexamine in normal and morphine-dependent rhesus monkeys: Observational studies. *J. Pharmacol. Exp. Ther.* 235: 296-301, 1985.

1764. Locke, K.W. and S.G. Holtzman. Behavioral effects of opioid peptides selective for Mu or Delta receptors. 1. Morphine-like discriminative stimulus effects. *J. Pharmacol. Exp. Ther.* 238: 990-996, 1986.

1765. Sandström, P.-E. Probenecid potentiates the hyperglycaemic effect but reduces the diuretic effect of frusemide in mice. *Brit. J. Pharmacol.* 89: 307-312, 1986.

1766. Christensen, S., *et al.* Dose dependence of proximal and distal tubular effects of furosemide in conscious rats. *J. Pharmacol. Exp. Ther.* 241: 987-993, 1987.

1767. Babini, R. and P. du Sovich. Furosemide pharmacodynamics: Effect of respiratory and acid-base disturbances. *J. Pharmacol. Exp. Ther.* 237: 623-628, 1986.

1768. Friedman, P.A. and F. Roch-Ramel. Hemodynamic and natriuretic effects of bumetanide and furosemide in the cat. *J. Pharmacol. Exp. Ther.* 203: 82-91, 1977.

1769. Lambert, C., *et al.* Nonrenal clearance of furosemide as a cause of diuretic response variability in the rat. *J. Pharmacol. Exp. Ther.* 222: 232-236, 1982.

1770. Gerkens, J.F. and R.A. Branch. The influence of sodium status and furosemide on canine acute amphotericin B nephrotoxicity. *J. Pharmacol. Exp. Ther.* 214: 306-311, 1980.

1771. Carbon, C., *et al.* Effects of furosemide on extravascular diffusion, protein binding and urinary excretion of cephalosporins and aminoglycosides in rabbits. *J. Pharmacol. Exp. Ther.* 213: 600-606, 1980.

1772. Fine, B.P., *et al.* Diuretic-induced growth failure in rats and its reversal by sodium repletion. *J. Pharmacol. Exp. Ther.* 242: 85-89, 1987.

Bibliography

1773. Bourland, W.A., *et al.* The role of the kidney in the early nondiuretic action of furosemide to reduce elevated left atrial pressure in the hypervolemic dog. *J. Pharmacol. Exp. Ther.* 202: 221-229, 1977.

1774. Anwer, M.S. Furosemide choleresis in isolated perfused rat liver: Partial dependency on perfusate sodium and chloride. *J. Pharmacol. Exp. Ther.* 235: 313-318, 1985.

1775. Tran, M., *et al.* Is adrenal medulla involved in the antihypertensive effect of nicardipine? *J. Pharmacol. Exp. Ther.* 244: 1116-1120, 1988.

1776. Williams, P.D., *et al.* Inhibition of renal Na^+, K^+-adenosine triphosphatase by gentamicin. *J. Pharmacol. Exp. Ther.* 231: 248-253, 1984.

1777. Elliot, W. C., *et al.* Experimental gentamicin nephrotoxicity: Effect of streptozocin-induced diabetes. *J. Pharmacol. Exp. Ther.* 233: 264-270, 1985.

1778. Patterson, E., *et al.* Cardiac electrophysiologic actions of KB-944 (fostedil), a new calcium antagonist, in the anesthetized dog. *J. Pharmacol. Exp. Ther.* 230: 632-640, 1984.

1779. Strandhoy, J.W., *et al.* Renal effects of the antihypertensive, guanabenz, in the dog. *J. Pharmacol. Exp. Ther.* 221: 347-352, 1982.

1780. Meacham, R.H., *et al.* Relationship of guanabenz concentrations in brain and plasma to antihypertensive effect in the spontaneously hypertensive rat. *J. Pharmacol. Exp. Ther.* 214: 594-598, 1980.

1781. Galligan, J.J., *et al.* Effects of cholinergic blockade, adrenergic blockade and sympathetic denervation on gastrointestinal myoelectric activity in guinea pig. *J. Pharmacol. Exp. Ther.* 238: 1114-1125, 1986.

1782. Gilder, D.A., *et al.* A comparison of the abilities of chlorpromazine and molindone to interact adversely with guanethidine. *J. Pharmacol. Exp. Ther.* 198: 255-263, 1976.

1783. Evans, B.K. Influence of neuronal activity levels on the cytotoxic effects of guanethidine. *J. Pharmacol. Exp. Ther.* 209: 205-214, 1979.

1784. McNEILAB, Inc. "Haldol (haloperidol): A summary of chemical, pharmacological, and clinical data." McNEILAB, Inc., Fort Washington, Pa. 1978.

1785. Consolo, S., *et al.* Effect of central stimulants and depressants on mouse brain acetylcholine and choline levels. *Eur. J. Pharmacol.* 18: 251-255, 1972.

1786. Sherman, K.A., *et al.* The effect of neuroleptics on acetylcholine concentration and choline uptake in striatum: Implications for regulation of acetylcholine metabolism. *J. Pharmacol. Exp. Ther.* 206: 677-686, 1978.

Bibliography

1787. Aulakh, C.S., *et al.* Long-term imipramine treatment enhances locomotor and food intake suppressant effects of m-chlorophenylpiperazine in rats. *Brit. J. Pharmacol.* 91: 747-752, 1987.

1788. Duncan, G.E., *et al.* Behavioral and neurochemical responses to haloperidol and SCH-23390 in rats treated neonatally or as adults with 6-hydroxydopamine. *J. Pharmacol. Exp. Ther.* 243: 1027-1034, 1987.

1789. McElroy, J.F. and J.M. O'Donnell. Discriminative stimulus properties of clenbuterol: Evidence for beta adrenergic involvement. *J. Pharmacol. Exp. Ther.* 245: 155-164, 1988.

1790. Harvey, J.A. and I. Gormezano. Effects of haloperidol and pimozide on classical conditioning of the rabbit nictitating membrane response. *J. Pharmacol. Exp. Ther.* 218: 712-719, 1981.

1791. Bacopoulos, N.G., *et al.* Chronic treatment with haloperidol on fluphenazine decanoate: Regional effects on dopamine and serotonin metabolism in primate brain. *J. Pharmacol. Exp. Ther.* 221: 22-28, 1982.

1792. Millington, W.R., *et al.* Dopaminergic agents selectively alter the post-translational processing of ß-endorphin in the intermediate pituitary of the rat. *J. Pharmacol. Exp. Ther.* 243: 160-170, 1987.

1793. Coates, G.H. and B. Cox. Harmine tremor after brain monoamine oxidase inhibition in the mouse. *Eur. J. Pharmacol.* 18: 284-286, 1972.

1794. Freeman, J.J., *et al.* Studies on the behavioral and biochemical effects of hemicholinium in vivo. *J. Pharmacol. Exp. Ther.* 210: 91-97, 1979.

1795. Gurll, N.J., *et al.* Naloxone without transfusion prolongs survival and enhances cardiovascular function in hypovolemic shock. *J. Pharmacol. Exp. Ther.* 220: 621-624, 1982.

1796. Lathers, C.M., *et al.* Correlation of ouabain-induced arrhythmia and nonuniformity in the histamine-evoked discharge of cardiac sympathetic nerves. *J. Pharmacol. Exp. Ther.* 203: 467-479, 1977.

1797. Lokhandwala, M.F. Inhibition of sympathetic nervous system by histamine: Studies with H_1- and H_2-receptor antagonists. *J. Pharmacol. Exp. Ther.* 206: 115-122, 1978.

1798. Yokotani, K. and Y. Osumi. Lack of direct splanchnic nerve inhibitory effects on histamine-induced gastric acid secretion in rats. *J. Pharmacol. Exp. Ther.* 236: 770-775, 1986.

1799. Gerkens, J.F., *et al.* Prostaglandin and histamine involvement in the gastric vasodilator action of pentagastrin. *J. Pharmacol. Exp. Ther.* 201: 421-426, 1977.

1800. Bergen, J. and E.A. Kroeger. Adrenoceptor-mediated mechanical responses of canine tracheal smooth muscle. *J. Pharmacol. Exp. Ther.* 238: 679-684, 1986.

Bibliography

1801.   Israel, E., *et al.* Differential effects of calcium channel blockers on leukotriene C_4- and D_4-induced contractions in guinea pig pulmonary parenchymal strips. *J. Pharmacol. Exp. Ther.* 243: 424-429, 1987.

1802.   Campbell, W.B. and H.D. Itskovitz. Effect of histamine and antihistamines on renal hemodynamics and functions in the isolated perfused canine kidney. *J. Pharmacol. Exp. Ther.* 198: 661-667, 1976.

1803.   Ogiso, T., *et al.* Pharmacokinetics of formation and excretion of some metabolites of hydralazine and their hypotensive effect in rats. *J. Pharmacol. Exp. Ther.* 233: 485-490, 1985.

1804.   Bolt, G.R. and P.R. Saxena. Interaction of atenolol with the systemic and regional hemodynamic effects of hydralazine in conscious renal hypertensive rabbits. *J. Pharmacol. Exp. Ther.* 230: 205-213, 1984.

1805.   Spokas, E.G. and H.-H. Wang. Regional blood flow and cardiac responses to hydralazine. *J. Pharmacol. Exp. Ther.* 212: 294-303, 1980.

1806.   Chelly, J.E., *et al.* Effects of hydralazine on regional blood flow in conscious dogs. *J. Pharmacol. Exp. Ther.* 238: 665-669, 1986.

1807.   Brown, N.L., *et al.* Pre- and postjunctional actions of hydralazine in vascular and nonvascular smooth muscle in vitro. *J. Pharmacol. Exp. Ther.* 226: 512-518, 1983.

1808.   Ferriola, P.C., *et al.* Thiazide diuretics inhibit chloride absorption by rabbit distal colon. *J. Pharmacol. Exp. Ther.* 238: 912-915, 1986.

1809.   Hofmann, L.M., *et al.* Aldosterone antagonism studies in the Rhesus monkey. *J. Pharmacol. Exp. Ther.* 202: 216-220, 1977.

1810.   Gerald, M.C. and T.K. Gupta. Catecholaminergic involvement in the effects of amphetamine isomers on seizure sensitivity. *Eur. J. Pharmacol.* 41: 231-234, 1977.

1811.   Fluharty, S.J., *et al.* Recovery of chronotropic responsiveness after systemic 6-hydroxydopamine treatment: Studies in the pithed rat. *J. Pharmacol. Exp. Ther.* 243: 415-423, 1987.

1812.   Maggi, C.A., *et al.* Dual effects of clonidine on micturition reflex in urethane anesthetized rats. *J. Pharmacol. Exp. Ther.* 235: 528-536, 1985.

1813.   Lautt, W.W. and M.C. Cote. Functional evaluation of 6-hydroxydopamine-induced sympathectomy in the liver of the cat. *J. Pharmacol. Exp. Ther.* 198: 562-567, 1976.

1814.   Slotkin, T.A., *et al.* Do sympathetic neurons coordinate cellular development in the heart and kidney? Effects of neonatal central and peripheral catecholaminergic lesions on cardiac and renal nucleic acids and proteins. *J. Pharmacol. Exp. Ther.* 244: 166-172, 1988.

Bibliography

1815. Criswell, H., *et al*. Assessment of purine-dopamine interactions in 6-hydroxydopamine-lesioned rats: Evidence for pre- and postsynaptic influences by adenosine. *J. Pharmacol. Exp. Ther.* 244: 493-500, 1988.

1816. Yokotani, K., *et al*. Sympathoadrenomedullary system mediation of the prostaglandin E_2-induced central inhibition of gastric acid output in rats. *J. Pharmacol. Exp. Ther.* 244: 335-340, 1988.

1817. Heffner, T.G. and L.S. Seiden. The effect of depletion of brain dopamine by 6-hydroxydopamine on tolerance to the anorexic effect of d-amphetamine to fenfluramine in rats. *J. Pharmacol. Exp. Ther.* 208: 134-143, 1979.

1818. Breese, G.R., *et al*. Behavioral differences between neonatal and adult 6-hydroxydopamine-treated rats to dopamine agonists: Relevance to neurological symptoms in clinical syndromes with reduced brain dopamine. *J. Pharmacol. Exp. Ther.* 231: 343-354, 1984.

1819. Muramatsu, I., *et al*. Nonadrenergic nature of prazosin-resistant, sympathetic contraction in the dog mesenteric artery. *J. Pharmacol. Exp. Ther.* 229: 532-538, 1984.

1820. Ice, K.S., *et al*. Sensitivity changes in the smooth muscles of the guinea-pig isolated vas deferens after treatment of animals with 6-hydroxydopamine. *J. Pharmacol. Exp. Ther.* 235: 349-353, 1985.

1821. DeOliveira, L.F. and A.D. Bretas. Effects of 5-hydroxytryptophan, isoniazid, and *p*-chlorophenylalanine on lidocaine seizure threshold of mice. *Eur. J. Pharmacol.* 29: 5-9, 1974.

1822. Clineschmidt, B.V. and J.C. McGuffin. Neurotensin administered intracisternally inhibits responsiveness of mice to noxious stimuli. *Eur. J. Pharmacol.* 46: 395-396, 1977.

1823. Maderazo, E.G., *et al*. Protective effects of ibuprofen and methylprednisolone on chemotactic factor-induced transcutaneous hypoxia. *J. Pharmacol. Exp. Ther.* 238: 453-456, 1986.

1824. Feigen, L.P., *et al*. Differential effects of ibuprofen and indomethacin in the regional circulation of the dog. *J. Pharmacol. Exp. Ther.* 219: 679-684, 1981.

1825. Romson, J.L., *et al*. The beneficial effects of oral ibuprofen on coronary artery thrombosis and myocardial ischemia in the conscious dog. *J. Pharmacol. Exp. Ther.* 215: 271-278, 1980.

1826. Zambraski, E.J., *et al*. Comparison of the effects of sulindac with other cyclooxygenase inhibitors on prostaglandin excretion and renal function in normal and chronic bile duct-ligated dogs and swine. *J. Pharmacol. Exp. Ther.* 228: 560-566, 1984.

Bibliography

1827.   Wise, W.C., *et al.* Ibuprofen improves survival from endotoxic shock in the rat. *J. Pharmacol. Exp. Ther.* 215: 160-164, 1980.

1828.   Apstein, C.S. and W.M. Vogel Coronary arterial vasodilator effect of ibuprofen. *J. Pharmacol. Exp. Ther.* 220: 167-171, 1982.

1829.   Seng, G.F. and B.M. Bayer. Inhibition of amino acid transport by nonsteroidal anti-inflammatory drugs: A model for predicting relative therapeutic potency. *J. Pharmacol. Exp. Ther.* 237: 496-503, 1986.

1830.   Harland, D. and M.J. Brown. Effects of acute and chronic administration of idazoxan on blood pressure and plasma catecholamine concentrations of rats. *J. Pharmacol. Exp. Ther.* 245: 265-273. 1988.

1831.   Curet, O., *et al.* Evidence for the involvement of presynaptic alpha-2 adrenoceptors in the regulation of norepinephrine metabolism in the rat brain. *J. Pharmacol. Exp. Ther.* 240: 327-336, 1987.

1832.   Kopia, G.A., *et al.* Alpha adrenoceptor regulation of coronary artery blood flow in normal and stenotic canine coronary arteries. *J. Pharmacol. Exp. Ther.* 239: 641-647, 1986.

1833.   Worms, P., *et al.* SR 95191, a selective inhibitor of type A monoamine oxidase with dopaminergic properties. 1. Psychopharmacological profile in rodents. *J. Pharmacol. Exp. Ther.* 240: 241-250, 1987.

1834.   Garcia Leme, J., *et al.* Pharmacological analysis of the acute inflammatory process induced in the rat's paw by local injection of carrageenin and by heat. *Brit. J. Pharmacol.* 48: 88-96, 1973.

1835.   Di Martino, M.J., *et al.* Antiarthritic and immunoregulatory activity of spirogermanium. *J. Pharmacol. Exp. Ther.* 236: 103-110, 1986.

1836.   Zukowska-Grojec, Z., *et al.*   Leukotriene D$_4$: Cardiovascular and sympathetic effects in spontaneously hypertensive rats (SHR) and Wistar-Kyoto (WKY) rats. *J. Pharmacol. Exp. Ther.* 223: 183-189, 1982.

1837.   Kimura, T. and S. Satoh. Inhibitory effect of quinacrine on myocardial reactive hyperemia in the dog. *J. Pharmacol. Exp. Ther.* 232: 269-274, 1985.

1838.   Iwatsuki, K., *et al.* Permissive role of prostaglandins in the action of bradykinin on the pancreas of anesthetized dogs. *J. Pharmacol. Exp. Ther.* 233: 700-706, 1985.

1839.   Quilley, C.P., *et al.* Failure of chronic aspirin treatment to inhibit urinary prostaglandin excretion in spontaneously hypertensive rats: Comparison with indomethacin and flurbiprofen. *J. Pharmacol. Exp. Ther.* 240: 916-921, 1987.

1840.   Baer, P.G., *et al.* Dissociation of effects of xanthine analogs on renal prostaglandins and renal excretory function in the awake rat. *J. Pharmacol. Exp. Ther.* 227: 600-604, 1983.

Bibliography

1841. Bidiville, J. and F. Roch-Ramel. Competition of organic anions for furosemide and p-amino-hippurate secretion in the rabbit. *J. Pharmacol. Exp. Ther.* 237: 636-643, 1986.

1842. Kirchner, K.A. Indomethacin antagonizes furosemide's intratubular effects during loop segment microperfusion. *J. Pharmacol. Exp. Ther.* 243: 881-886, 1987.

1843. Hial, V., *et al.* Alteration of tumor growth by aspirin and indomethacin: Studies with two transplantable tumors in mouse. *Eur. J. Pharmacol.* 37: 367-376, 1976.

1844. MSD PCM Report. "Poison Control Manual." Information supplied by MSD PCM as requested by author. MSD, Inc., West Point, Pa. 1979.

1845. Scheurer, U., *et al.* Cyclooxygenase inhibitors affect met-enkephalin- and acetylcholine-stimulated motility of the isolated rat colon. *J. Pharmacol. Exp. Ther.* 234: 742-746, 1985.

1846. Duncan, G.E., *et al.* Effects of antidepressant drugs injected into the amygdala on behavioral responses of rats in the forced swim test. *J. Pharmacol. Exp. Ther.* 238: 758-762, 1986.

1847. Peat, M.A., *et al.* Effects of single dose of methamphetamine and iprindole on the serotonergic and dopaminergic system of the rat brain. *J. Pharmacol. Exp. Ther.* 225: 126-131, 1983.

1848. Hayes, J.S., *et al.* Roles for Ca^{++} and cyclic AMP in mediating the cardiotonic actions of isomazole (LY 175326). *J. Pharmacol. Exp. Ther.* 237: 18-24, 1986.

1849. Schayer, R.W. and M.A. Reilly. Histamine catabolism in guinea pigs, rats and mice. *Eur. J. Pharmacol.* 25: 101-107, 1974.

1850. Fink, G.D. and J.W. Fisher. Stimulation of erythropoiesis by beta adrenergic agonists. I. Characterization of activity in polycythemic mice. *J. Pharmacol. Exp. Ther.* 202: 192-198, 1977.

1851. Nishimura, T.-I., *et al.* Effects of 1-(4-nitrophenyl)-2- isopropylaminoethanol (INPEA) and propranolol and their dextro-isomers on hemodynamic and metabolic responses to isoproterenol in dogs. *J. Pharmacol. Exp. Ther.* 226: 595-602, 1983.

1852. Hayes, J.S., *et al.* Effects of beta adrenoceptor down-regulation on the cardiovascular responses to the stereoisomers of dobutamine. *J. Pharmacol. Exp. Ther.* 235: 58-65, 1985.

1853. Thornhill, J.A. and M. Desautels. Is acute morphine hyperthermia of unrestrained rats due to selective activation of brown adipose tissue thermogenesis? *J. Pharmacol. Exp. Ther.* 231: 422-429, 1984.

1854. Karmazyn, M., *et al.* Comparative effects of acetylsalicyclic acid (ASA) and sulfinpyrazone on isoproterenol-induced heart damage. *J. Pharmacol. Exp. Ther.* 764-770, 1981.

Bibliography

1855. Fink, G.D. and J.W. Fisher. Stimulation of erythropoiesis by beta adrenergic agonists. I. Characterization of activity in polycythemic mice. *J. Pharmacol. Exp. Ther.* 202: 192-198, 1977.

1856. Hayes, J.S., *et al.* Effects of prolonged isoproterenol infusion on cardiac and vascular responses to adrenoceptor agents. *J. Pharmacol. Exp. Ther.* 237: 757-763, 1986.

1857. Hewett, K.W. and M.R. Rosen. Alpha and beta adrenergic interactions with ouabain-induced delayed afterdepolarizations. *J. Pharmacol. Exp. Ther.* 229: 188-192, 1984.

1858. Olson, R.D., *et al.* Beta adrenergically mediated release of renin in the dog is not confined to either beta-1 or beta-2 adrenoceptors. *J. Pharmacol. Exp. Ther.* 222: 606-611, 1982.

1859. Khanna, O.P., *et al.* The effect of adrenergic agonists and antagonists on vesicourethral smooth muscle of rabbits. *J. Pharmacol. Exp. Ther.* 216: 95-100, 1981.

1860. Olney, J.W., *et al.* Kainic acid: A Powerful neurotoxic analogue of glutamate. *Brain Res.* 77: 507-512, 1974.

1861. Vaupel, D.B., *et al.* Phencyclidine analogs and precursors: Rotarod and lethal dose studies in the mouse. *J. Pharmacol. Exp. Ther.* 230: 20-27, 1984.

1862. Little, H.J., *et al.* Ketamine and the guniea-pig ileum: Possible opiate agonist and antagonists actions and effects of peptidase inhibition. *J. Pharmacol. Exp. Ther.* 225: 206-212, 1983.

1863. Winters, W.D., *et al.* Ketamine and morphine-induced analgesia and catalepsy. I. Tolerance, cross-tolerance, potentiation, residual morphine levels and naloxone action in the rat. *J. Pharmacol. Exp. Ther.* 244: 51-57, 1988.

1864. Risner, M.E. Intravenous self-administration of phencyclidine and related compounds in the dog. *J. Pharmacol. Exp. Ther.* 221: 637-644, 1982.

1865. Moreton, J.E., *et al.* Ketamine self-administration by the Rhesus monkey. *J. Pharmacol. Exp. Ther.* 203: 303-309, 1977.

1866. Beardsley, P.M. and R.L. Balster. Behavioral dependence upon phencyclidine and ketamine in the rat. *J. Pharmacol. Exp. Ther.* 242: 203-211, 1987.

1867. Conolan, S., *et al.* In vivo and in vitro activity of selective 5-hydroxytryptamine$_2$ receptor antagonists. *Brit. J. Pharmacol.* 89: 129-135, 1986.

1868. McCall, R.B. and L.T. Harris. Characterization of the central sympathoinhibitory action of ketanserin. *J. Pharmacol. Exp. Ther.* 241: 736-740, 1987.

Bibliography

1869.   Hollenberg, N.K., *et al.* Endothelial injury provokes collateral arterial vasoconstriction: Response to a serotonin$_2$ antagonist, thromboxane antagonist or synthetase inhibition. *J. Pharmacol. Exp. Ther.* 244: 1164-1168, 1988.

1870.   Jaffe, B.M., *et al.* Comparative effects of ketanserin, atropine and methysergide on the gastrointestinal effects of hyperserotoninemia in the awake dog. *J. Pharmacol. Exp. Ther.* 238: 536-541, 1986.

1871.   Marek, G.J. and L.S. Seiden. Effects of selective 5-hydroxytryptamine-2 and nonselective 5-hydroxytryptamine antagonists on the differential -reinforcement of low-rate 72-second schedule. *J. Pharmacol. Exp. Ther.* 244: 650-658, 1988.

1872.   VanNueten, J.M., *et al.* Vascular effects of ketanserin (R41468), a novel antagonist of 5-HT$_2$ serotonergic receptors. *J. Pharmacol. Exp. Ther.* 218: 217-230, 1981.

1873.   Antonaccio, M.J., *et al.* Antihypertensive effects of 12 beta adrenoceptor antagonists in conscious spontaneously hypertensive rats: Relationship to changes in plasma renin activity, heart rate and sympathetic nerve function. *J. Pharmacol. Exp. Ther.* 238: 378-387, 1986.

1874.   Mostaghim, R., *et al.* Endothelial potentiation of relaxation response to beta adrenoceptor blocking agents. *J. Pharmacol. Exp. Ther.* 239: 797-801, 1986.

1875.   Hahn, R.A. and B.R. MacDonald. Primate myocardial and systemic hemodynamic responses to leukotriene D$_4$: Antagonism by LY171883. *J. Pharmacol. Exp. Ther.* 242: 62-69, 1987.

1876.   Feigen, L. Differential effects of leukotrienes C$_4$, D$_4$ and E$_4$ in the canine renal and mesenteric vascular beds. *J. Pharmacol. Exp. Ther.* 225: 682-687, 1983.

1877.   Hattori, Y. and R. Levi. Negative inotropic effect of leukotrienes: Leukotrienes C$_4$ and D$_4$ inhibit calcium-dependent contractile responses in potassium-depolarized guinea-pig myocardium. *J. Pharmacol. Exp. Ther.* 230: 646-651, 1984.

1878.   Roche Report. Information supplied by Roche as requested by author. 1979.

1879.   Judson, B.A. and A. Goldstein. Genetic control of opiate-induced locomotor activity in mice. *J. Pharmacol. Exp. Ther.* 206: 56-60, 1978.

1880.   Howell, L.L., *et al.* Effects of levorphanol and several kappa-selective opioids on respiration and behavior in rhesus monkeys. *J. Pharmacol. Exp. Ther.* 245: 364-372, 1988.

1881.   McGilliard, K.L. and A.E. Takemori. Antagonism by naloxone of narcotic-induced respiratory depression and analgesia. *J. Pharmacol. Exp. Ther.* 207: 494-503, 1978.

1882.   Martin, J.R. and A.E. Takemori. Modification of the development of acute opiate tolerance by increased dopamine receptor sensitivity. *J. Pharmacol. Exp. Ther.* 241: 48-55, 1987.

Bibliography

1883. Eisenberg, R.M. and S.B. Sparber. Changes in plasma corticosterone levels as a measure of acute dependence upon levorphanol in rats. *J. Pharmacol. Exp. Ther.* 211: 364-369, 1979.

1884. Pickworth, W.B. and L.G. Sharpe. Morphine-induced mydriasis and inhibition of pupillary light reflex and fluctuations in the cat. *J. Pharmacol. Exp. Ther.* 234: 603-606, 1985.

1885. Varro, A., *et al.* Effect of antiarrhythmic drugs on the premature action potential duration in canine cardiac purkinje fibers. *J. Pharmacol. Exp. Ther.* 233: 304-311, 1985.

1886. Coyle, D.E. and N. Sperelakis. Bupivacaine and lidocaine blockade of calcium-mediated slow action potentials in guinea pig ventricular muscle. *J. Pharmacol. Exp. Ther.* 242: 1001-1005, 1987.

1887. Matsumura, N., *et al.* Effect of lidocaine on the myocardial acidosis induced by coronary artery occlusion in dogs. *J. Pharmacol. Exp. Ther.* 242: 1114-1119, 1987.

1888. Horowski, R. and H. Wachtel. Direct dopaminergic action of lisuride hydrogen maleate, an ergot derivative, in mice. *Eur. J. Pharmacol.* 36: 373-383, 1976.

1889. Beatty, O. III., *et al.* Action of lithium on the adrenergic nerve ending. *J. Pharmacol. Exp. Ther.* 218: 309-317, 1981.

1890. Ozawa, H., *et al.* Potentiating effect of lithium chloride on aggressive behavior induced in mice by nialamide plus l-dopa and by clonidine. *Eur. J Pharmacol.* 34: 169-179, 1975.

1891. Hong, J.-S., *et al.* Effects of lithium and haloperidol administration on the rat brain levels of substance P. *J. Pharmacol. Exp. Ther.* 224: 590-593, 1983.

1892. Wettstein, J.G. and R.D. Spealman. Behavioral effects of the ß-carboline derivatives ZK93423 and ZK91296 in squirrel monkeys: Comparison with lorazepam and suriclone. *J. Pharmacol. Exp. Ther.* 240: 471-475, 1987.

1893. McNicholas, L.F., *et al.* Physical dependence on diazepam and lorazepam in the dog. *J. Pharmacol. Exp. Ther.* 226: 783-789, 1983.

1894. Neilsen, E.B. Discriminative stimulus properties of lysergic acid diethylamide in the monkey. *J. Pharmacol. Exp. Ther.* 234: 244-249, 1985.

1895. Gimpl, M.P., *et al.* Effects of LSD on learning as measured by classical conditioning of the rabbit nictitating membrane response. *J. Pharmacol. Exp. Ther.* 208: 330-334, 1979.

1896. Matta, S.G., *et al.* Nicotine elevates rat plasma ACTH by a central mechanism. *J. Pharmacol. Exp. Ther.* 243: 217-226, 1987.

Bibliography

1897. Sprague, R.S., *et al*. Differential responses of the pulmonary circulation to prostaglandins E_2 and $F_{2\alpha}$ in the presence of unilateral alveolar hypoxia. *J. Pharmacol. Exp. Ther.* 229: 38-43, 1984.

1898. Blasingham, M.C., *et al*. The effect of meclofenamate on renal blood flow in the unanesthetized dog: Relation to renal prostaglandins and sodium balance. *J. Pharmacol. Exp. Ther.* 214: 1-4, 1980.

1899. Umans, J.G. and C.E. Inturrisi. Antinociceptive activity and toxicity of meperidine and normeperidine in mice. *J. Pharmacol. Exp. Ther.* 223: 203-206, 1982.

1900. Witkin, J.M., *et al*. Modification of behavioral effects of morphine meperidine and normeperidine by naloxone and by morphine tolerance. *J. Pharmacol. Exp. Ther.* 225: 275-283, 1983.

1901. Ciofalo, V.B., *et al*. Flunixin meglumine: A non-narcotic analgesic. *J. Pharmacol. Exp. Ther.* 200: 501-507, 1977.

1902. LeFur, G., *et al*. Relationships between plasma corticosteroids and benzodiazepines in stress. *J. Pharmacol. Exp. Ther.* 211: 305-308, 1979.

1903. Higuchi, T., *et al*. Studies on the effects of phenobarbital and endotoxin on the toxicity and metabolism of 6-mercaptopurine in mice. *Experientia* 33: 940-941, 1977.

1904. Reimers, T.J. and P.M. Sluss. 6-Mercaptopurine treatment of pregnant mice: Effects on second and third generations. *Science* 201: 65-67, 1978.

1905. Lucki, I., *et al*. Differential actions of serotonin antagonists on two behavioral models of serotonin receptor activation in the rat. *J. Pharmacol. Exp. Ther.* 228: 133-139, 1984.

1906. Torphy, T.J., *et al*. Inhibitory effects of methacholine on drug-induced relaxation, cyclic AMP accumulation, and cyclic AMP-dependent protein kinase activation in canine tracheal smooth muscle. *J. Pharmacol. Exp. Ther.* 233: 409-417, 1985.

1907. Olsen, G.D. and S.C. Schlitt. Theophylline effect upon respiration and ventilation in the dog: Interaction with methodone. *J. Pharmacol. Exp. Ther.* 217: 278-284, 1981.

1908. McMillan, D.E., *et al*. Effects of drugs on behavior in rats maintained on morphine, methadone or pentobarbital. *J. Pharmacol. Exp. Ther.* 215: 9-14, 1980.

1909. Shah, N.S. and A.G. Donald. Pharmacological effects and metabolic fate of levo-methadone during postnatal development in rat. *J. Pharmacol. Exp. Ther.* 208: 491-497, 1979.

1910. Bero, L.A. and C.M. Kuhn. Catecholaminergic regulation of opiate-stimulated growth hormone secretion in the developing rat. *J. Pharmacol. Exp. Ther.* 237: 137-142, 1986.

Bibliography

1911. Kuhn, C.M. and M.B. Bartolome. Effect of chronic methadone administration on neuroendocrine function in young adult rats. *J. Pharmacol. Exp. Ther.* 234: 204-210, 1985.

1912. Hurwitz, A., *et al.* Opioid effects on hepatic disposition of dyes in mice. *J. Pharmacol. Exp. Ther.* 232: 617-623, 1985.

1913. Sprague, G.L. and A.E. Takemori. Enhancement of morphine analgesia and brain levels by methamphetamine in mice. *J. Pharmacol. Exp. Ther.* 207: 485-493, 1978.

1914. Harrigan, S.E. and D.A. Downs. Continuous intravenous naltrexone effects on morphine self-administration in rhesus monkeys. *J. Pharmacol. Exp. Ther.* 204: 481-486, 1978.

1915. Fischman, M.W. and C.R. Schuster. Long term behavioral changes in the Rhesus monkey after multiple daily injections of d-methylamphetamine. *J. Pharmacol. Exp. Ther.* 201: 593-605, 1977.

1916. Ritter, J.K., *et al.* Increases of substance P-like immunoreactivity within striatal-nigral structures after subacute methamphetamine treatment. *J. Pharmacol. Exp. Ther.* 229: 487-492, 1984.

1917. Johnson, J.H. and J.A. Rosecrans. Blockade of ovulation by methadone in the rat: A central nervous system-mediated acute effect. *J. Pharmacol. Exp. Ther.* 213: 110-113, 1980.

1918. Shewell, J. The effect of methotrexate on spontaneous memory adenocarcinomata in female C_3H mice. *Br. J. Cancer* 33: 210-216, 1976.

1919. Medzihradsky, J., *et al.* Time limitations in the reversal by citrovorum factor of methotrexate-induced immunosuppression in mice. *Biochem. Pharmacol.* 26: 203-206, 1977.

1920. Freeman-Narrod, M. and S.A. Narrod. Chronic toxicity of methotrexate in mice. *JNCI, J. Natl. Cancer Inst.* 58: 735-739, 1977.

1921. Zaharko, D.S., *et al.* Tolerance of long-term methotrexate infusions by mice. *Biochem. Pharmacol.* 25: 1317-1321, 1976.

1922. Shebuski, R.J., *et al.* Enhanced pulmonary alpha-2 adrenoceptor responsiveness under conditions of elevated pulmonary vascular tone. *J. Pharmacol. Exp. Ther.* 242: 158-165, 1987.

1923. Kalkman, H.O., *et al.* Characterization of the antihypertensive properties of ketanserin (R41468) in rats. *J. Pharmacol. Exp. Ther.* 222: 227-231, 1982.

1924. Fouin-Fortunet, H., *et al.* Inactivation of cytochrome P-450 by the drug methoxsalen. *J. Pharmacol. Exp. Ther.* 236: 237-247, 1986.

Bibliography

1925. Mays, D.C., *et al*. Inhibition and induction of drug biotransformation in vivo by 8-methoxypsoralen: Studies of caffeine, phenytoin and hexobarbital metabolism in the rat. *J. Pharmacol. Exp. Ther.* 243: 227-233, 1987.

1926. Jovic, R. and M. Milosevic. Effective doses of some cholinolytics in the treatment of anticholinesterase poisoning. *Eur. J. Pharmacol.* 12: 85-93, 1970.

1927. von Eick, A.J. and J. Bock. The effect of atropine and methylatropine on the sweat secretion of unrestrained mice, measured with radioactive saline. *Eur. J. Pharmacol.* 27: 263-265, 1974.

1928. Van Giersbergen, P.L.M. and W. de Jong. Antagonism by naltrexone of the hypotension and bradycardia induced by α-methyldopa in conscious normotensive rats. *J. Pharmacol. Exp. Ther.* 244: 341-347, 1988.

1929. Frankel, R.J., *et al*. Role of central and peripheral mechanisms in the action of α-methyldopa on blood pressure and renin secretion. *J. Pharmacol. Exp. Ther.* 201: 400-405, 1977.

1930. Forsyth, R.P. Hemodynamic effects of systemic and central administration of α-methyldopa. *J. Pharmacol. Exp. Ther.* 205: 675-682, 1978.

1931. Wiggins, J.F., *et al*. Effects of α-methyldopa and its metabolites on prolactin release: In vivo and in vitro studies. *J. Pharmacol. Exp. Ther.* 212: 304-308, 1980.

1932. Jenner, P. and C.D. Marsden. The influence of piribedil (ET 495) on components of locomotor activity. *Eur. J. Pharmacol.* 33: 211-215, 1975.

1933. Commins, D.L., *et al*. Biochemical and histological evidence that methylenedioxymethylamphetamine (MDMA) is toxic to neurons in the rat brain. *J. Pharmacol. Exp. Ther.* 241: 338-345, 1987.

1934. Schmidt, C.J. Neurotoxicity of the psychedelic amphetamine, methylenedioxymethamphetamine. *J. Pharmacol. Exp. Ther.* 240: 1-7, 1987.

1935. Johnson, M., *et al*. Effects of 3,4-methylenedioxyamphetamine and 3,4-methylenedioxymethamphetamine isomers on central serotonergic, dopaminergic and nigral neurotensin systems of the rat. *J. Pharmacol. Exp. Ther.* 244: 977-983, 1988.

1936. Nash, J.F., Jr., *et al*. Elevation of serum prolactin and corticosterone concentrations in the rat after the administration of 3,4-methylenedioxymethamphetamine. *J. Pharmacol. Exp. Ther.* 245: 873-879, 1988.

1937. Greely, G.H., Jr. and J.S. Kizer. The effects of chronic methylphenidate treatment on growth and endocrine function in the developing rat. *J. Pharmacol. Exp. Ther.* 215: 545-551, 1980.

1938. Hall, E.D., *et al*. A nonglucocorticoid steroid analog of methylprednisolone duplicates its high-dose pharmacology in models of central nervous system trauma and neuronal membrane damage. *J. Pharmacol. Exp. Ther.* 242: 137-142, 1987.

Bibliography

1939. Sonsalla, P.K., *et al.* Characteristics of 1-Methyl-4-(2'-methylphenyl)-1,2,3,6-tetrahydropyridine-induced neurotoxicity in the mouse. *J. Pharmacol. Exp. Ther.* 242: 850-857, 1987.

1940. Fuller, R.W. and S.K. Hemrick-Luecke. Inhibition of types A & B monoamine oxidase by 1-methyl-4-phenyl-1,2,3,6-tetrahydropyridine. *J. Pharmacol. Exp. Ther.* 232: 696-701, 1985.

1941. Gerhardt, G., *et al.* Dopaminergic neurotoxicity of 1-methyl-4-phenyl-1,2,3,6-tetrahydropyridine (MPTP) in the mouse: An in vivo electrochemical study. *J. Pharmacol. Exp. Ther.* 235: 259-265, 1985.

1942. Kuschinsky, K. and O. Hornykiewicz. Effects of morphine on striatal dopamine metabolism: Possible mechanism of its opposite effect on locomotor activity in rats and mice. *Eur. J. Pharmacol.* 26: 41-50, 1974.

1943. Wigdor, S. and G.L. Wilcox. Central and systemic morphine-induced antinociception in mice: Contribution of descending serotonergic and noradrenergic pathways. *J. Pharmacol. Exp. Ther.* 242: 90-95, 1987.

1944. Wigdor, S. and G.L. Wilcox. Central and systemic morphine-induced antinociception in mice: Contribution of descending serotonergic and noradrenergic pathways. *J. Pharmacol. Exp. Ther.* 242: 90-95, 1987.

1945. Ozawa, H. and T. Miyauchi. Potentiating effect of lithium chloride on methamphetamine-induced stereotype in mice. *Eur. J. Pharmacol.* 41: 213-216, 1977.

1946. Brady, L.S. and J.E. Barrett. Effects of serotonin receptor antagonists on punished responding maintained by stimulus-shock termination or food presentation in squirrel monkeys. *J. Pharmacol. Exp. Ther.* 234: 106-112, 1985.

1947. Lee, R.W., *et al.* Beta-2 adrenoceptor control of the venous circulation in intact dogs. *J. Pharmacol. Exp. Ther.* 242: 1138-1143, 1987.

1948. Neal, B.S. and S.B. Sparber. Mianserin attenuates naloxone-precipitated withdrawal signs in rats acutely or chronically dependent upon morphine. *J. Pharmacol. Exp. Ther.* 236: 157-165, 1986.

1949. Dwoskin, L.P. and S.B. Sparber. Behaviorally inactive doses of mianserin antagonize the suppressant effect of lysergic acid diethylamide on a fixed ratio operant. *J. Pharmacol. Exp. Ther.* 225: 77-84, 1983.

1950. Lee, R.W., *et al.* Dog model to study the effects of pharmacologic agents on the peripheral circulation: Effects of milrinone. *J. Pharmacol. Exp. Ther.* 240: 1014-1019, 1987.

1951. Meller, E. and E. Friedman. Differential dose- and time-dependent effects of molindone on dopamine neurons of rat brain: Mediation by irreversible inhibition of monoamine oxidase. *J. Pharmacol. Exp. Ther.* 220: 609-615, 1982.

Bibliography

1952. Schindler, C.W., *et al.* Effects of morphine, ethylketocyclazocine, U-50, 488H and naloxone on the acquisition of a classically conditioned response in the rabbit. *J. Pharmacol. Exp. Ther.* 243: 1010-1017, 1987.

1953. Stewart, J.J., *et al.* Centrally mediated intestinal stimulation by morphine. *J. Pharmacol. Exp. Ther.* 202: 174-181, 1977.

1954. Sweeney, M.I., *et al.* Involvement of adenosine in the spinal antinociceptive effects of morphine and noradrenaline. *J. Pharmacol. Exp. Ther.* 243: 657-665, 1987.

1955. DeLander, G.E., *et al.* Role of spinal mu opioid receptors in the development of morphine tolerance and dependence. *J. Pharmacol. Exp. Ther.* 231: 91-96, 1984.

1956. Simpkins, J.W., *et al.* Evidence for the delivery of narcotic antagonists to the colon as their glucuronide conjugates. *J. Pharmacol. Exp. Ther.* 244: 195-205, 1988.

1957. Walker, L.A. and J.C. Murphy. Effect of renal denervation on the antinatriuretic response to morphine administration in conscious rats. *J. Pharmacol. Exp. Ther.* 237: 799-802, 1986.

1958. Danesh, S. and L.A. Walker. Effects of central administration of morphine on renal function in conscious rats. *J. Pharmacol. Exp. Ther.* 244: 640-645, 1988.

1959. Garty, M. and A. Hurwitz. Tolerance to morphine effects on renal disposition of xenobiotics in mice. *J. Pharmacol. Exp. Ther.* 239: 346-350, 1986.

1960. Hovav, E. and M. Weinstock. Temporal factors influencing the development of acute tolerance to opiates. *J. Pharmacol. Exp. Ther.* 242: 251-256, 1987.

1961. Weinstock, M., *et al.* Hypersensitivity of morphine-tolerant rabbits to the respiratory stimulant effect of a cholinergic agonist. *J. Pharmacol. Exp. Ther.* 226: 232-237, 1983.

1962. van den Hoogen, R.H.W.M. and F.C. Colpaert. Respiratory effects of morphine in awake unrestrained rats. *J. Pharmacol. Exp. Ther.* 237: 252-259, 1986.

1963. Ling, G.S.F., *et al.* Separation of opioid analgesia from respiratory depression: Evidence for different receptor mechanisms. *J. Pharmacol. Exp. Ther.* 232: 149-155, 1985.

1964. Klemfuss, H., *et al.* Morphine-induced mydriasis and fluctuation in the rat: Time and dose relationships. *J. Pharmacol. Exp. Ther.* 208: 91-95, 1979.

1965. Manara, L., *et al.* Inhibition of gastrointestinal transit by morphine in rats results primarily from direct drug action on gut opioid sites. *J. Pharmacol. Exp. Ther.* 237: 945-949, 1986.

1966. Johnson, E.E. Morphine: A dual effect at the canine choledochoduodenal junction. *J. Pharmacol. Exp. Ther.* 219: 274-280, 1981.

Bibliography

1967.   Porreca, F. and T.F. Burks.   The spinal cord as a site of opioid effects on gastrointestinal transit in the mouse.   *J. Pharmacol. Exp. Ther.*   227: 22-27, 1983.

1968.   Adler, M.W., *et al.*   Anticonvulsant action of acute morphine administration in rats.   *J. Pharmacol. Exp. Ther.*   198: 655-660, 1976.

1969.   Tagashira, E., *et al.*   Pentazocine-tripelennamine ("T's and Blues") substitution studies in morphine-dependent rodents.   *J. Pharmacol. Exp. Ther.*   231: 97-101, 1984.

1970.   Rosow, C.E., *et al.*   Opiates and thermoregulation in mice.   II.   Effects of opiate antagonists.   *J. Pharmacol. Exp. Ther.*   220: 464-467, 1982.

1971.   Tallarida, R.J., *et al.*   Miosis and fluctuation in the rabbit pupil: Effects of morphine and naloxone.   *J. Pharmacol. Exp. Ther.*   201: 587-592, 1977.

1972.   Mello, N.K., *et al.*   Naltrexone effects on morphine and food self-administration in morphine-dependent Rhesus monkeys.   *J. Pharmacol. Exp. Ther.*   218: 550-557, 1981.

1973.   Rosenfeld, G.C. and T.F. Burks.   Single dose tolerance to morphine hypothermia in the rat: Differentiation of acute from long-term tolerance.   *J. Pharmacol. Exp. Ther.*   202: 654-659, 1977.

1974.   Schaefer, G.J. and S.G. Holtzman.   Discriminative effects of morphine in the squirrel monkey.   *J. Pharmacol. Exp. Ther.*   201: 67-75, 1977.

1975.   Hurwitz, A. and H.R. Fischer.   Narcotic effects on hepatic disposition of sulfobromophthalein in rats.   *J. Pharmacol. Exp. Ther.*   227: 68-72, 1983.

1976.   Bero, L.A. and C.M. Kuhn.   Role of serotonin in opiate-induced prolaction secretion and antinociception in the developing rat.   *J. Pharmacol. Exp. Ther.*   240: 831-836, 1987.

1977.   Cicero, T.J., *et al.*   Morphine-induced supersensitivity to the effects of naloxone on luteinizing hormone secretion in the male rat.   *J. Pharmacol. Exp. Ther.*   225: 35-41, 1983.

1978.   Dray, A. and R. Metsch.   Inhibition of urinary bladder contractions by a spinal action of morphine and other opioids.   *J. Pharmacol. Exp. Ther.*   231: 254-260, 1984.

1979.   Yaksh, T.L. and G.J. Harty.   Pharmacology of the allodynia in rats evoked by high dose intrathecal morphine.   *J. Pharmacol. Exp. Ther.*   244: 501-507, 1988.

1980.   Lux, F., *et al.*   Differential effects of subcutaneous and intrathecal morphine administration on blood glucose in mice: Comparison with intracerebroventricular administration.   *J. Pharmacol. Exp. Ther.*   245: 187-194, 1988.

1981.   Fox, D.A. and T.F. Burks.   Roles of central and peripheral mu, delta and kappa opioid receptors in the mediation of gastric acid secretory effects in the rat.   *J. Pharmacol. Exp. Ther.*   244: 456-462, 1988.

Bibliography

1982. Platt, K., *et al.* Evidence implicating alpha-2-adrenergic receptors in the anticonvulsant action of intranigral muscimol. *J. Pharmacol. Exp. Ther.* 241: 751-754, 1987.

1983. Blaker, W.D., *et al.* Simultaneous modulation of hippocampal cholinergic activity of extinction by intraseptal muscimol. *J. Pharmacol. Exp. Ther.* 225: 361-365, 1983.

1984. Blanquet, F., *et al.* Action of trimebutine in cat and rabbit colon: Evidence of an opioid-like effect. *J. Pharmacol. Exp. Ther.* 234: 708-712, 1985.

1985. Ueda, N., *et al.* Effects of met-enkephalin on the substance P-ergic and cholinergic responses in the rabbit iris sphincter muscle. *J. Pharmacol. Exp. Ther.* 226: 507-511, 1983.

1986. Faden, A.I. and J.W. Holaday. Naloxone treatment of endotoxin shock: Stereospecificity of physiologic and pharmacologic effects in the rat. *J. Pharmacol. Exp. Ther.* 212: 441-447, 1980.

1987. Vasko, M.R. and E.F. Domino. Tolerance development to the biphasic effects of morphine on locomotor activity and brain acetylcholine in the rat. *J. Pharmacol. Exp. Ther.* 207: 848-858, 1978.

1988. Koob, G.F., *et al.* Effects of opiate antagonists and their quaternary derivatives on heroin self-administration in the rat. *J. Pharmacol. Exp. Ther.* 229: 481-486, 1984.

1989. Leander, J.D. Further study of kappa opioids on increased urination. *J. Pharmacol. Exp. Ther.* 227: 35-41, 1983.

1990. Krivoy, W., *et al.* Actions of morphine on the segmental reflex of the decerebrate-spinal cat. *Brit. J. Pharmacol.* 47: 457-464, 1973.

1991. Spiehler, V.R. and L.O. Randall. Agonist-antagonist properties of phenoxybenzamine in antinociception and opiate dependence tests. *Eur. J. Pharmacol.* 55: 389-395, 1979.

1992. Dunham, E.W. and R. Vince. Hypotensive and renal vasodilator effects of carbocyclic adenosine (aristeromycin) in anesthetized spontaneously hypertensive rats. *J. Pharmacol. Exp. Ther.* 238: 954-959, 1986.

1993. Primi, M.P. and L. Bueno. Effects of centrally administered naloxone on gastrointestinal myoelectrical activity in morphine-dependent rats. *J. Pharmacol. Exp. Ther.* 240: 320-326, 1987.

1994. Snyder, E.W., *et al.* Naloxone epileptogenesis in monkeys. *J. Pharmacol. Exp. Ther.* 217: 299-305, 1981.

1995. Nabeshima, T., *et al.* Inhibition of enkephalin degradation attenuated stress-induced motor suppression (conditioned suppression of motility). *J. Pharmacol. Exp. Ther.* 244: 303-309, 1988.

Bibliography

1996.   Valentino, R.J. and R.G. Wehby.   Morphine effects on locus ceruleus neurons are dependent on the state of arousal and availability of external stimuli: Studies in anesthetized and unanesthetized rats.   *J. Pharmacol. Exp. Ther.*   244: 1178-1186, 1988.

1997.   Mastrianni, J.A. and A.J. Ingenito.   On the relationship between clonidine hypotension and brain ß-endorphin in the spontaneously hypertensive rat: Studies with alpha adrenergic and opiate blockers.   *J. Pharmacol. Exp. Ther.*   242: 378-387, 1987.

1998.   Nance, P.W. and J. Sawynok.   Substance P-induced long term blockade of spinal adrenergic analgesia: Reversal by morphine and naloxone.   *J. Pharmacol. Exp. Ther.*   240: 972-977, 1987.

1999.   Powell-Jones, K., *et al*.   Skeletal muscle thermogenesis: Its role in the hyperthermia of conscious rats given morphine or ß-endorphin.   *J. Pharmacol. Exp. Ther.*   243: 322-332, 1987.

2000.   Moerschbaecher, J.M., *et al*.   Differential antagonism by naltrexone of the effects of opioids on a fixed-ratio discrimination in rats.   *J. Pharmacol. Exp. Ther.*   244: 237-246, 1988.

2001.   Rosella-Dampman, L.M., *et al*.   Naltrexone effects on plasma vasopressin concentration elevated and lowered by various stimuli.   *J. Pharmacol. Exp. Ther.*   226: 373-381, 1983.

2002.   Gurll, N.J., *et al*.   Naltrexone improves survival rate and cardiovascular function in canine hemorrhagic shock.   *J. Pharmacol. Exp. Ther.*   220: 625-628, 1982.

2003.   Chang, E.B.   An antiabsorptive basis for precipitated withdrawal diarrhea in morphine-dependent rats.   *J. Pharmacol. Exp. Ther.*   228: 364-369, 1984.

2004.   Wynsen, J.C., *et al*.   Differential effects of nifedipine, nicorandil and nitroglycerin on the pressor responses elicited by selective alpha-1 and alpha-2 adrenoceptor agonists in conscious dogs.   *J. Pharmacol. Exp. Ther.*   241: 846-854, 1987.

2005.   Imanishi, S., *et al*.   Effects of SG-75 (nicorandil) on electrical activity of canine cardiac purkinje fibers: Possible increase in potassium conductance.   *J. Pharmacol. Exp. Ther.*   225: 198-205, 1983.

2006.   Miner, L.L., *et al*.   Classical genetic analysis of nicotine-induced seizures and nicotinic receptors.   *J. Pharmacol. Exp. Ther.*   231: 545-554, 1984.

2007.   Sybertz, E.J. and B.J. Zimmerman.   Facilitation of chemoreceptor-induced reflex vasoconstriction by intravertebral arterial administration of clonidine.   *J. Pharmacol. Exp. Ther.*   203: 56-63, 1977.

2008.   Miner, L.L., *et al*.   Genetic analysis of nicotine-induced seizures and hippocampal nicotinic receptors in the mouse.   *J. Pharmacol. Exp. Ther.*   239: 853-860, 1986.

Bibliography

2009. Spealman, R.D. Maintenance of behavior by postponement of scheduled injection of nicotine in squirrel monkeys. *J. Pharmacol. Exp. Ther.* 227: 154-160, 1983.

2010. Aubert, J.F., *et al.* Nicotine-induced release of vasopressin in the conscious rat: Role of opioid peptides and hemodynamic effects. *J. Pharmacol. Exp. Ther.* 243: 681-685, 1987.

2011. Marks, M.J., *et al.* Dose-response analysis of nicotine tolerance and receptor changes in two inbred mouse strains. *J. Pharmacol. Exp. Ther.* 239: 358-364, 1986.

2012. Marks, M.J., *et al.* Effects of chronic nicotine infusion on the tolerance development and nicotinic receptors. *J. Pharmacol. Exp. Ther.* 226: 817-825, 1983.

2013. Tripathi, H.L., *et al.* Nicotine-induced antinociception in rats and mice: Correlation with nicotine brain levels. *J. Pharmacol. Exp. Ther.* 221: 91-96, 1982.

2014. Sharp, B.M. and S. Beyer. Rapid desensitization of the acute stimulatory effects of nicotine on rat plasma adrenocorticotropin. *J. Pharmacol. Exp. Ther.* 238: 486-491, 1986.

2015. Sharp, B.M., *et al.* Attenuation of the plasma prolactin response to restraint stress after acute and chronic administration of nicotine to rats. *J. Pharmacol. Exp. Ther.* 241: 438-442, 1987.

2016. Morita, T., *et al.* Undifferentiated effects of calcium antagonists on pressor responses to selective alpha-1 and alpha-2 adrenoceptor agonists in anesthetized dogs. *J. Pharmacol. Exp. Ther.* 234: 728-734, 1985.

2017. Woodman, O.L., *et al.* Nifedipine attenuates both alpha-1 and alpha-2 adrenoceptor-mediated pressor and vasoconstrictor responses in conscious dogs and primates. *J. Pharmacol. Exp. Ther.* 239: 648-653, 1986.

2018. Kanda, K. and S.F. Flaim. Effects of nifedipine on total cardiac output distribution in conscious rat. *J. Pharmacol. Exp. Ther.* 228: 711-718, 1984.

2019. Timmermans, P.B.M.W.M., *et al.* Sensitivity of alpha-1 adrenoceptor-mediated pressor responses to inhibition by Ca^{++} entry blockers in the pithed rat: Arguments against the role of receptor reserve. *J. Pharmacol. Exp. Ther.* 240: 864-870, 1987.

2020. Barone, F.C., *et al.* Effects of calcium channel entry blockers, nifedipine and nilvadipine, on colonic motor activity. *J. Pharmacol. Exp. Ther.* 237: 99-106, 1986.

2021. Fitzpatrick, D.B. and M. Karmazyn. Comparative effects of calcium channel blocking agents and varying extracellular calcium concentration on hypoxia/reoxygenation and ischemia/reperfusion-induced cardiac injury. *J. Pharmacol. Exp. Ther.* 228: 761-768, 1984.

2022. Marre, M., *et al.* Diuretic and natriuretic effects of nifedipine on isolated perfused rat kidneys. *J. Pharmacol. Exp. Ther.* 223: 263-270, 1982.

Bibliography

2023. Khatter, J.C., *et al.* Digitalis-induced mechanical toxicity: Protection by slow
Ca^{++} channel blockers. *J. Pharmacol. Exp. Ther.* 239: 206-210, 1986.

2024. Kanda, K. and S.F. Flaim. Effects of nimodipine on cerebral blood flow in
conscious rats. *J. Pharmacol. Exp. Ther.* 236: 41-47, 1986.

2025. Haws, C.W., *et al.* Effects of nimodipine on cerebral blood flow. *J.
Pharmacol. Exp. Ther.* 225: 24-28, 1983.

2026. McCalden, T.A., *et al.* In vivo actions for a calcium channel blocker
(nimodipine) on the cerebrovascular response to infused 5-hydroxy-tryptamine.
J. Pharmacol. Exp. Ther. 237: 36-39, 1986.

2027. Taylor, D.G. and T.E. Kowalski. Comparison of calcium channel inhibitors on
vagal heart rate responses elicited by arterial baroreceptor reflexes in anesthetized
dogs. *J. Pharmacol. Exp. Ther.* 228: 491-499, 1984.

2028. Malo, P.E., *et al.* Effects of intravenous and aerosol nifedipine on prostaglandin
F2a and histamine-induced bronchoconstriction in anesthetized dogs. *J.
Pharmacol. Exp. Ther.* 221: 410-415, 1982.

2029. Cooke, J.P., *et al.* Nimodipine and inhibition of alpha adrenergic activation of
the isolated canine saphenous vein. *J. Pharmacol. Exp. Ther.* 234: 598-602, 1985.

2030. Drexler, H., *et al.* Effects of nisoldipine on cardiocirculatory dynamics and
cardiac output distribution in conscious rats at rest and during treadmill
exercise. *J. Pharmacol. Exp. Ther.* 232: 376-381, 1985.

2031. Schipke, J.D., *et al.* Effect of nisoldipine on coronary resistance, contractility
and oxygen consumption of the isolated blood-perfused canine left ventricle. *J.
Pharmacol. Exp. Ther.* 244: 1000-1004, 1988.

2032. Higuchi, M. Effects of nitroglycerin on transmural energy metabolism in the
underperfused canine heart. *J. Pharmacol. Exp. Ther.* 222: 694-698, 1982.

2033. Gross, G.J. and D.C. Warltier. Endocardial viability ratio on effect of
nitroglycerin and propranolol on regional myocardial blood flow in intact canine
hearts. *J. Pharmacol. Exp. Ther.* 203: 664-674, 1977.

2034. Duncan, G.E., *et al.* Rapid down regulation of beta adrenergic receptors by
combining antidepressant drugs with forced swim: A model of
antidepressant-induced neural adaptation. *J. Pharmacol. Exp. Ther.* 234:
402-408, 1985.

2035. Muraki, T., *et al.* Mechanism of morphine in increasing plasma cyclic GMP
level in male mice. *J. Pharmacol. Exp. Ther.* 224: 431-435, 1983.

2036. Risner, M.E., *et al.* Effects of the stereoisomers of nicotine and nornicotine on
schedule-controlled responding and physiological parameters of dogs. *J.
Pharmacol. Exp. Ther.* 244: 807-813, 1988.

Bibliography

2037. Goldman, S., *et al.* Effects of verapamil on positive inotropic stimulation in the left atrium and ventricle of conscious dogs. *J. Pharmacol. Exp. Ther.* 222: 270-275, 1982.

2038. Tackett, R.L. and J.E. Holl. Histaminergic mechanisms involved in the centrally mediated effects of ouabain. *J. Pharmacol. Exp. Ther.* 215: 552-556, 1980.

2039. Hayashi, S. and M.K. Park. Neurogenic and myogenic contractile responses of dog mesenteric arteries to reduced K^+ concentration and their interactions with ouabain. *J. Pharmacol. Exp. Ther.* 230: 527-533, 1984.

2040. Wyeth Report. Information supplied by Wyeth as requested by author. 1979.

2041. Shannon, H.E., *et al.* Interactions between narcotic analgesics and benzodiazepine derivatives on behavior in the mouse. *J. Pharmacol. Exp. Ther.* 199: 389-399, 1976.

2042. Shannon, H.E. and S.G. Holtzman. Blockage of the specific lethal effects of narcotic analgesics in the mouse. *Eur. J. Pharmacol.* 39: 295-303, 1976.

2043. Pircio, A.W. and J.A. Gylys. Oxilorphan (1-*N*-cyclopropylmethyl-3,14-dihydroxy-morphinan): A new synthetic narcotic antagonist. *J. Pharmacol. Exp. Ther.* 193: 23-34, 1975.

2044. Cheymol, G., *et al.* Pharmacological effects of two new ß-adrenoceptor blocking drugs: Kö 1366 and Kö 1313. *Eur. J. Pharmacol.* 17: 341-351, 1972.

2045. Fisher, A., *et al.* A new probe for heterogeneity in muscarinic receptors: 2-methyl-spiro-4-(1,3-dioxolane-4,3')-quinuclidine. *Eur. J. Pharmacol.* 37: 329-338, 1976.

2046. Witkin, J.M., *et al.* Nonmuscarinic neurotoxicity of oxotremorine. *J. Pharmacol. Exp. Ther.* 241: 34-41, 1987.

2047. Weinstock, M., *et al.* The role of peripheral catecholamines in oxotremorine tremor in the rat and its antagonism by beta adrenoceptor blocking agents. *J. Pharmacol. Exp. Ther.* 206: 91-96, 1978.

2048. Brown, D.M., *et al.* Some initial animal and human pharmacological studies with benapryzine (BRL 1288). *Brit. J. Pharmacol.* 47: 476-486, 1973.

2049. Slater, P. Effect of 6-hydroxydopamine on some actions of tremorine and oxotremorine. *Eur. J. Pharmacol.* 25: 130-137, 1974.

2050. Bhargava, H.N. and E.L. Way. Morphine tolerance and physical dependence: Influence of cholinergic agonists and antagonists. *Eur. J. Pharmacol.* 36: 79-88, 1976.

2051. Ringdahl, B., *et al.* Regional differences in receptor reserve for analogs of oxotremorine in vivo: Implications for development of selective muscarinic agonists. *J. Pharmacol. Exp. Ther.* 242: 464-471, 1987.

Bibliography

2052. Miller, R.D., *et al.* Hypothermia and the pharmacokinetics and pharmacodynamics of pancuronium in the cat. *J. Pharmacol. Exp. Ther.* 207: 532-538, 1978.

2053. Sanguinetti, M.C. and T.C. West. Influence of papaverine on spontaneous activity of isolated right atria from small mammals. *J. Pharmacol. Exp. Ther.* 228: 500-509, 1984.

2054. Nawrath, H. Action potential, membrane currents and force of contraction in cat ventricular heart muscle treated with papaverine. *J. Pharmacol. Exp. Ther.* 218: 544-549, 1981.

2055. Langley, A.E. and N. Weiner. The effect of pargyline pretreatment on the enhancement of the exocytic release of norepinephrine during nerve stimulation which is induced by a benzoquinolizine compound with reserpine-like properties. *J. Pharmacol. Exp. Ther.* 213: 534-538, 1980.

2056. Yeh, S.Y., *et al.* Potentiation of the analgesia of meperidine in the rat by pargyline. *J. Pharmacol. Exp. Ther.* 209: 125-134, 1979.

2057. Khanna, N.K. Effect of some ß-adrenergic blocking agents on the acetylcholine content of heart. An experimental study in mice. *Eur. J. Pharmacol.* 17: 309-311, 1972.

2058. Rogers, K.J. Role of brain monoamines in the interaction between pethidine and tranylcypromine. *Eur. J. Pharmacol.* 14: 86-88, 1971.

2059. Airoldi, L., *et al.* Distribution of penfluridol in rats and mice. *Eur. J. Pharmacol.* 25: 291-295, 1974.

2060. Yokotani, K. and Y. Osumi. Alpha-1 adrenoceptors mediate splanchnic nerve inhibition of pentagastrin-induced gastric acid secretion and mucosal blood flow in rats. *J. Pharmacol. Exp. Ther.* 236: 743-747, 1986.

2061. White, J.M. and S.G. Holtzman. Properties of pentazocine as a discriminative stimulus in the squirrel monkey. *J. Pharmacol. Exp. Ther.* 223: 396-401, 1982.

2062. Yeh, S.Y. Potentiation of pentazocine antinociception by tripelennamine in the rat. *J. Pharmacol. Exp. Ther.* 235: 683-689, 1985.

2063. Ankier, S.I. New hot plate tests to quantify antinociceptive and narcotic antagonist activity. *Eur. J. Pharmacol.* 27: 1-4, 1974.

2064. Pircio, A.W., *et al.* The pharmacology of butorphanol, a 3,14-dihydroxymorphinan narcotic antagonist analgesic. *Arch. Int. Pharmacodyn. Ther.* 220: 231-257, 1976.

2065. Dunwiddie, T.V., *et al.* Facilitation of recurrent inhibition in rat hippocampus by barbiturate and related nonbarbiturate depressant drugs. *J. Pharmacol. Exp. Ther.* 238: 564-575, 1986.

2066.   Yutrzenka, G.J., *et al*. Continuous intraperitoneal infusion of pentobarbital: A model of barbiturate dependence in the rat. *J. Pharmacol. Exp. Ther.* 232: 111-118, 1985.

2067.   Okamoto, M., *et al*. Effect of dosing frequency on the development of physical dependence and tolerance to pentobarbital. *J. Pharmacol. Exp. Ther.* 238, 1004-1008, 1986.

2068.   Walker, L.A., *et al*. Renal response to pentobarbital anesthesia in rats: Effect of interrupting the renin-angiotensin system. *J. Pharmacol. Exp. Ther.* 236: 721-728, 1986.

2069.   Commissaris, R.L., *et al*. Dispositional without functional tolerance to the hypothermic effects of pentobarbital in the rat. *J. Pharmacol. Exp. Ther.* 220: 536-539, 1982.

2070.   Sofia, R.D., *et al*. Anticonvulsant activity of Δ^9-tetrahydrocannabinol compared with three other drugs. *Eur. J. Pharmacol.* 35: 7-16, 1976.

2071.   Cavero, I., *et al*. Pharmacological, hemodynamic and autonomic nervous system mechanisms responsible for the blood pressure and heart rate lowering effects of pergolide in rats. *J. Pharmacol. Exp. Ther.* 228: 779-791, 1984.

2072.   Lorrain, J., *et al*. Effects of pergolide on the cardiovascular responses to sinoaortic deafferentation in dogs with intact or surgically decentralized adrenal glands. *J. Pharmacol. Exp. Ther.* 240: 288-293, 1987.

2073.   Daniell, H.B., *et al*. Effects of perhexiline or survival time and infarct size in experimental myocardial infarction. *J. Pharmacol. Exp. Ther.* 200: 155-165, 1977.

2074.   Greeley, G.J., Jr., *et al*. Effects of chronic perphenazine treatment on growth and endocrine function in developing rats. *J. Pharmacol. Exp. Ther.* 220: 133-138, 1982.

2075.   Squibb Report. Information supplied by Squibb as requested by author. 1979.

2076.   Kapetanovic, I.M. and J.J. Mieyal. Inhibition of acetaminophen-induced hepatotoxicity by phenacetin and its alkoxy analogs. *J. Pharmacol. Exp. Ther.* 209: 25-30, 1979.

2077.   Brocco, M.J., *et al*. Effects of chronic phencyclidine administration on the schedule-controlled behavior of rats. *J. Pharmacol. Exp. Ther.* 226: 449-454, 1983.

2078.   Beardsley, P.M. and R.L. Balster. Evaluation of antagonists of the discriminative stimulus and response rate effects of phencyclidine. *J. Pharmacol. Exp. Ther.* 244: 34-40, 1988.

2079.   Byrd, L.D. Comparison of the behavioral effects of phencyclidine, ketamine, d-amphetamine and morphine in the squirrel monkey. *J. Pharmacol. Exp. Ther.* 220: 139-144, 1982.

Bibliography

2080. Spain, J.W. and G.I. Klingman. Continuous intravenous infusion of phenycyclidine in unrestrained rats results in the rapid induction of tolerance and physical dependence. *J. Pharmacol. Exp. Ther.* 234: 415-424, 1985.

2081. Slifer, B.L., *et al.* Behavioral dependence produced by continuous phencyclidine infusion in rhesus monkeys. *J. Pharmacol. Exp. Ther.* 230: 399-406, 1984.

2082. Itoh, Y., *et al.* Phencyclidine and the dynamics of mouse brain histamine. *J. Pharmacol. Exp. Ther.* 235: 788-792, 1985.

2083. Murray, T.F. and D.L. Cheney. The effect of phencyclidine on the turnover rate of acetylcholine in various regions of rat brain. *J. Pharmacol. Exp. Ther.* 217: 733-737, 1981.

2084. Hadley, R.W. and J.R. Hume. Actions of phencyclidine on the action potential and membrane currents of single guinea-pig myocytes. *J. Pharmacol. Exp. Ther.* 237: 131-136, 1986.

2085. Temma, K., *et al.* Negative chronotropic and positive inotropic actions of phencyclidine on isolated atrial muscle in guinea pigs and rats. *J. Pharmacol. Exp. Ther.* 226: 885-892, 1983.

2086. Faraj, B.A., *et al.* Similarity between tyramine-induced neurotoxicity and the coma of Reye's syndrome. *J. Pharmacol. Exp. Ther.* 226: 608-615, 1983.

2087. Botting, R., *et al.* Modification by monoamine oxidase inhibitors of the analgesic, hypothermic and toxic actions of morphine and pethidine in mice. *J. Pharm. Pharmacol.* 30: 36-40, 1978.

2088. Lew, C., *et al.* Effects of imipramine, desipramine and monoamine oxidase inhibitors on the metabolism and psychomotor stimulant action of d-amphetamine in mice. *Eur. J. Pharmacol.* 14: 351-359, 1971.

2089. VonVoightlander, P.F., *et al.* U-54494A: A unique anticonvulsant related to kappa opioid agonists. *J. Pharmacol. Exp. Ther.* 243: 542-547, 1987.

2090. Chauvelot-Moachon, L., *et al.* Alpha-1-acid glycoprotein concentrations and protein binding of propranolol in Sprague-Dawley and Dark Agouti rat strains treated by phenobarbital. *J. Pharmacol. Exp. Ther.* 244: 1103-1108, 1988.

2091. Elrod, S.V. and S.W. Leslie. Acute and chronic effects of barbiturates on depolarization-induced calcium influx into synaptosomes from rat brain regions. *J. Pharmacol. Exp. Ther.* 212: 131-136, 1980.

2092. Vorhees, C.V. Fetal anticonvulsant syndrome in rats: Dose- and period-response relationships of prenatal diphenylhydantoin, trimethadione and phenobarbital exposure on the structural and functional development of the offspring. *J. Pharmacol. Exp. Ther.* 227: 274-287, 1983.

Bibliography

2093. Douidar, S.M. and A.E. Ahmed. A novel mechanism for the enhancement of acetaminophen hepatotoxicity by phenobarbital. *J. Pharmacol. Exp. Ther.* 240: 578-583, 1987.

2094. Bai, S. and F.P. Abramson. Interaction of phenobarbital with propranolol in the dog. 3. Beta blockade. *J. Pharmacol. Exp. Ther.* 224: 62-67, 1983.

2095. Nichols, A.J., *et al.* Comparison of the effects of the novel inotropic agent, ibopamine, with epinine, dopamine and fenoldopam on renal vascular dopamine receptors in the anesthetized dog. *J. Pharmacol. Exp. Ther.* 242: 573-578, 1987.

2096. Weiss, H.R., *et al.* Effect of alpha and beta adrenergic blockade on oxygen transport in rat skeletal muscle and brain. *J. Pharmacol. Exp. Ther.* 198: 403-411, 1976.

2097. Downey, H.F., *et al.* Regional renal and splanchnic blood flows during nicotine infusion: Effects of alpha and of combined alpha and beta adrenergic blockage. *J. Pharmacol. Exp. Ther.* 220: 375-381, 1982.

2098. Jones, C.E., *et al.* Cardiac and coronary effects of prazosin and phenoxybenzamine during coronary hypotension. *J. Pharmacol. Exp. Ther.* 236: 205-211, 1986.

2099. Fluharty, S.J., *et al.* Tyrosine hydroxylase activity and catecholamine biosynthesis in the adrenal medulla of rats during stress. *J. Pharmacol. Exp. Ther.* 233: 32-38, 1985.

2100. Garland, C.J. and J.A. Bevan. Alpha adrenoceptor antagonists selectively reduce thrombin-stimulated contraction in rabbit arteries. *J. Pharmacol. Exp. Ther.* 238: 947-953, 1986.

2101. Helke, C.J., *et al.* Intrathecal administration of a substance P receptor antagonist: Studies on peripheral and central nervous system hemodynamics and on specificity of action. *J. Pharmacol. Exp. Ther.* 242: 131-136, 1987.

2102. Hamed, A.T., *et al.* Evaluation of the role of alpha-1 and alpha-2 adrenoceptors in the maintenance of neurogenic tone to the hindlimb vasculature. *J. Pharmacol. Exp. Ther.* 238: 599-605, 1986.

2103. Chang, Y.-H. Adjuvant polyarthritis. II. Suppression by tilorone. *J. Pharmacol. Exp. Ther.* 203: 156-161, 1977.

2104. Williamson, H.E., *et al.* Phenylbutazone-induced decrease in renal blood flow. *J. Pharmacol. Exp. Ther.* 204: 130-134, 1978.

2105. Gengo, P.J., *et al.* Effects of prolonged phenylephrine infusion on cardiac adrenoceptors and calcium channels. *J. Pharmacol. Exp. Ther.* 244: 100-105, 1988.

2106. Baggot, J.D. Disposition and fate of drugs in the body. In: *Veterinary Pharmacology and Therapeutics*, 6th ed., N.H. Booth and L.E. McDonald, eds., Iowa St. Univ. Press, Ames, IA, 1988, pp. 38-71.

Bibliography

2107. Rosen, M.R., *et al*. Effect of alpha adrenergic agonists and blockers on purkinje fiber transmembrane potentials and automaticity in the dog. *J. Pharmacol. Exp. Ther*. 231: 566-571, 1984.

2108. Field, E. and L. Tyrey. Tolerance to the luteinizing hormone and prolactin suppressive effects of Δ-9-tetrahydrocannabinol develops during chronic prepuberal treatment of female rats. *J. Pharmacol. Exp. Ther*. 238: 1034-1038, 1986.

2109. Shapiro, B.H., *et al*. Persistent defects in the hepatic monooxygenase system of adult rats exposed, perinatally, to maternally administered phenytoin. *J. Pharmacol. Exp. Ther*. 238: 68-75, 1986.

2110. Martz, F., *et al*. Phenytoin teratogenesis: Correlation between embryopathic effect and covalent binding of putative arene oxide metabolite in gestational tissue. *J. Pharmacol. Exp. Ther*. 203: 231-239, 1977.

2111. Tucker, A.N., *et al*. Alterations of bone marrow cell cycle kinetics by diphenylhydantoin: Relationship to folate utilization and immune function. *J. Pharmacol. Exp. Ther*. 234: 57-62, 1985.

2112. Raines, A., *et al*. Description and analysis of the myotonolytic effects of phenytoin in the decerebrate cat: Implications for potential utility of phenytoin in spastic disorders. *J. Pharmacol. Exp. Ther*. 232: 283-294, 1985.

2113. Jaillon, P. and R.E. Kates. Phenytoin-induced changes in quinidine and 3-hydroxyquinidine pharmacokinetics in conscious dogs. *J. Pharmacol. Exp. Ther*. 213: 33-37, 1980.

2114. Buccafusco, J.J. Mechanism of the clonidine-induced protection against acetylcholinesterase inhibitor toxictity. *J. Pharmacol. Exp. Ther*. 222: 595-599, 1982.

2115. Varagic, V.M. and V. Stojanavic. The effect of enkephalins and of ß-endorphin on the hypertensive response to physostigmine in the rat. *Brit. J. Pharmacol*. 92: 197-202, 1987.

2116. Caputi, A.P., *et al*. Modulatory effect of brain acetylcholine on reflex-induced bradycardia and tachycardia. *J. Pharmacol. Exp. Ther*. 215: 309-316, 1980.

2117. Weinstock, M., *et al*. Antagonism of the cardiovascular and respiratory depressant effects of morphine in the conscious rabbit by physostigmine. *J. Pharmacol. Exp. Ther*. 218: 504-508, 1981.

2118. Carter, R.B. and L.A. Dykstra. Effects of picenadol (LY150720) and its stereoisomers on electric shock titration. *J. Pharmacol. Exp. Ther*. 234: 299-306, 1985.

2119. Lotti, V.J., *et al*. The anticonvulsant action of methazolamide in mice: Antagonism by various inhibitors of dopamine ß-hydroxylase. *Eur. J. Pharmacol*. 44: 387-390, 1977.

Bibliography

2120. Barman, S.M. and G.L. Gebber. Picrotoxin- and bicuculline-sensitive inhibition of cardiac vagal reflexes. *J. Pharmacol. Exp. Ther.* 209: 67-72, 1979.

2121. DiMicco, J.A., *et al.* Central nervous system sites involved in the cardiovascular effects of picrotoxin. *J. Pharmacol. Exp. Ther.* 203: 64-71, 1977.

2122. Rosenkranz, R.P. and K.F. Killam, Jr. Effects of intracerebroventricular administration of prostaglandins E_1 and E_2 on chemically induced convulsions in mice. *J. Pharmacol. Exp. Ther.* 209: 231-237, 1979.

2123. Tulanay, F.C., *et al.* The effect of dopaminergic stimulation and blockade on the nociceptive and antinociceptive responses in mice. *Eur. J. Pharmacol.* 33: 65-70, 1975.

2124. McMillen, B.A., *et al.* Pimozide: Delayed onset of action at rat striatal pre- and postsynaptic dopamine receptors. *J. Pharmacol. Exp. Ther.* 215: 150-155, 1980.

2125. Manders, W.T., *et al.* Cardio-selective beta adrenergic stimulation with prenalterol in the conscious dog. *J. Pharmacol. Exp. Ther.* 215: 266-270, 1980.

2126. Tanaka, N., *et al.* Evaluation of ocular toxicity of two beta blocking drugs, carteolol and practolol, in beagle dogs. *J. Pharmacol. Exp. Ther.* 224: 424-430, 1983.

2127. Basil, B., *et al.* ß-adrenoceptor blocking properties and cardioselectivity of M&B 17,803 A. *Brit. J. Pharmacol.* 48: 198-211, 1973.

2128. Prokocimer, P.G., *et al.* Role of the sympathetic nervous system in the maintenance of hypertension in rats harboring pheochromocytoma. *J. Pharmacol. Exp. Ther.* 241: 870-874, 1987.

2129. Bache, R.J., *et al.* Differences in the effects of alpha-1 adrenergic blockade with prazosin and indoramin on coronary blood flow during exercise. *J. Pharmacol. Exp. Ther.* 245: 232-237, 1988.

2130. Shebuski, R.J. and B.G. Zimmerman. Suppression of reflex tachycardia by central administration of the alpha-1 adrenoceptor antagonists urapidil and prazosin in anesthetized dogs. *J. Pharmacol. Exp. Ther.* 234: 456-462, 1985.

2131. Mostaghim, R., *et al.* Endothelial potentiation of relaxation response to phentolamine in rat thoracic aorta. *J. Pharmacol. Exp. Ther.* 244: 475-478, 1988.

2132. Smith, R.D., *et al.* Acute tolerance to prazosin in conscious hypertensive rats: Involvement of the renin-angiotensin system. *J. Pharmacol. Exp. Ther.* 217: 397-405, 1981.

2133. Marco, J., *et al.* Enhanced glucagon secretion by pancreatic islets from prednisolone-treated mice. *Diabetologia* 12: 307-311, 1976.

2134. Blyth, W. and G.E. Stewart. Systemic candidiasis in mice treated with prednisolone and amphotericin B. 1. Morbidity, mortality and inflammatory reaction. *Mycopathologia* 66: 41-50, 1978.

2135. Schilling, W. and S.-E. Svehag. Synergistic effect of alloantibodies $F(ab^1)_2$ and prednisone on murine split heart allograft survival. *Acta Pathol. Microbiol. Scand. Sect. C* 84: 325-332, 1976.

2136. Abbott Laboratories. Personal communication.

2137. Horton, R.W., *et al*. Monoamine and GABA metabolism and the anticonvulsant action of di-n-propylacetate and ethanolamine-o-sulfate. *Eur. J. Pharmacol.* 41: 387-397, 1977.

2138. Ehring, G.R., *et al*. Quantitative structure activity studies of antiarrhythmic properties in a series of lidocaine and procainamide derivatives. *J. Pharmacol. Exp. Ther.* 244: 479-492, 1988.

2139. Maden, B.R. and F.S.K. Farar. Anticonvulsant activity of some ß-adrenoceptor blocking agents in mice. *Eur. J. Pharmacol.* 29: 1-4, 1974.

2140. Nickander, R., *et al*. Propoxyphene and norpropoxyphene: Pharmacologic and toxic effects in animals. *J. Pharmacol. Exp. Ther.* 200: 245-253, 1977.

2141. Boissier, J.R., *et al*. Studies on 1-(O-cyclopropylphenoxy)-3-iso-propylamino-2-propanol, a new ß-adrenergic blocking drug. *Eur. J. Pharmacol.* 15: 151-159, 1971.

2142. Joselevitz-Goldman, J., *et al*. Effects of propranolol on regional O_2 supply and O_2 consumption in reperfused dog myocardium. *J. Pharmacol. Exp. Ther.* 242: 102-107, 1987.

2143. Smits, J.F.M., *et al*. Is the antihypertensive effect of propranolol caused by an action within the central nervous system? *J. Pharmacol. Exp. Ther.* 215: 221-225, 1980.

2144. Rimele, T.J., *et al*. Pharmacology of bucindolol in isolated canine vascular smooth muscle. *J. Pharmacol. Exp. Ther.* 231: 317-325, 1984.

2145. Saelens, D.A., *et al*. Studies on the contribution of active metabolites to the anticonvulsant effects of propranolol. *Eur. J. Pharmacol.* 42: 39-46, 1977.

2146. Levy, A., *et al*. Disposition of propranolol isomers in mice. *Eur. J. Pharmacol.* 40: 93-100, 1976.

2147. Zivny, J., *et al*. Effect of beta adrenergic blocking agents on erythropoiesis in rats. *J. Pharmacol. Exp. Ther.* 226: 222-225, 1983.

2148. Powell, J.R. Increased total and regional vascular resistance produced by propranolol. *J. Pharmacol. Exp. Ther.* 213: 64-69, 1980.

2149. Corbett, H., *et al*. Interaction between oral hydralazine and propranolol. II. Assessment of altered splanchnic blood flow as the determinant of altered presynaptic extraction. *J. Pharmacol. Exp. Ther.* 239: 517-521, 1986.

2150. Schneider, S.M., *et al*. Beta-blockade for acute theophylline-induced seizures. *Vet. Hum. Toxicol.* 29: 451-453, 1987.

2151. Young, S.L. and R.A. Silbajoris. Type II cell response to chronic beta adrenergic agonist and antagonists infusions. *J. Pharmacol. Exp. Ther.* 233: 271-276, 1985.

2152. Lindenschmidt, R.C. and H.P Witschi. Propranolol-induced elevation of pulmonary collagen. *J. Pharmacol. Exp. Ther.* 232: 346-350, 1985.

2153. Aucoin, D.P., *et al*. Propylthiouracil-induced immune-mediated disease in the cat. *J. Pharmacol. Exp. Ther.* 234: 13-18, 1985.

2154. Lau, C. and T.A. Slotkin. Maturation of sympathetic neurotransmission in the rat heart. VIII. Slowed development of noradrenergic synapses resulting from hypothyroidism. *J. Pharmacol. Exp. Ther.* 220: 629-636, 1982.

2155. Panzenbeck, M.J., *et al*. 6-keto-prostaglandin E_1 is a potent coronary vasodilator and stimulates a vagal reflex in dogs. *J. Pharmacol. Exp. Ther.* 244: 814-819, 1988.

2156. Baer, P.G., *et al*. Prostacyclin effects on renal hemodynamic and excretory functions in the rat. *J. Pharmacol. Exp. Ther.* 208: 294-297, 1979.

2157. Susic H. and K.U. Malik. Prostacyclin and prostaglandin E_2 effects on adrenergic transmission in the kidney of anesthetized dog. *J. Pharmacol. Exp. Ther.* 218: 588-592, 1981.

2158. Nelson, P.K., *et al*. Erythropoietic effects of prostacyclin (PGI_2) and its metabolite 6-keto-prostaglandin (PG)E_1. *J. Pharmacol. Exp. Ther.* 226: 493-499, 1983.

2159. Simpson, P.J., *et al*. Reduction of experimental canine myocardial infarct size with prostaglan E_1: Inhibition of neutrophil migration and activation. *J. Pharmacol. Exp. Ther.* 244: 619-624, 1988.

2160. Lin, M.T. Systemic administration of prostaglandin E_1 produces hypothermic effects in unanesthetized rats. *J. Pharmacol. Exp. Ther.* 209: 349-351, 1979.

2161. Lin, M.T. Effects of intravenous and intraventricular prostaglandin E_1 on thermoregulatory responses in rabbits. *J. Pharmacol. Exp. Ther.* 204: 39-45, 1978.

2162. Hayashi, S., *et al*. Relaxant and contractile responses to prostaglandins in premature, newborn and adult baboon cerebral arteries. *J. Pharmacol. Exp. Ther.* 233: 628-635, 1985.

2163. Bouman, L.N., *et al*. Electrophysiological effects of alinidine on nodal and atrial fibers in the guinea-pig heart. *J. Pharmacol. Exp. Ther.* 229: 551-556, 1984.

2164. Saito, A., *et al.* Pharmacological analysis of autonomic innervation of the right atria of rats and guinea pigs: Demonstration of nonadrenergic noncholinergic nerves. *J. Pharmacol. Exp. Ther.* 238: 713-719, 1986.

2165. Fukushima, K. Experimental studies on the drugs of antishock. *Kagoshima Daigaku Igaku Zasshi* 13: 416-437, 1961.

2166. Allan, G. and R. Levi. The cardiac effects of prostaglandins and their modification by the prostaglandin antagonist N-0164. *J. Pharmacol. Exp. Ther.* 214: 45-49, 1980.

2167. Gross, D.M., *et al.* Effects of prostaglandins A_2, E_2 and F_2 alpha on erythropoietin production. *J. Pharmacol. Exp. Ther.* 198: 489-496, 1976.

2168. Wasserman, M.A., *et al.* Inhibition of bronchoconstriction by aerosols of prostaglandins E_1 and and E_2. *J. Pharmacol. Exp. Ther.* 214: 68-73, 1980.

2169. Zook, T.E. and J.W. Strandhoy. Mechanisms of the natriuretic and diuretic effects of prostaglandin $F_{2\alpha}$ *J. Pharmacol. Exp. Ther.* 217: 674-680, 1981.

2170. Gessner, P.K. Failure of diphenylhydantoin to prevent alcohol withdrawal convulsions in mice. *Eur. J. Pharmacol.* 27: 120-129, 1974.

2171. Harralson, J.D., *et al.* Inhibition of dopamine ß-hydroxylase by 4-hydoxypyrazole: Ethanol-pyrazole effects on serum dopamine ß-hydroxylase in vivo. *J. Pharmacol. Exp. Ther.* 206: 69-74, 1978.

2172. Chiariello, M., *et al.* Inhibition of ischemia-induced phospholipase activation by quinacrine protects jeopardized myocardium in rats with coronary artery occlusion. *J. Pharmacol. Exp. Ther.* 241: 560-568, 1987.

2173. Morikawa, Y. and M.R. Rosen. Effects of quinidine on the transmembrane potentials of young and adult canine cardiac purkinje fibers. *J. Pharmacol. Exp. Ther.* 236: 832-838, 1986.

2174. Nawrath, H. Action potential, membrane currents and force of contraction in mammalian heart muscle fibers treated with quinidine. *J. Pharmacol. Exp. Ther.* 216: 176-182, 1981.

2175. Nishimura, M., *et al.* Membrane actions of quinidine sulfate in the rabbit atrioventricular node studied by voltage clamp method. *J. Pharmacol. Exp. Ther.* 244: 780-788, 1988.

2176. Chassaing, C., *et al.* Mechanism of action of quinidine on heart rate in the dog. *J. Pharmacol. Exp. Ther.* 222: 688-693, 1982.

2177. Clohisy, D.R., *et al.* Effect of quinidine on the renal clearance of digoxin in the presence of low and high serum digoxin concentrations. *J. Pharmacol. Exp. Ther.* 222: 49-51, 1982.

2178. Wilkerson, R.D. and B.L. Beck. Increase in serum digoxin concentration produced by quinidine does not increase the potential for digoxin-induced ventricular arrhythmias in dogs. *J. Pharmacol. Exp. Ther.* 240: 548-553, 1987.

2179. Nagahama, S., *et al.* Mechanism of the pressor action of LY 171555, a specific dopamine D_2 receptor agonist, in the conscious rat. *J. Pharmacol. Exp. Ther.* 236: 735-742, 1986.

2180. Hahn, R.A. and B.R. MacDonald. Primate cardiovascular responses mediated by dopamine receptors: Effects of N,N-di-n-propyldopamine and LY 171555. *J. Pharmacol. Exp. Ther.* 229: 132-138, 1984.

2181. Freidman, R.L., *et al.* Discriminative stimulus properties of quipazine: Mediation by serotonin$_2$ binding sites. *J. Pharmacol. Exp. Ther.* 228: 628-635, 1984.

2182. Alper, R.H. and J.M. Snider. Activation of serotonin$_2$ (5-HT$_2$) receptors by Quipazine increases arterial pressure and renin secretion in conscious rats. *J. Pharmacol. Exp. Ther.* 243: 829-833, 1987.

2183. Hawthorn, M.H., *et al.* Characteristics of adaptive supersensitivity in the left atrium of the guinea pig. *J. Pharmacol. Exp. Ther.* 241: 453-457, 1987.

2184. London, E.D. and G.G. Buterbaugh. Modification of electroshock convulsive response in thresholds in neonatal rats after brain monoamine reduction. *J. Pharmacol. Exp. Ther.* 206: 81-90, 1978.

2185. Kitagawa, H., *et al.* Dissociation between acid secretion and mucosal blood flow after treatment of rats with reserpine. *J. Pharmacol. Exp. Ther.* 236: 784-788, 1986.

2186. Stewart, J.J. and P.C. Jobe. Effects of reserpine on monoamines and intestinal transit in the rat. *J. Pharmacol. Exp. Ther.* 217: 357-362, 1981.

2187. Nasseri, A., *et al.* Reserpine-induced postjunctional supersensitivity in rat vas deferens and caudal artery without changes in alpha adrenergic receptors. *J. Pharmacol. Exp. Ther.* 234: 350-357, 1985.

2188. Abel P.W., *et al.* Chronic reserpine treatment alters sensitivity and membrane potential of the rabbit saphenous artery. *J. Pharmacol. Exp. Ther.* 217: 430-439, 1981.

2189. Hyttel, J. and B. Fjallard. Central 5-HTP decarboxylase inhibiting properties of RO4-4602 in relation to 5-HTP potentiation in mice. *Eur. J. Pharmacol.* 19: 112-114, 1972.

2190. Fink, G.D. and J.W. Fisher. Stimulation of erythropoiesis by beta adrenergic agonists. II. Mechanism of action. *J. Pharmacol. Exp. Ther.* 202: 199-208, 1977.

2191. Morris, M.E., *et al.* Sulfate homeostasis. I. Effect of salicylic acid and its metabolites on inorganic sulfate in rats. *J. Pharmacol. Exp. Ther.* 244: 945-949, 1988.

Bibliography

2192. Bruner, C.A., *et al.* Will chronic intracerebroventricular saralasin infusion produce selective blockade of brain angiotensin II receptors in the rat? *J. Pharmacol. Exp. Ther.* 226: 13-18, 1983.

2193. Solomon, R.E. and G.F. Gebhart. Mechanisms of effects of intrathecal serotonin on nociception and blood pressure in rats. *J. Pharmacol. Exp. Ther.* 245: 905-912, 1988.

2194. Sofia, R.D. The lethal effects of Δ^9-tetrahydrocannabinol in mice enhanced by pretreatment with SKF 525-A or chloramphenicol. *Eur. J. Pharmacol.* 26: 383-385, 1974.

2195. Patterson, E., *et al.* Antiarrhythmic and antifibrillatory actions of the beta adrenergic receptor antagonist, dl-sotalol. *J. Pharmacol. Exp. Ther.* 230: 519-526, 1984.

2196. Carmeliet, E. Electrophysiologic and voltage clamp analysis of the effects of sotalol on isolated cardiac muscle and purkinje fibers. *J. Pharmacol. Exp. Ther.* 232: 817-825, 1985.

2197. Ku, D.D. and E. Meezan. Increased renal tubular sodium pump and Na^+, K^+-adenosine triphosphatase in streptozotocin-diabetic rats. *J. Pharmacol. Exp. Ther.* 229: 664-670, 1984.

2198. Mathison, R. and J.S. Davison. Modified smooth muscle responses of jejunum in streptozotocin-diabetic rats. *J. Pharmacol. Exp. Ther.* 244: 1045-1050, 1988.

2199. Maggi, C.A., *et al.* Activation of micturition reflex by substance P and substance K: Indirect evidence for the existence of multiple tachykinin receptors in the rat urinary bladder. *J. Pharmacol. Exp. Ther.* 238: 259-266, 1986.

2200. Murray, C.W., *et al.* Neurokinin-induced salivation in the anesthetized rats: A three receptor hypothesis. *J. Pharmacol. Exp. Ther.* 242: 500-506, 1987.

2201. Hedner, J., *et al.* Interaction of substance P with the respiratory control system in the rat. *J. Pharmacol. Exp. Ther.* 228: 196-201, 1984.

2202. Kachur, J.F., *et al.* Neurohumoral control of ileal electrolyte transport. II. Neurotensin and Substance P. *J. Pharmacol. Exp. Ther.* 220: 456-463, 1982.

2203. Huizinga, J.D., *et al.* Electrophysiological basis of excitation of canine colonic circular muscle by cholinergic agents and substance P. *J. Pharmacol. Exp. Ther.* 231: 692-699, 1984.

2204. Malo, P.E., *et al.* Characterization of substance P-induced contractions of guinea-pig trachea. *J. Pharmacol. Exp. Ther.* 237: 782-786, 1986.

2205. Starr, M.S., *et al.* Behavioral depressant and antinociceptive properties of substance P in the mouse: Possible implication of brain monoamines. *Eur. J. Pharmacol.* 48: 203-212, 1978.

2206. Stern, P. and S. Hukovic. Pharmacological analysis of central actions of synthetic substance P. *Arch. Int. Pharmacodyn. Ther.* 202: 259-262, 1960.

2207. O'Keefe, R.J., *et al.* Local and neurally mediated effects of sufentanil on canine skeletal muscle vascular resistance. *J. Pharmacol. Exp. Ther.* 242: 699-706, 1987.

2208. Lau, Y.S., *et al.* Role of calmodulin-dependent phosphorylation in chronic sulpiride-induced striated dopamine receptor supersensitivity. *J. Pharmacol. Exp. Ther.* 229: 32-37, 1984.

2209. Gnegy, M.E., *et al.* Chronic sulpiride treatment produces supersensitivity of striatal adenylate cyclase to dopamine in sexually immature or adult castrated rats. *J. Pharmacol. Exp. Ther.* 224: 627-633, 1983.

2210. Johnson, C.E., *et al.* Dopamine antagonist effect of verapamil on isolated perfused rabbit ear artery. *J. Pharmacol. Exp. Ther.* 226: 802-805, 1983.

2211. Feuerstein, G., *et al.* Cardiorespiratory, sympathetic and biochemical responses to T-2 toxin in the guinea pig and rat. *J. Pharmacol. Exp. Ther.* 232: 786-794, 1985.

2212. Verbeuren, T.J., *et al.* Effects of tertatol on post- and prejunctional beta adrenoceptors. *J. Pharmacol. Exp. Ther.* 233: 801-809, 1985.

2213. Butcher, L.L., *et al.* Behavioral and biochemical effects of preferentially protecting monoamines in the brain against the action of reserpine. *Eur. J. Pharmacol.* 18: 204-212, 1972.

2214. Sofia, R.D. and H. Barry III. Depressant effect of Δ^l - tetrahydrocannabinol enhanced by inhibition of its metabolism. *Eur. J. Pharmacol.* 13: 134-137, 1970.

2215. Sofia, R.D. Lethal effects of Δ^l-tetrahydrocannabinol in aggregated and isolated mice following single dose administration. *Eur. J. Pharmacol.* 20: 139-142, 1972.

2216. Stark, P. and P.B. Dews. Cannabinoids. II. Cardiovascular effects. *J. Pharmacol. Exp. Ther.* 214: 131-138, 1980.

2217. Fredericks, A.B., *et al.* The cardiovascular and autonomic effects of repeated administration of Δ-9-tetrahydrocannabinol to Rhesus monkeys. *J. Pharmacol. Exp. Ther.* 216: 247-253, 1981.

2218. Stark, P. and P.B. Dews. Cannabinoids. I. Behavioral effects. *J. Pharmacol. Exp. Ther.* 214: 124-130, 1980.

2219. Campbell, K.A., *et al.* Δ^9-tetrahydrocannabinol differentially effects sensory-evoked potentials in the rat dentate gyrus. *J. Pharmacol. Exp. Ther.* 239: 936-940, 1986.

2220. Schulze, G.E., *et al.* Acute effects of Δ-9-tetrahydrocannabinol in rhesus monkeys as measured by performance in a battery of complex operant tests. *J. Pharmacol. Exp. Ther.* 245: 178-186, 1988.

Bibliography

2221. Frederickson, R.C.A., *et al*. Correlation between the in vivo and an in vitro expression of opiate withdrawal precipitated by naloxone: Their antagonism by 1-(-)-Δ^9-tetrahydrocannabinol. *J. Pharmacol. Exp. Ther.* 199: 375-384, 1976.

2222. Johnson, K.M. and W.L. Dewey. The effects of Δ^9-tetrahydro-cannabinol on the conversion of [^{3}H]tryptophan to 5-[^{3}H]hydroxytryptamine in mouse brain. *J. Pharmacol. Exp. Ther.* 207: 140-150, 1978.

2223. Lindamood, C. III and B.K. Colasanti. Effects of Δ^9-tetrahydrocannabinol and cannabinol on sodium-dependent high affinity choline uptake in the rat hippocampus. *J. Pharmacol. Exp. Ther.* 213: 216-221, 1980.

2224. Tyrey, L. Δ^9-tetrahydrocannabinol: A potent inhibitor of episodic luteinizing hormone secretion. *J. Pharmacol. Exp. Ther.* 213: 306-308, 1980.

2225. Bhargava, H.N. Inhibition of naloxone induced withdrawal in morphine dependent mice by 1-trans-Δ^9-tetrahydrocannabinol. *Eur. J. Pharmacol.* 36: 259-262, 1976.

2226. Beardsley, P.M., *et al*. Dependence on tetrahydrocannabinol in rhesus monkeys. *J. Pharmacol. Exp. Ther.* 239: 311-319, 1986.

2227. Bloom, A.S., *et al*. 9-nor-9ß-hydroxyhexahydrocannabinol, a cannabinoid with potent antinociceptive activity: Comparisons with morphine. *J. Pharmacol. Exp. Ther.* 200: 263-270, 1977.

2228. Doherty, P.A., *et al*. Respiratory and cardiovascular depressant effects of nabilone, N-methyllevonantradol and Δ^9-tetrahydrocannabinol in anesthetized cats. *J. Pharmacol. Exp. Ther.* 227: 508-516, 1983.

2229. Poddar, M.K. and W.L. Dewey. Effects of cannabinoids on catecholamine uptake and release in hypothalamic and striatal synaptosomes. *J. Pharmacol. Exp. Ther.* 214: 63-67, 1980.

2230. Churchill, P.C., *et al*. Action and mechanism of action of veratrine on renin secretion from rat kidney slices. *J. Pharmacol. Exp. Ther.* 229: 27-31, 1984.

2231. Frederickson, R.C.A., *et al*. A comparison of thalidomide and pentobarbital-new methods for identifying novel hypnotic drugs. *J. Pharmacol. Exp. Ther.* 203: 240-251, 1977.

2232. Denenberg, V.H., *et al*. Effects of theophylline on behavioral state development in the newborn rabbit. *J. Pharmacol. Exp. Ther.* 221: 604-608, 1982.

2233. Katims, J.J., *et al*. Interactions in the behavioral effects of methylxanthines and adenosine derivatives. *J. Pharmacol. Exp. Ther.* 227: 167-173, 1983.

2234. Ramzan, I.M. and G. Levy. Kinetics of drug action in disease states. XVII. Effect of experimental renal failure on the pharmacodynamics of theophylline-induced seizures in rats. *J. Pharmacol. Exp. Ther.* 240: 584-588, 1987.

Bibliography

2235. Kafiluddi, R., *et al*. Effects of theophylline on inotropic and arrhythmogenic actions of cardiotonic steroids in guinea pig cardiac muscle. *J. Pharmacol. Exp. Ther*. 244: 556-563, 1988.

2236. Allen, D.O., *et al*. Relationships between cyclic AMP levels and lipolysis in fat cells after isoproterenol and forskolin stimulation. *J. Pharmacol. Exp. Ther*. 238: 659-664, 1986.

2237. Katsuragi, T. and C. Su. Augmentation by theophylline of [^{3}H] purine release from vascular adrenergic nerves: Evidence for presynaptic autoinhibition. *J. Pharmacol. Exp. Ther*. 220: 152-156, 1982.

2238. Vogel, R.A., *et al*. Effects of thyrotropin-releasing hormone on locomotor activity operant performance and ingestive behavior. *J. Pharmacol. Exp. Ther*. 208: 161-168, 1979.

2239. Yarbrough, G.G. Studies on the neuropharmacology of thyrotropin releasing hormone (TRH) and a new TRH analog. *Eur. J. Pharmacol*. 48: 19-27, 1978.

2240. Helke, C.J. and E.T. Phillips. Thyrotropin-releasing hormone receptor activation in the spinal cord increases blood pressure and sympathetic tone to the vasculature and the adrenals. *J. Pharmacol. Exp. Ther*. 245: 41-46, 1988.

2241. Mailman, R.B., *et al*. Change in brain guanosine 3',5'-monophosphate (cGMP) content by thyrotropin-releasing hormone. *J. Pharmacol. Exp. Ther*. 208: 169-175, 1979.

2242. Breese, G.R., *et al*. Effects of thyrotropin-releasing hormone (TRH) on the actions of pentobarbital and other centrally acting drugs. *J. Pharmacol. Exp. Ther*. 193: 11-22, 1975.

2243. Hall, E.D., *et al*. Glucocorticoid effects on spinal cord function. *J. Pharmacol. Exp. Ther*. 206: 361, 370, 1978.

2244. Zenoble, R.D. and R.J. Kemppainen. Adrenocortical suppression by topically applied corticosteroids in healthy dogs. *J. Am. Vet. Med. Assoc*. 191: 685-688, 1987.

2244. Zenoble, R.D. and R.J. Kemppainen. Adrenocortical suppression by topically applied corticosteroids in healthy dogs. *J. Am. Vet. Med. Assoc*. 191: 685-688, 1987.

2245. Slizgi, G.R., *et al*. Effects of the highly selective kappa opioid, U-50,488, on renal function in the anesthetized dog. *J. Pharmacol. Exp. Ther*. 230: 641-645, 1984.

2246. Goering, J. and B.G. Zimmerman. Analysis of adrenoceptor blockade and hypotension elicited by urapidil and prazosin in conscious rats. *J. Pharmacol. Exp. Ther*. 237: 553-557, 1986.

2247. Zelis, R. Relative presynaptic and postsynaptic effects of urapidil on adrenoceptors in the rabbit pulmonary artery. *J. Pharmacol. Exp. Ther*. 237: 746-749, 1986.

Bibliography

2248. Churchill, P.C. and M.C. Churchill. Vanadate inhibits renin secretion from rat kidney slices. *J. Pharmacol. Exp. Ther.* 213: 144-149, 1980.

2249. Kumar, A. and C.N. Corder. Diuretic and vasoconstrictor effects of sodium orthovanadate on the isolated perfused rat kidney. *J. Pharmacol. Exp. Ther.* 213: 85-90, 1980.

2250. Berkowitz, B.A. and S. Sherman. Characterization of vasopressin analgesia. *J. Pharmacol. Exp. Ther.* 220: 329-334, 1982.

2251. Dersham, G.H. and J. Han. Actions of verapamil on purkinje fibers from normal and infarcted heart tissues. *J. Pharmacol. Exp. Ther.* 216: 261-264, 1981.

2252. Adachi, H., *et al.* Effects of verapamil and nitroglycerin on coronary and systemic hemodynamics in conscious dogs. *J. Pharmacol. Exp. Ther.* 241: 1072-1078, 1987.

2253. Chelly, J.E., *et al.* Pharmacodynamic and pharmacokinetic interactions between lidocaine and verapamil. *J. Pharmacol. Exp. Ther.* 243: 211-216, 1987.

2254. McGonigle, R.J.S., *et al.* Enhanced erythropoitin production by calcium entry blockers in rats exposed to hypoxia. *J. Pharmacol. Exp. Ther.* 241: 428-432, 1987.

2255. McAllister, R.G., Jr., *et al.* The pharmacology of verapamil. I. Elimination kinetics in dogs and correlation of plasma levels with effect on the electrocardiogram. *J. Pharmacol. Exp. Ther.* 202: 38-44, 1977.

2256. Howard-Butcher, S., *et al.* Differential effects of xylamine on extracellular concentrations of norepinephrine and dopamine in rat central nervous system: An in vivo electrochemical study. *J. Pharmacol. Exp. Ther.* 233: 58-63, 1985.

2257. Fischer, J.B. and A.K. Cho. Release of norepinephrine from organ-cultured superior cervical ganglia: Effects of the norepinephrine uptake inhibitor xylamine. *J. Pharmacol. Exp. Ther.* 225: 623-629, 1983.

2258. Arbel, E.R. and G. Glick. Effects of veratrine on the in situ dog heart: Evidence for increased ventricular fibrillation threshold. *J. Pharmacol. Exp. Ther.* 208: 314-318, 1979.

2259. Lucot, J.B. and G.H. Crampton. Xylazine emesis, yohimbine and motion sickness susceptibility in the cat. *J. Pharmacol. Exp. Ther.* 237: 450-455, 1986.

2260. Plunkett, L.M. and R.L. Tackett. Central alpha receptors and their role in digoxin cardiotoxicity. *J. Pharmacol. Exp. Ther.* 227: 683-686, 1983.

2261. Scatton, B., *et al.* Antidopaminergic properties of Yohimbine. *J. Pharmacol. Exp. Ther.* 215: 494-499, 1980.

2262. Kanda, A., *et al.* Enhancement by Yohimbine of nicotine- and dimethylphenylpiperadinium-induced release of norepinephrine from cardiac sympathetic nerves of the dog: Interaction of presynaptic alpha and nicotinic receptors. *J. Pharmacol. Exp. Ther.* 243: 1095-1100, 1987.

Bibliography

2263. Sanger, D.J., *et al.* Behavioral effects of non-benzodiazepine anxiolytic drugs: A comparison of CGS 9896 and zopiclone with chlordiazepoxide. *J. Pharmacol. Exp. Ther.* 232: 831-837, 1985.

2264. Barrett, J.E., *et al.* Behavioral studies with anxiolytic drugs. II. Interactions of zopiclone with ethyl-ß-carboline-3-carboxylate and RO 15-1788 in squirrel monkeys. *J. Pharmacol. Exp. Ther.* 236: 313-319, 1986.

2265. Lin, J.H., *et al.* Differential effects of phenobarbital on ester and ether glucuronidation of diflunisal in rats. *J. Pharmacol. Exp. Ther.* 242: 1013-1018, 1987.

2266. Kalivas, P. and P. Duffy. Sensitization to repeated morphine injection in the rat: Possible involvement of A10 dopamine neurons. *J. Pharmacol. Exp. Ther.* 241: 204-212, 1987.

2267. Long, J.B., *et al.* Neurologic deficits and neuronal injury in rats resulting from nonopioid action of the delta opioid receptor antagonist ICI 174864. *J. Pharmacol. Exp. Ther.* 244: 1169-1177, 1988.

2268. Brown, B.S., *et al.* Antiarrhythmic, electrophysiologic and hemodynamic effects of ACC-9358. *J. Pharmacol. Exp. Ther.* 243: 1225-1234, 1987.

2269. Kitzen, J.M., *et al.* Cardiac electrophysiologic and hemodynamic activity of pimobendan (UD-CG 115 BS), a new inotropic agent. *J. Pharmacol. Exp. Ther.* 244: 929-939, 1988.

2270. Takeshita, A., *et al.* Phentolamine and isoproterenol: Comparison of effects on vascular resistance and oxygen uptake in skeletal muscle during hypotension. *J. Pharmacol. Exp. Ther.* 199: 353-359, 1976.

2271. Schumacher, W.A., *et al.* Effect of thromboxane receptor antagonists on renal artery thrombosis in the cynomologus monkey. *J. Pharmacol. Exp. Ther.* 243: 460-466, 1987.

2272. Davis, L.E. ed. *Handbook of Small Animal Therapeutics*, Churchill Livingstone, N.Y. 1985.

2273. Stamathis, G., ed. *Veterinary Drug Formulary*, Cornell Research Foundation, Inc., Williams and Wilkins, Baltimore, 1985.

2274. Booth, N.H. and L.E. McDonald, eds. *Veterinary Pharmacology and Therapeutics*, 6th ed, Iowa State Univ. Press, Ames, IA, 1988.

2275. Rossoff, I.S. *Handbook of Veterinary Drugs*, Springer Publishing Co., N.Y., 1974.

2276. Hsu, W.H. and Z.-X. Lu. Effect of Yohimbine on xylazine-ketamine anesthesia in cats. *JAVMA* 185: 886-888, 1984.

2277. Hatch, R.C., *et al.* Antagonism of ketamine anesthesia in cats by 4-aminopyridine and yohimbine. *Am. J. Vet. Res.* 44: 417-423, 1983.

Bibliography

2278. Hatch, R.C., *et al.* Antagonism of xylazine sedation with yohimbine, 4-aminopyridine, and doxapram in dogs. *Am. J. Vet. Res.* 46: 371-376, 1985.

2279. Hughes, H.C. Anesthesia of Laboratory Animals. *Lab. Animal* Sep 81: 40-56, 1981.

2280. Baggot, J.D. *Principles of Drug Disposition in Domestic Animals: The Basis of Veterinary Clinical Pharmacology*, W.B. Saunders Co., Philadelphia, 1979.

INDEX

Cafergot - *see* Ergotamine
Caffeine, 72-73
Cafron - *see* Benactyzine
Calciparin - *see* Heparin
Calcium Disodium Versenate - *see*
    Edetate, Calcium Disodium
Calcium chloride, 74
Cantil - *see* Mepenzolate
Cantril - *see* Mepenzolate
Capoten - *see* Captopril
Capsaicin, 75, 212
Captopril, 76
Carbachol, 77
Carbamazepine, 78
Carbamylcholine - *see* Carbachol
Carbamylhydrazine - *see* Semicarbazide
Carbidopa, 79, 239
Carbostesin - *see* Bupivacaine
Carbrital - *see* Pentobarbital
Carbuten - *see* Mebutamate
Carcholin - *see* Carbachol
Cardiac, 1, 3, 6, 8, 12-13, 17, 19-20,
    22, 24-26, 28-29, 32-34, 36, 38,
    40, 43, 45, 49, 54-56, 58, 60-61,
    64, 69, 73-74, 77, 83, 86-87, 91,
    93-94, 96, 100, 103, 105-106,
    115-117, 122, 124-126, 130-138,
    140-141, 143-144, 147, 149,
    154-159, 163, 165-169, 174-175,
    179, 181-182, 184, 189-192, 194,
    199-202, 204-209, 213, 217-218,
    221, 223, 226, 228-229, 231-237,
    240, 242, 244, 246-247, 250-252,
    254-255, 257, 259-260, 266, 268,
    270, 272, 275-276, 278-279, 282,
    285, 288, 290, 292, 297-298, 303,
    305-306, 309, 311-312, 314-315,
    317-321, 323-325, 327-328, 332,
    336, 343, 345, 349, 354, 358, 360,
    362-364, 367, 369, 373, 378-379,
    381, 383, 388-390, 393, 399,
    401-402, 406, 408, 411-413,
    415-416, 419-420, 423, 428, 431,
    434, 436, 438, 440-444, 446-447,
    449-450, 453, 458, 460, 462,
    465-467, 469-470, 475, 477-480,
    486-489, 491-494, 496, 499-504,
    507
Cardiazol - *see* Pentylenetetrazol
Cardidigin - *see* Digitoxin
Cardiovascular, 8-9, 16-17, 19-22, 27,
    32, 34-35, 38-39, 41-42, 44-45,

Cardiovascular (continued)
    49, 54, 57, 63, 66-68, 72, 75-77,
    81-82, 87-88, 90, 92, 94, 99, 102,
    106, 119, 123, 128, 130, 132, 134,
    138, 140-141, 145, 151-153, 156,
    160, 162, 164, 166-167, 173,
    179-180, 193, 197-198, 205,
    207-208, 212, 214, 216-220, 222,
    225, 229, 234, 236-239, 243,
    252-253, 256, 259, 261, 265-266,
    269, 275, 279, 283, 289-290, 292,
    295, 298, 300, 307, 313, 315,
    317-319, 322, 355-357, 359, 361,
    364, 366, 368, 372, 376, 380, 382,
    386, 391-392, 394, 405, 408,
    411-413, 416-417, 420-421, 424,
    428, 432, 437, 442, 444, 448, 451,
    453-456, 461, 464, 470, 473, 480,
    482, 491-493, 497, 500-502,
    505-506
Cardizem - *see* Diltiazem
Cardoxin - *see* Dipyridamole
Carisoma - *see* Carisoprodol
Carisoprodol, 80
Catapres - *see* Clonidine
Catatonic, 68, 210, 249, 295, 392, 398,
    428, 487
Catechol - *see* Pyrocatechol
Catral - *see* Pheniprazine
Catron - *see* Pheniprazine
Catroniazid - *see* Pheniprazine
Centchroman, 81
Centedrin - *see* Methylphenidate
Centrac - *see* Profadol
Central nervous system - *see* CNS
Cerespan - *see* Papaverine
Cerucal - *see* Metoclopramide
Chinacrin - *see* Quinacrine
Chlor-PZ - *see* Chlorpromazine
Chlor-Trimeton - *see* Chlorpheniramine
Chloral hydrate, 82
A-Chloralose, 83
Chloralosane - *see* α-Chloralose
Chlordiazepoxide, 84-85
Chlorimipramine, 52, 86
Chlorisondamine, 87
Chlormeprazine - *see* Prochlorperazine
p-Chloroamphetamine, 88
p-Chlorophenylalanine, 89
Chlorothiazide, 90
Chlorpheniramine, 91
Chlorpromazine, 92-93, 468
Cholinergic, 55, 77, 158, 268, 299, 309,
    368, 373

678

Reudox - *see* Phenylbutazone
Revertina - *see* Mecamylamine
Revivon - *see* Diprenorphine
Rexitene - *see* Guanabenz
Rioprostil, 429
Ritalin - *see* Methylphenidate
Ritanserin, 430
Ro1-6794 - *see* Dextrorphan
Ro11-1163/000 - *see* Moclobemide
Ro15-1788/000 - *see* Flumazenil
Rogitine - *see* Phentolamine
Rompun - *see* Xylazine
SB7505 - *see* Ibopamine
SG-75 - *see* Nicorandil
SK-65 - *see* Propoxyphene
SK-79.229-00 - *see* Fengabine
SK-Bamate - *see* Meprobamate
SK-Lygen - *see* Chlordiazepoxide
SK-Pramine - *see* Imipramine
SKF-525-A - *see* Proadifen
SKF-82526-J - *see* Fenoldopam
SKF92058 - *see* Metiamide
SL76002 - *see* Progabide
SQ11725 - *see* Nadolol
SU-3088 - *see* Chlorisondamine
Sal Ammoniac - *see* Ammonium
    Chloride
Salbutamol - *see* Albuterol
Salicylic acid, 431
Salisan - *see* Chlorothiazide
Salmiac - *see* Ammonium Chloride
Saluric - *see* Chlorothiazide
Sandimmune - *see* Cyclosporine
Sandril - *see* Reserpine
Sanedrine - *see* Ephedrine
Sansert - *see* Methysergide
Sar - *see* Saralasin
Saralasin, 432
Sarenin - *see* Saralasin
Scopolamine, 433-434
Secobarbital, 435
Seconal - *see* Secobarbital
Sedantoinal - *see* Mephenytoin
Sedative, 30, 62, 65, 71, 84, 92, 137,
    173, 180, 261, 307, 330, 333, 342,
    370, 395, 398, 404, 410, 427, 433,
    435, 440, 455, 459, 474, 497, 505
Sedoneural - *see* Sodium Bromide
Semap - *see* Penfluridol
Semicarbazide, 436

Sensorcaine - *see* Bupivacaine
Seotal - *see* Secobarbital
Serax - *see* Oxazepam
Serenid - *see* Oxazepam
Sernyl - *see* Phencyclidine
Sernylan - *see* Phencyclidine
Serotonin, 82-84, 86, 89, 203, 221, 267,
    279, 287, 344, 422, 427, 435,
    437-438, 508
Serpasil - *see* Reserpine
Serpasol - *see* Reserpine
Sertraline, 439
Servier 2395 - *see* Tertatol
Sigmart - *see* Nicorandil
Sinarest - *see* Oxymetazoline
Sinetens - *see* Prazosin
Singoserp - *see* Syrosingopine
Siringina - *see* Syrosingopine
6-Hydroxydopa, 211
6-Hydroxydopamine, 212-213
Skopolate - *see* Scopolamine
Skopyl - *see* Scopolamine
Sodium Orthovanadate - *see* Vanadate
Sodium bromide, 440
Sodium fluoride, 441
Sodium nitrite, 442
Sofarin - *see* Warfarin
Solfoton - *see* Phenobarbital
Solgol - *see* Nadolol
Soma - *see* Carisoprodol
Somadril - *see* Carisoprodol
Sombulex - *see* Hexobarbital
Somio - *see* α-Chloralose
Somnos - *see* Chloral Hydrate
Somophyllin - *see* Theophylline
Sotacor - *see* Sotalol
Sotalex - *see* Sotalol
Sotalol, 443
Sparine - *see* Promazine
Sparteine, 444
Spartocin - *see* Sparteine
Spheroidine - *see* Tetrodotoxin
Spiropent - *see* Clenbuterol
St 567-BR - *see* Alinidine
Stadol - *see* Butorphanol
Stelazine - *see* Trifluoperazine
Stemetil - *see* Prochlorperazine
Sterane - *see* Prednisolone
Stimolag Fortis - *see* Pipradrol
Straub tail reaction, 102, 334, 342